The Lung in Health and Disease

The Lung
in Health and Disease

Charles F. Geschickter, M.D.

Professor of Pathology and Chairman
Department of Research Pathology
Georgetown University Medical Center
Washington, D.C.

With a chapter on Pulmonary Mechanics by

Robert E. Snell, M.D.

Associate Staff in Internal Medicine
Cape Cod Hospital
Hyannis, Massachusetts
Formerly Assistant Professor of Pediatrics and Physiology
Georgetown University School of Medicine
Washington, D. C.

J. B. Lippincott Company
Philadelphia   Toronto

ISBN 0-397-50311-3
Library of Congress Catalog Card Number 73-1947

Printed in the United States of America
1   3   4   2

Library of Congress Cataloging in Publication Data

Geschickter, Charles Freeman

   The lung in health and disease.

   Bibliography: p.
   1. Lungs—Diseases. 2. Respiration.
I. Title. [DNLM: 1. Lung—Physiology. 2. Lung diseases.
WF 600 G389L 1973]
RC756.G47   616.2'4   73-1947
ISBN 0-397-50311-3

Preface

This book brings together the clinical and pathologic aspects of diseases of the lungs and the modern methods for evaluating the physiologic responses that accompany them. Methods for determining lung volumes and blood gases are presented, as well as current radiological diagnostic techniques, including radioisotopic scanning.

The book is intended for medical students, residents, and general practitioners and, throughout the text, brevity and clarity have been sought to facilitate utility from the standpoint of the nonspecialist. The indicated treatment is given in general terms but is not detailed for therapeutic application. The range of lung diseases discussed is inclusive, and the ever-present interrelationship between pulmonary and cardiovascular disease is emphasized.

The author gratefully acknowledges the assistance and generosity of the Department of Radiology at Georgetown University Medical Center for the roentgenograms that have been reproduced in the text. The assistance of the editorial staff of J. B. Lippincott Company in providing some of the line drawings and preparing the index is appreciated, as is the assistance of Martha E. Norton, who typed and edited the manuscript.

Contents

Contents

1
Structure and Function

DEVELOPMENT AND STRUCTURE OF THE LUNGS

In the fourth week of embryonic life, an evagination in the pharynx, known as the laryngotracheal groove, forms a tubular outgrowth of endoderm from which the larynx, trachea, bronchi and the lungs subsequently develop. This outgrowth (or "lung bud") at first has an extensive communication with the pharynx and is surrounded by mesenchyme that will form the tracheal cartilages and musculature. As the upper part of the primitive trachea elongates, it forms two bronchial buds, pushing them caudally in front of the esophagus. The right bud or bronchus is larger than the left and its course more directly downward. The left bronchus is directed more laterally. By the fifth week, the right bronchus forms two buds while only one forms on the left.

These mainstem bronchi branch and rebranch to form the bronchial tree of the adult; they supply five pulmonary lobes—three on the right and two on the left. Ultimately on the right, there is an upper apical bronchus, a main or middle bronchus and a right lower bronchus. The last does not have a symmetrical mate on the left, but the first two are paired. The early branches of right and left bronchi appear successively from a single main stem. Later, the branches divide and subdivide in dichotomous fashion (Fig. 1-1). These bronchial passages are semirigid tubes, their walls being reinforced by cartilagenous rings. Nevertheless, the diameters of the larger and smaller branches dilate with inspiration and contract partially with expiration.

The bronchial buds are surrounded by mesenchyme that attaches the adult lung to the mediastinum and ultimately forms the walls of the pleural cavities. These cavities are lined by mesothelium from the coelomic lining. During the first five months of development, there is no distinction between

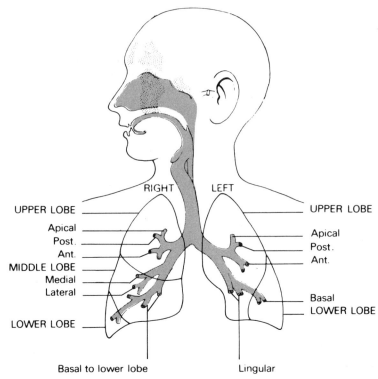

UPPER LOBE

Apical
Post.
Ant.
MIDDLE LOBE
Medial
Lateral

LOWER LOBE

RIGHT   LEFT

UPPER LOBE

Apical
Post.
Ant.

Basal
LOWER LOBE

Basal to lower lobe   Lingular

Fig. 1-1. Distribution of mainstem bronchi to lobes of the lung.

the columnar epithelial lining of the bronchi and alveolar ducts (which are extensions of the bronchioles) and the buds of the future alveoli. However in the sixth month, the alveolar lining changes from columnar to simple squamous epithelium and extensive vascularization of the interalveolar mesenchyme (characteristic of the adult lung) occurs (Fig. 1-2).

The nasal air passages, the respiratory portion of the larynx and the trachea are lined by ciliated columnar epithelium interspersed with goblet cells. Beneath the lamina propia supporting these cells are both mucus and serum secreting glands embedded in the submucosa. The wall of the trachea is supported by cartilagenous rings bound together by smooth muscle fibers. These histologic components of the trachea are continued into the main-stem bronchi into which it divides and into the subsequent bronchial branches until the terminal bronchioles are reached. These bronchioles are less than 1 mm. in diameter and have no cartilage in their walls. They serve as interlobular ducts for the pulmonary parenchyma, which is composed of innumerable lobules 1 to 2 cm. in diameter. At its apex, each of these lobules receives a bronchiole. The base of the lobule is

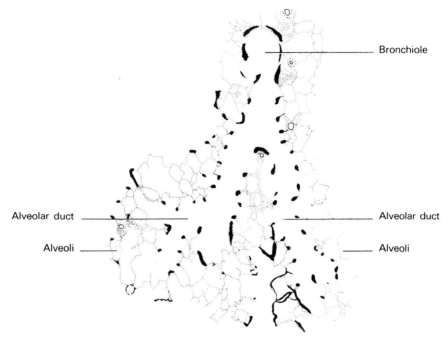

Bronchiole

Alveolar duct

Alveoli

Alveolar duct

Alveoli

Fig. 1-2. Histology of pulmonary alveoli. The musculature is deeply
stained (Redrawn after Baltisberger).

usually directed toward the pleura, with a lesser number of lobules having
their base directed toward the mediastinum.

Within the lobule, the bronchiole opens into an alveolar duct containing
fibers of smooth muscle in its wall. This duct enters into a common space
or atrium from which multiple alveoli radiate. The partitions that separate
the alveoli contain the capillary network. These air spaces and their
capillaries provide for the gaseous exchange between blood and air and,
together, comprise the pulmonary functional units. However, the alveolar
ducts and alveoli, including the capillary network, are usually referred to
collectively as the "sponge work" or parenchyma of the lung. In addition
to being connected via the atria,* the individual alveoli are also connected
by a minute airway, the "alveolar pores," which permit air to pass from
one alveolus to another. In one form of emphysema (panacinar) in which
the alveoli are dilated and their walls ruptured, cross-ventilation of entrapped air from one alveolus to another is considered a major factor in the
progress of the disease.

The structure of the alveolar walls and their capillaries has been defined

---

* Most histology texts consider the atria as a part of the alveolar ducts.

by electronmicroscopy. A continuous thin layer of epithelial cytoplasm lines the alveoli, bulging to enclose nuclei. Beneath this layer is a basement membrane covering the capillaries, which are lined by a single layer of endothelium, which also has a basement membrane. Gaseous diffusion between the alveolar space and the capillary blood must traverse the epithelial lining and its basement membrane, the endothelial basement membrane and the endothelial cytoplasm (Fig. 1-3). In addition, a non-cellular surfactant fluid lines the alveoli. This fluid is secreted by Type II alveolar pneumocytes * and contains dipalmityl lecithin. This secretion is present within these cells as dense inclusions in newborn mammals.

At intervals, the alveolar and capillary walls divide to enclose fibrils of connective and elastic tissue which are extensions from similar and more abundant fibrils surrounding the alveolar ducts. These fibrils protect the alveolar structures from overexpansion. Within the meshes of the fibrils are phagocytes and granulocytes. The macrophages are increased and contain hemosiderin in heart failure. Both the macrophages and granulocytes are much increased in pneumonitis.

The adult human lung contains about 300 million alveoli and, if the air passages are patent, these provide an abundant reserve capacity. Surgical

---

* In the adult, the majority of alveolar lining cells are Type I pneumocytes with thin cytoplasm devoid of secretory inclusions. The Type II granular pneumocytes are plump cells with microvilli and contain secretory inclusions (Nash, G. *et al.:* Alveolar cell carcinoma: does it exist? Cancer *29*:322, 1972).

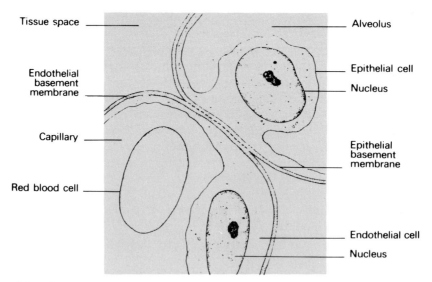

Fig. 1-3. Diagram of electron micrograph of human lung showing diffusion surfaces.

removal of a lung is well tolerated if the opposite lung is free of disease. Dyspnea and hypoxia are more often the result of an impeded airway (by asthma or bronchitis), of restricted expansion, or the result of circulatory failure than of the loss of alveolar diffusion surface.

BLOOD SUPPLY OF THE LUNGS

The blood supply of the lungs differs from the circulation of other organs in three important respects: (1) The pulmonary artery delivers the entire output of the right heart to the lungs, but these vessels carry venous blood that is incompetent to maintain the aeration and nourishment of pulmonary structures. (2) The pulmonary veins carry oxygenated blood from the lungs to the left atrium for distribution to the entire body by the left ventricle. Only a small portion of this aerated blood supply is available for the nourishment of the pulmonary structures via the bronchial arteries. (3) The vascular bed of the lungs passes blood from the small arteries to the alveolar capillaries at low pressure (approximately 25/10 mm. Hg) without an intervening group of arterioles for regulating this pressure, which normally varies directly with the output of the right ventricle.

The pulmonary artery subdivides at the hilum into branches which follow the bronchial tree so that each main branch of bronchus is accompanied by a branch of the pulmonary artery. The subdivisions which reach the respiratory bronchioles break up into the capillaries supplying alveolar ducts and alveoli (Fig. 1-4).

The returning aerated blood from the capillaries is collected into the branches of the pulmonary veins, which lie anteriorly and below the main stem bronchi, which they parallel.

The bronchi and interstitial tissues of the lung and the alveolar wall receive oxygenated blood via the bronchial arteries branching from the thoracic aorta. These are relatively small and are closely bound to the bronchi. Branches of these vessels traverse the interlobular septum to supply the pleura. These vessels are enlarged in bronchiectasis.

The lymphatic drainage of the lungs begins in the visceral pleura and drains via the interlobular septa into branches that travel in the connective tissue surrounding the bronchioles and bronchi and the various arteries and veins. Small lymphatics have been described in tissue bordering the alveolar ducts and bronchioles but not between the alveoli (Fig. 1-5).

During strenuous exercise, the return of blood via the superior and inferior venae cavae to the right atrium and ventricle is aided by the increased negative intrathoracic pressure that accompanies the increased respiratory movements. During periods of severe hypoxia, the capillary

Tracheobronchial tree

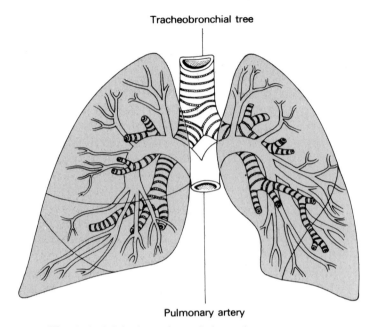

Pulmonary artery

Fig. 1-4. Main branches of the pulmonary artery.

bed of the lungs leaks fluid, which is drained back to the right atrium via the lymphatics and subclavian veins (Drinker).[31]

In patients with severe bronchitis or pneumonia, the inflammatory hyperemia increases the width of the pulmonary arteries through distention and they pursue a straighter course. With passive congestion due to left ventricular failure and with mitral stenosis, the venous pressure causes them to pursue a more tortuous course. These changes in vascular patterns are often discernible in the roentgenogram of the chest. In long standing mitral stenosis, there is secondary arterial constriction that is attributable to a protective mechanism which inhibits pulmonary edema. A number of diseases accompanied by pulmonary fibrosis tend to obliterate the capillary channels and produce pulmonary hypertension with ultimate right ventricular failure. These include long standing emphysema, silicosis and other forms of pneumoconiosis and so-called collagen diseases such as scleroderma (progressive systemic sclerosis).

In the fetus, blood from the superior and the inferior venae cavae that enters the right atrium passes predominantly to the left atrium via the foramen ovale to bypass the nonfunctioning lungs. However, some gains access to the right ventricle and passes into the pulmonary artery to proceed to the lungs. Again, a major portion of this blood bypasses the lungs

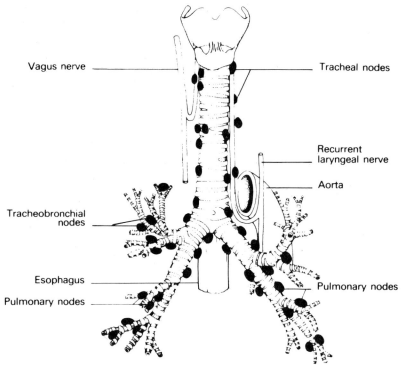

Vagus nerve

Tracheal nodes

Recurrent
laryngeal nerve

Aorta

Tracheobronchial
nodes

Esophagus

Pulmonary nodes

Pulmonary nodes

Fig. 1-5. Lymph nodes of the tracheobronchial tree.

via the ductus arteriosus, this time to enter the aorta immediately distal to the arch (Potter, E. L.: Pathology of the Fetus and the Newborn, Year Book, Chicago, 1953).

PULMONARY FUNCTIONS

Ventilatory Volumes

The spongelike structure of the lungs provides an interface between air and blood flow permitting a continuous exchange of the respiratory gases in the blood with the environment. Air flow is accomplished by the bellows action of the chest wall and diaphragm aided by the elastic recoil of the lungs during expiration. Blood flow is accomplished by the pumping action of the right ventricle, whose filling is aided by negative intrathoracic pressure during inspiration. The amounts of air and blood passing in and out of the lungs are approximately equal—about 5 liters/minute. Air flow or ventilation at the alveolar level is 350 ml. per breath at 14 breaths per minute, whereas cardiac output is 70 ml. per contraction at 70 per minute.

This ratio of air flow (V) to blood flow (Q) is called the Ventilatory Perfusion or V/Q Ratio.

Normal respiration is defined as that which brings sufficient air in the alveoli into contact with sufficient pulmonary circulation to maintain the blood gases within physiologic limits. Most diseases of the lungs alter ventilatory capacity, but because pulmonary blood flow can be shunted away from nonaerated tissue and because the rate of respirations is increased via chemical stimuli, changes in the blood O_2 and CO_2 concentrations are not correspondingly altered. For this reason, abnormal variations in respiration that accompany disease are not adequately reflected by the level of the blood gases, and techniques have been developed for evaluating pulmonary functions in accordance with three separate components: (1) by spirometry to measure air volumes and flow; (2) by isotopic scanning to determine blood flow and its distribution * aided at times by the use of angiograms of the pulmonary vessels; and, (3) by chemical analysis of blood gases for O_2 and CO_2 content.

In clinical practice, the patient's capacity to inflate the lungs during inspiration and deflate them with expiration can be roughly estimated by fluoroscopic examination. More accurate measurement requires spirometry, which permits the determination of air flow during inspiration and expiration, during a given time period, and during breathing at normal and maximum levels of effort.

During quiet breathing, the normal adult inhales and exhales 500 ml of air at a rate of 12 to 14 breaths per minute for an average breathing capacity of 6 to 7 liters per minute. This exchange of 500 ml. per breath is known as *tidal volume* (V_t).† Deep breathing increases tidal volume but slows respirations; shallow breathing decreases the tidal volume but increases the respiratory rate. In clinical practice, rapid shallow breathing suggests diminished lung capacity.

The *vital capacity* (VC) is the maximum volume of air that can be exhaled after a forced inspiration. The normal adult averages 4,000 to 5,000 ml. This capacity may be reduced by obstruction of the air passages, by restricted respiratory excursions, by loss of elastic recoil in the lungs or by actual loss of lung parenchyma (Fig. 1-6).

During quiet breathing, tidal volume (V_t) is distributed chiefly to the centrally located alveoli; with deep breathing, the central and lower portion of the lungs are included; with maximal breathing (VC), the entire capacity of both lungs is used (Fig. 1-7). After normal inspiration and expiration

---

* Isotopic scanning with ^{133}Xe is also used to measure air flow and its distribution.

† Tidal volume minus anatomic dead space gives the volume of alveolar ventilation. The dead space refers to the airway between the nasopharynx and alveoli where no exchange of respiratory gases with blood occurs and is roughly equivalent to one milliliter of dead space for each pound of body weight (Chap. 2).

CAUSES OF DIMINISHED VITAL CAPACITY

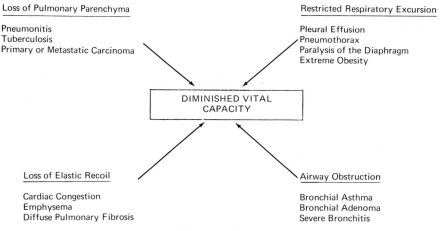

Loss of Pulmonary Parenchyma

Pneumonitis
Tuberculosis
Primary or Metastatic Carcinoma

Restricted Respiratory Excursion

Pleural Effusion
Pneumothorax
Paralysis of the Diaphragm
Extreme Obesity

DIMINISHED VITAL CAPACITY

Loss of Elastic Recoil

Cardiac Congestion
Emphysema
Diffuse Pulmonary Fibrosis

Airway Obstruction

Bronchial Asthma
Bronchial Adenoma
Severe Bronchitis

Figure 1-6.

of tidal air (V_t), a maximum forced expiration measures expiratory reserve volume (ERV). This is equal to the VC minus V_t (Fig. 1-7).

After exhaling the maximum forced volume of air, an additional volume of 1,500 ml. of residual air remains in the lungs (normal adults). This is known as residual volume (RV) and can be exchanged only by diffusion

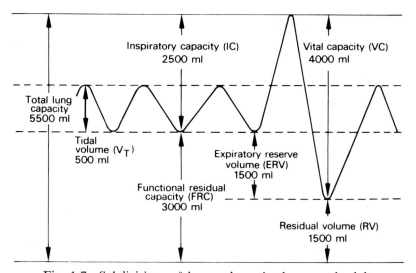

Inspiratory capacity (IC)
2500 ml

Vital capacity (VC)
4000 ml

Total lung capacity
5500 ml

Tidal volume (V_T)
500 ml

Expiratory reserve volume (ERV)
1500 ml

Functional residual capacity (FRC)
3000 ml

Residual volume (RV)
1500 ml

Fig. 1-7. Subdivisions of lung volume in the normal adult.

and not by ventilation. The VC plus the RV is known as the total lung capacity (TLC), which approximates 6,000 ml. in the normal adult.

Vital Capacity (VC)	4,000 ml.
+Residual Air (RV)	1,500 ml.
Total Lung Capacity (TLC)	5,500 ml.

Usually in asthma and emphysema, the expiratory reserve volume (ERV) is decreased, indicating either diminished rate of air flow in the bronchial passages (asthma) or increased residual air (RV) (exchanged only by diffusion) as in emphysema.

Residual air cannot be measured directly. It can be calculated by having the patient (after a forced expiration) breathe pure oxygen for seven minutes and collecting the expired air in a nitrogen-free spirometer. At the end of this time, the collected nitrogen derived from the residual air represents 80 percent of the residual volume. Thus, if the volume of nitrogen is 1,000 ml., residual air equals $1,000 \times \dfrac{100}{80} = 1,250$ ml. In healthy young adults, the N_2 of residual air is replaced by oxygen in 2 minutes. In patients with asthma and/or emphysema, this may require 7 minutes. When carried out at the end of a complete expiration, the test measures residual volume; when performed after a full inspiration, total lung capacity is measured (residual volume equals TLC minus VC) (Fig. 1-7). Chronic infiltrating disease of the lung (silicosis, sarcoidosis or radiation fibrosis) and deformity of the thoracic cage affecting its size or excursions (kyphoscoliosis or marked obesity) diminish the total capacity (TLC). Forms of emphysema and pulmonary cysts may increase TLC.

By prolonging expiration in the presence of ventilatory impairment such as airway obstruction, a normal vital capacity can be achieved with

TABLE 1-1. Predicted Maximum Breathing Capacity in Children in Relation to Height

Height in cm.	Maximum Breathing Capacity (liters/min.) *
100	23
120	47
140	71
160	95
180	119

* Based on the formula FEV $0.75 \times 40 =$ breathing capacity in l (liters) min.
† Values refer to the subject in upright position (seated or standing) and are 5 percent lower in recumbancy.
Modified from Bates & Christie.[9]

maximum effort. For this reason, a more reliable estimate of the patient's ventilation is achieved by measuring the volume of forced expiration in the first second (after a forced inspiration). The normal adult can expire 83 percent of his vital capacity in the first second. This *timed vital capacity* (FEV_1) approximates 3,000 ml. When multiplied by 30, it gives an estimate of the maximum breathing capacity per minute, which approximates 80 to 100 liters per minute in adults. When forced expiratory volume is measured for ¾ second ($FEV_{0.75}$), multiplying by 40 gives a similar estimate. The forced expiratory volume in one second, when divided by the vital capacity, should equal 80 percent under normal conditions. When the quotient is diminished, obstruction to normal air flow is presumed *provided* that the vital capacity is in the normal range. Pulmonary fibrosis or destruction of lung tissue may reduce vital capacity by one half and thus raise the quotient within the normal 75 to 83 percent range.

In children, the FEV_1 (or $FEV_{0.75}$) increases with their height as age advances (see Table 1-1). Increase in the various subdivisions of lung

INCREASED LUNG VOLUME WITH GROWTH IN CHILDREN

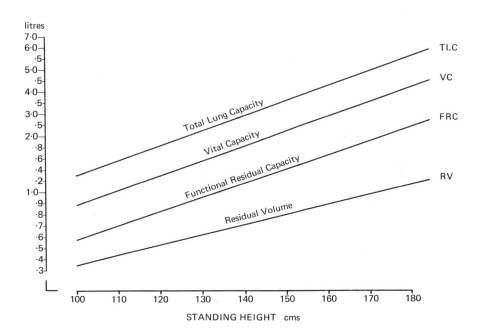

Fig. 1-8. Increased lung volume with growth in children. (Bates, D. and Christie, R.: Respiratory Function in Disease. Philadelphia, W. B. Saunders.)

volume with increased height are shown graphically in Figure 1-8. The subdivisions of lung volume also shift with age. Total lung capacity and vital capacity decline progressively from 20 to 60 years. Conversely, residual volume (air that cannot be exchanged during respiration) shows a corresponding increase. This increased storage of residual air results from progressive loss of elasticity in the lungs with advancing age. As described subsequently, expiration depends chiefly upon passive recoil of tissues expanded during the muscular effort of inspiration.

The subdivisions of lung volume during childhood increase with height from a total lung volume of 1.2 liters at 100 cm. at age 4 years to 5 liters at adolescence (age 15 to 16). Vital capacity ranges from 0.9 liter to 3.7 liters and reserve volume from 0.3 liter to 1 liter. These values are achieved with maximum height or growth (160 to 180 cm.) and are maintained through adulthood, with total lung volume and vital capacity decreasing noticeably after the age of 50 to 60 years. They are diminished with obesity and with loss of lung compliance or elasticity in disease (Fig. 1-6).

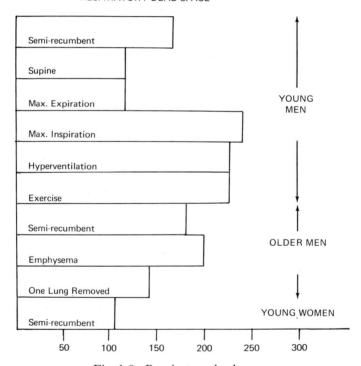

Fig. 1-9. Respiratory dead space.

2

Respiratory Mechanics

PULMONARY MECHANICS

During inspiration, the muscles of respiration (the diaphragm in particular) produce differences in pressure between mouth, alveoli and pleural space to move air into the chest and expand the lungs and chest wall. This muscular force is opposed within the respiratory system by the resistance of its elastic properties and the frictional resistance of gas and tissues. During expiration, the energy which has been applied to the system to expand its elastic components now aids in the movement of air from the lungs using the "elastic recoil" of the lungs to overcome frictional resistance.

In measuring pulmonary function, it is possible to separate those forces related to elastic deformation from those associated with frictional resistance. The elastic properties are measured by the ratio between a volume change (ΔV) within the system and the related pressure changes (ΔP), known as compliance (C). The resistance (R), on the other hand, represents the ratio between a pressure change and the associated volume change per unit time of flow ($\Delta \dot{V}$). Measurements for compliance can be made during either inspiration or expiration in the normal tidal range but expiration is preferred. The equation for calculation is:

$$\text{Static Compliance } (C_{st}) = \frac{\dot{V}}{P} = \frac{0.500 \text{ liter}}{2.5 \text{ cm.}} = 0.200 \text{ liter/cm. } H_2O$$
(Normal Adult)

The volume change results from a pressure sufficient to overcome: (1) airway resistance; (2) tissue resistance; (3) chest wall tissue resistance; and (4) gas inertia. The intrapleural pressure is not measured directly but is measured by a manometer attached to an intraesophageal balloon. Compliance, indicating the elasticity of the lung in mathematical terms is the

13

approximate reciprocal of the tissue resistance (known as elastance) overcome by breathing. In other words, resistance equals pressure divided by
air flow or $R = \dfrac{P}{V}$.

The esophageal balloon for measuring intrathoracic pressure is made of
thin rubber and measures 15 cm. in length and 2 cm. in circumference,
sealed to a polyethylene catheter. Balloon pressure equals intrapleural
pressure in subjects in the upright position if the balloon is filled without
stretching. Volume changes with pressure differ in inspiration and expiration because of changes in airway resistance. During inspiration, negative
pressure expands the tracheobronchial tree, but the positive pressure during
expiration narrows it, as pointed out by Einthoven in 1892.[35]

STATIC BEHAVIOR OF THE LUNGS

Shown in Figure 2-1 is a static volume—pressure curve for the intact
human lung. The pressure difference is that between the mouth and the
pleural space (assumed from pressure changes in the esophageal balloon).
The slope of this curve ($\Delta V/\Delta P$) is the compliance of the lung (C_1). As
can be seen, this slope varies according to the level of inflation of the lung;
at the extremes of inflation and deflation, the lung is "stiffer" than in the
midvolume range. At the volume level of usual quiet breathing, C_1 is

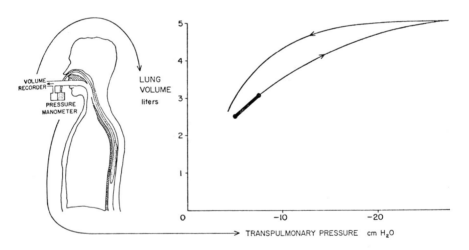

$$\text{STATIC COMPLIANCE} = \frac{\Delta V}{\Delta P} = \frac{0.500}{2.5} = 0.200 \ \text{liter/cm}$$

Fig. 2-1. Static pressure-volume relationships in a normal subject.
(Bates, D. V., and Christie, R. V.: Respiratory Function in Disease.
Philadelphia, Saunders)

about 0.2 L per cm. H_2O. Diseases such as emphysema can produce increases in compliance as previously noted, while patients with interstitial fibrosis have decreased lung compliance.

The clinician ordinarily does not measure lung compliance, but assesses the elasticity of pulmonary tissues from lung volumes and capacities (see Fig. 1-7). Normally, a young adult male with a total lung capacity of 6 liters can move three fourths of this volume from his chest starting from a point of complete inflation and utilizing maximum exhalation. The remaining one fourth of total lung capacity, representing residual volume, is increased as vital capacity is diminished. Such an alteration of ratios is usually indicative of loss of compliance.

As previously noted, calculation of residual capacity and total lung volume require the wash-out of nitrogen by breathing oxygen for 7 minutes. The wash-out method (and similar ones such as helium dilution) for calculating residual air in the lungs determines the volume in communication with the open airway. If air is contained in a pulmonary cyst without a bronchus communication, oxygen cannot enter nor is nitrogen washed out. The same applies in varying degrees to air in portions of the lung with obstructive airways that are poorly ventilated. Thus, these techniques usually underestimate the true volume of air in the chest when significant pulmonary disease is present.

THE BODY PLETHYSMOGRAPH

More accurate measurements are obtained with the body plethysmograph (Fig. 2-2). In this device, the patient sits completely enclosed in an airtight box and pants at FRC (functional reserve volume or maximal expiration after normal inspiration) against an external obstruction. This obstruction prevents the movement of air through the airways during the action of the respiratory muscles with panting, which produces alternate expansion and compression of air in the chest. Measurements of pressure and volume changes in the box permit the calculation of the volume of air in the patient's chest by the application of Boyle's law. This law states that at a constant temperature, the pressure exerted by a particular amount of gas is inversely proportional to the volume occupied by the gas. The volume determined by this method includes all the air subject to the action of the respiratory muscles and not just the well-ventilated volumes. In chronic obstructive disease, measurements of FRC are significantly higher by this method than by the gas wash-out technique. Using both methods the discrepancy gives an estimate of the amount of air trapped in poorly ventilated portions of the patient's lungs.

Definite limits to expansion and inflation of the lung in the intact chest

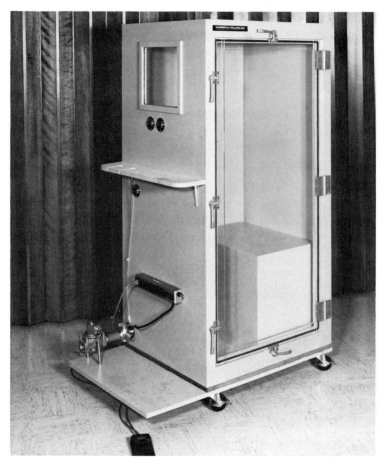

Fig. 2-2. Body plethysmograph. (Courtesy Warren E. Collins Inc.)

(indicated by relatively fixed total lung capacity and residual volume) imply mechanisms for maintaining alveolar stability so that the normal lung neither overinflates nor collapses. One important factor in maintaining this stability is the secretion of pulmonary surfactant, a fluid of mixed lipids and polysaccharides secreted by Type II alveolar pneumocytes. Surfactant reduces surface tension at the air-liquid boundary in the alveolus. When the alveoli are deflated, concentration of surfactant rises, surface tension is reduced and the tendency toward further collapse is inhibited. When the lung inflates, surfactant concentration diminishes, surface tension increases and retards further inflation. By such means, surface tension varies with the degree of inflation or deflation of the lungs. In infants born with respiratory immaturity, lack of surfactant secretion produces the syndrome of idiopathic respiratory distress in which the lungs tend to collapse and resist inflation because of increased surface tension in the alveoli. Low levels of surfactant after the 30th week of gestation increase the risk of the respiratory distress syndrome in the newborn.* (Chap. 11)

More important than this secretion in providing alveolar stability at high volumes is the tensile strength of the supporting tissues. The interalveolar pulmonary connective tissues limit expansion. When this tissue is damaged, overinflation occurs as in emphysema, where total lung capacity is increased with high residual volume.

DYNAMIC BEHAVIOR OF THE LUNG AND AIRWAY RESISTANCE

The dynamics of pulmonary ventilation can be described in different ways. Resistance to air flow represents the ratio between the pressure applied to the system and the resultant flow achieved. According to the site where the pressure measurements are made, it is possible to determine values for resistance of the airway, pulmonary (air plus lung tissue) or total respiratory (airway plus lung tissue plus thoracic wall) resistance. Airway resistance measured by the body plethysmograph is 1.5 cm. H_2O per L per sec. in the young adult male.

Clinically, the presence of increased resistance to air flow is estimated from the forced expiratory volume (FEV) curve. As previously noted (Chap. 1), the normal individual, during forced expiration, can exhale 80 percent of his vital capacity in one second (FEV_1). The patient with obstructive pulmonary disease may have a normal total vital capacity, but because of increased resistance to air flow, will require a longer time to move an equivalent air volume from his lungs. His FEV_1 expressed as a percentage of vital capacity will be less than 80 percent.

VARIATIONS IN AIR FLOW WITH VARYING DEGREES OF EFFORT

Just as there are limits to volume change in the lungs, so there are limits to the flow rates that can be achieved during a maximum forced expiration. During a series of forced expiratory efforts by a normal individual, the subject first inhales to his total lung capacity and then exhales with varying degrees of effort to his residual volume. At similar volumes, expressed as "% TLC," measurements are made of the applied pressure and the resultant flow.

As shown, when a large volume of air is still in the lung, (90% TLC) the flow rates achieved will increase as the driving pressure increases,

* Clements, J. A. *et al.:* Respiratory-distress syndrome: rapid test for surfactant in amniotic fluid, New England J. Med. *286:*1077, 1972.

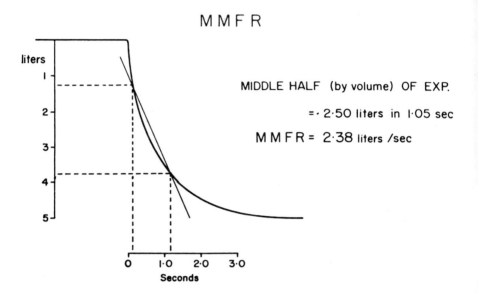

Fig. 2-3. Maximal midexpiratory flow rates. (Bates, D. V. and Christie, R. V.: Respiratory Function in Disease. Philadelphia, W. B. Saunders, 1964)

although not in a linear fashion. The flow rates at such high lung volumes are said to be "effort dependent." However, at lower lung volumes (below 70% TLC), the highest flow rates are achieved at pressures well below maximum and increases in pressure above the level do not result in a further increase in flow. Such flows are "effort independent." Thus, the limiting factors to the maximum flow rates achieved at low lung volumes are related to the anatomic state of the lung and airways and not to the muscular effort supplied by the individual.

Since only submaximal pressures are required to achieve maximum flow rates at lower lung volumes, it is possible to ignore pressure measurement and instead, describe flow-volume relationships during a forced expiratory maneuver. An example of a maximum expiratory flow volume (MEFV) curve is shown in Figure 2-3. As can be seen, peak expiratory flow is reached while the volume of air in the chest is still high; this is in the effort dependent area of the curve. Maximum expiratory flow rates, measured at specific volume points when the amount of air in the chest is lower, are independent of effort and can be used to quantitate degrees of obstruction. Flow measurements at the point where one half the vital capacity has been exhaled are commonly used. In a normal subject, these range between 2.5 to 5.3 L per sec. Patients with asthma, cystic fibrosis, emphysema and

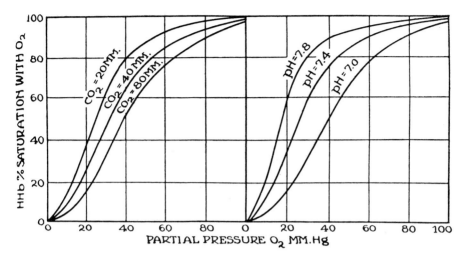

Fig. 2-4. HbO_2 dissociation curve. Note that with normal CO_2, hemoglobin remains 90% to 95% saturated although P_{O_2} diminishes to 80%. (Grollman, A.: Clinical Physiology. New York, Blakiston, 1957)

other chronic obstructive pulmonary diseases usually have values well below this level.

VENTILATORY PERFUSION RELATIONS

Inhaled air contains roughly 80 percent nitrogen and 20 percent oxygen. In respiratory physiology, these are translated into partial pressures in terms of mm. Hg pressure. The oxygen pressure of inhaled air at sea level is roughly 150 mm. Hg. This is arrived at by the barometric pressure of room air (at 20° C.) of 760 mm. Hg, subtracting water vapor pressure of 17 mm. Hg and multiplying by 20.9 percent, which represents the percentage of oxygen to give roughly 155 mm. Hg of P_{O_2} (oxygen pressure). During inhalation, the P_{O_2} reaching the alveoli is lowered by saturation with water vapor at body temperature and by mixing with air in the dead space, which contains a residuum from prior exhalations.

The effect of normal respiration at normal oxygen pressure and normal pulmonary perfusion (assuming normal alveolar-capillary diffusion) upon the blood gases is indicated in the following tabulation:

Venous	Lungs	Arterial
P_{O_2} 40 mm. Hg	Min. Vol. ventilation$=6$ L. (500 ml. tidal air $\times$ 12 R/min.)	P_{O_2} 100 mm. Hg
P_{CO_2} 46 mm. Hg	Alveolar ventilation$=4$ L./min. Pulmonary blood flow$=5$ L. Ventilation/Perfusion (V/Q) Ratio$=0.8$	P_{CO_2} 40 mm. Hg

With oxygen tension in the alveoli and in the arterial blood in equilibrium at 100 mm. Hg, the arterial oxygen tension is 97.4 percent. In the above table, the alveolar ventilation per minute is 2 liters less than the minute volume supplied by ventilation. This difference is due to the anatomic dead space where the passage of air through the tracheobronchial tree and naso-pharynx fails to contact the capillary pulmonary blood flow and effect gaseous exchange. The dead space can be read from the chart reproduced from Comroe *et al.* (Fig. 1-9) and varies between 150 and 200 ml. in the adult. In another method of calculation, the dead space in milliliters is assumed to equal the patient's ideal weight in pounds.

When the volume of anatomic dead space (150 ml.) is subtracted from the tidal volume (500 ml.), the remaining 350 ml. of inspired air entering the alveoli equals *alveolar ventilation* (V_A).

With rapid shallow breathing (tidal volume 250 ml. and a rate of 32 per min.), a minute volume of 8000 ml. is achieved but the V_A is only 3200 ml. On the other hand, with slow deep respirations a tidal volume of 100 ml. at 8 per minute gives a minute volume of 800 ml. and a V_A of 6800 ml., because dead space remains practically constant under both conditions. Theoretically, with shallow ventilation equal in volume only to dead space, breathing would be ineffectual; but even with tidal volume reduced to 70 ml. and a dead space of 150 ml., diffusion may permit enough alveolar ventilation for survival.

Alveolar ventilation is difficult to measure and is determined by dividing the volume of CO_2 in expired gas by the percent of CO_2 in alveolar air (determined by catheter). This, when multiplied by 100 equals V_A in milliliters.

$$\text{Alveolar ventilation (ml.)} = \frac{\text{volume of expired } CO_2 \text{ (ml.)}}{\text{Percent } CO_2 \text{ in alveolar gas}} \times 100$$

For practical purposes, a patient is assumed to have normal alveolar venti-lation when arterial P_{CO_2} is within the range of 35 to 45 mm. Hg. When P_{CO_2} is greater than 45, alveolar hypoventilation is indicated; when the value is below 35 mm. Hg, alveolar hyperventilation is indicated.

PULMONARY CIRCULATION AND PERFUSION

Regardless of the efficiency or adequacy of alveolar ventilation, a corre-spondingly adequate blood supply to the alveolar capillaries is required to ensure the uptake of oxygen and release of CO_2 in environmental exchange. The appropriate matching of adequate alveolar ventilation to pulmonary capillary circulation provides a normal ventilation-perfusion ratio ($\dot{V}/\dot{Q}$). Imbalance between the two produces inequality in ventila-tion-perfusion or abnormal $\dot{V}/\dot{Q}$ ratios. However, in the normal adult in the upright position, there is a vertical gradient of pulmonary blood supply with the apices receiving relatively less blood flow than the bases of the lung (West).[96, 97] Similarly, inspired air is not equally distributed to all alveoli and $\dot{V}/\dot{Q}$ inequalities result. Such inequalities in the normal adult usually result in a 5 mm. Hg difference between alveolar P_{O_2} and arterial P_{O_2}. In a number of diseases such as emphysema and pulmonary fibrosis, this difference is pronounced and arterial hypoxemia develops.

Disturbances in ventilation and perfusion can be demonstrated in a number of fashions.* One of the more recent approaches uses scanning with radioactive xenon to document defects in both perfusion and ventilation (Fig. 4-12). Such defects are probably the most common cause of hypoxemia seen in patients with chronic obstructive pulmonary disease. Gas transfer at the alveolar level between blood and air proceeds from high to low concentrations by passive diffusion without the aid of active transport mechanisms. Normally, blood entering the pulmonary capillaries has a P_{O_2} of 40 mm. Hg and a P_{CO_2} of 46 mm. Hg. It is separated by the alveolar epithelium and capillary endothelium from alveolar air with a P_{O_2} of 100 mm. Hg and a P_{CO_2} of 40 mm. Hg. These gases then diffuse across this barrier until the partial pressures are equalized on either side. Thus, blood leaves the pulmonary capillaries with gas tensions identical to those in the alveolus (P_{O_2} 100 mm. Hg; P_{CO_2} 40 mm. Hg).

In pulmonary disease, the efficiency of diffusion is frequently measured, but whether this represents thickening or changes in the permeability of the alveolar wall or inequalities in the $\dot{V}/\dot{Q}$ ratio cannot be determined. Theoretically, the blood uptake of oxygen by diffusion and the clearance of CO_2 from the blood should be measured, but this is not practical. Instead, the uptake of small amounts of inhaled carbon monoxide is measured or the wash-out from the lungs of intravenously administered [133]Xe. In a number of pulmonary diseases such as pneumoconiosis, sarcoidosis or scleroderma, progressive dyspnea followed by cyanosis eventually decreases total lung volume (TLC) and restricts both ventilatory and perfusion capacities. Because in the earlier stages, hypoxemia and hypercapnia exceed the degree of fibrosis visible in the roentgenogram, these were classed as "alveolar-capillary block" syndromes. These are now considered examples of ventilatory–perfusion inequality with increased physiologic dead space. This is the conclusion of Holland[50] and also Finley et al.[40] in patients with the "alveolar–capillary block" syndrome and also of Read and Williams,[75] who studied the Hamman-Rich syndrome and asbestosis. Nevertheless, in pa-

---

* Evidence of mismatching or unequal $\dot{V}/\dot{Q}$ ratios can be obtained by recording continuous percentages of CO_2 during expiration. Normally, after evacuating dead space, CO_2 values rise to a plateau and then remain constant during forced expiration. In inadequately ventilated lungs, the CO_2 concentration continues to rise.

tients with this syndrome a reduced CO uptake may occur while there is still normal vital capacity and the measurement aids in diagnosis. In these conditions, the degree of impairment in effective diffusion is indicated by the reduced capacity of the pulmonary circulation to absorb carbon monoxide, when the patient inhales air containing 0.2 percent CO. The affinity of hemoglobin for CO keeps plasma levels minimal, ensuring a constant rate of diffusion. The amount of CO passing from the alveoli to the blood in one minute is calculated by subtracting expired CO from the inspired amount, the analysis of CO being performed with an infra-red analyzer. The calculation is:

$$\text{Fractional CO Uptake } (\%) = \frac{\text{CO absorbed/minute}}{\text{CO inspired/minute}} \times 100 = D_{Lco}$$

An index of 50 percent is normal; 30 percent or less indicates impaired diffusion.

Diffusion measured by the carbon monoxide technique is a measurement of the rate at which pulmonary blood flow clears a diffusible gas from the

TABLE 2-1. Average Standard Respiratory Values in Adults

Vital Capacity (VC)	5 liters
FEV′=80% of VC	
Maximum Breathing Capacity (FEV L/min.)	
FEV .75×40	120-150 L./min.
Expiratory Reserve Capacity (ERV)	3.5 liters
Residual Volume (RV)	1.5 liters
Total Lung Capacity (TLC)	6-7 liters
Tidal Volume (VT)	500 ml.
Alveolar Ventilation (Va)	350 ml.
Dead Space (V_{DS})	150 ml.
Maximal Midexpiratory Flow Rate (MMFR)	4 L./sec.
Alveolar Ventilation/Minute ($\dot{V}$)	5 L./min.
Cardiac Output/Minute ($\dot{Q}$)	5 L./min.
Ventilation/Perfusion Ratio ($\dot{V}/\dot{Q}$)	0.8−1.0
Diffusion Constant (DLcoSB)	34 ml./min./mm. Hg
Maximal Intrapeural Negative Pressure	−30 cm. H_2O
Lung Compliance (static)	0.200 L./cm. H_2O
pH (blood)	7.4
Arterial P_{O_2}	80-100 mm. Hg
Venous P_{O_2}	25-40 mm. Hg
Arterial O_2 Saturation	95-97%
P_{CO_2} after oxygenating venous blood or arterial	40 mm. Hg
HCO_3^- (standard Bicarbonate, plasma)	22-26 m. Eq./L.
Buffer Base ($HCO_3 \times 2$) +phosphate and serum proteins (Whole Blood)	48 m. Eq./L. (46-54 arterial)

alveoli. A similar measurement in the opposite direction can be made by injecting intravenously the radioactive gas ^{133}Xe and determining by scintillation detectors or camera, the extent to which the lungs are contaminated by the gas and in turn, the rate of clearance or wash-out after equilibrium has been obtained by perfusion. Scanning of the lungs with ^{133}Xe is a more useful procedure, since it gives a visualized distribution of perfusion as the intravenously administered gas appears in the lung and also gives a measurement of ventilatory capacity at wash-out time, determined one minute after perfusion has reached equilibrium.

PULMONARY CIRCULATION

Blood flows through the lungs at low pressure (25/10 mm. Hg) through a vascular bed of low resistance with a pressure drop from pulmonary artery to left atrium averaging 10 mm. Hg. Since capillary pressure is 15 mm. Hg lower than the plasma osmotic pressure, fluid transudation into the alveolar spaces is averted. This contrasts sharply with the renal circulation. One fourth of the cardiac output circulates through the kidney at a glomerular hydrostatic pressure of 40 mm. Hg which is approximately 15 mm. *higher* than osmotic pressure to produce the urinary filtrate. In the lungs, the entire cardiac output of the right ventricle passes through the capillary bed for a maximum exposure to alveolar gases, but without intercellular or intraalveolar transudation. Pulmonary edema is a pathologic event. It follows damage to the capillary walls by irritant gases, by severe asphyxia or by viral infection. Back pressure during left ventricular failure is a common cause and the rapid infusion of hypotonic fluids with dilution of plasma proteins may also cause edema.

The pulmonary blood volume in the normal adult averages 1.2 liters, of which 30 percent is intraarterial and 65 percent venous. The remainder in the capillaries (about 60 ml.) makes this circuit in 0.73 seconds at rest and with exercise, 95 ml. circuits in 0.34 seconds.[79]

Pulmonary perfusion rates and arterial pressures are measured by catheter introduced via the brachial vein through the right heart into the pulmonary artery. This type of test is not without hazard and may disturb cardiac rhythm or produce brachial phlebitis. With the catheter in place, angiopneumograms are usually obtained, outlining the vascular tree with radiopaque solution. The degree of pulmonic hypertension can be measured, pulmonary emboli or hemangioma with venous-arterial shunt and abnormalities of the great vessels may be demonstrated by these techniques. Increased pressure in the pulmonic circuit occurs with congenital pulmonic stenosis, with emphysema, with mitral stenosis and with acute left ventricular failure.[24]

VARIATIONS IN PULMONARY PERFUSION

Numerous observations indicate that the pulmonary circulation adjusts to either an oxygen-poor or carbon dioxide-enriched environment without the stimulus of vasomotor nerves. Under these circumstances, there is increased blood flow and also pulmonary vasoconstriction suggesting the intervention of sympathomimetic hormones. To test the adaptation of pulmonary perfusion to hypoxia, human subjects were given a 5 percent oxygen mixture in a single lung and 3 of 5 subjects showed a shift of blood away from the hypoxic side.[11] This unilateral hypoxia provokes increased ipsilateral resistance to blood flow. The site at which vasoconstriction occurs has not been determined but it appears that the pulmonary vascular smooth muscle (regardless of its location) undergoes indiscriminate constriction at low oxygen tensions. The response seems to be direct. This vasoconstriction is accompanied by increased pulmonary arterial pressure. Such circulatory redistribution is minor compared to the mechanical effects of venous-arterial fistula or emboli.

With chronic hypoxia at high altitudes, there is right ventricular hypertrophy with increased output, suggesting high resistance to pulmonic flow, but the significance of high resistance is uncertain. The thickness of the precapillary vessels is increased, and the polycythemic blood is more viscous. These changes at high altitude are not influenced by breathing a 35 percent oxygen mixture.

Measurements made in pulmonary blood flow during the breathing of 100 percent oxygen show no appreciable effect on pulmonic pressure or blood flow. In emphysema and pulmonic hypertension breathing 30 percent oxygen only occasionally lowers pressure. Rogers, R. M. *et al.,* using saline bronchopulmonary lavage in patients, showed that increased alveolar pressure in the liquid-filled lung shifted blood flow to the contralateral lung.[77b]

Increased carbon dioxide, (acute hypercapnia) produces no marked change in pulmonary vascular resistance or blood flow, since hydrogen ion concentration is combated by increased minute ventilation. However, it is believed that local acidosis exerts a vasoconstricting effect, but the means by which this is accomplished is obscure. In combined chronic hypoxia and hypercapnia resulting from lung diseases which cause hypoventilation, the accumulation of carbon dioxide is proportional to the metabolic rate. In patients with chronic bronchitis and pulmonary emphysema, the carbon dioxide retention reflects an imbalance between ventilation and perfusion. In patients with malfunctioning of chest bellows with this combined disturbance, severe pulmonary hypertension may develop resulting in cor pulmonale and in turn heart failure. This is usually an acute response and does not occur with chronic acidosis. However, the two together (hypercapnia and hypoxia) have only a slightly greater effect in raising pulmonary arterial pressure than hypoxia per se.[41]

In the majority of ventilatory disturbances, pulmonic perfusion is capable of adapting to decreased ventilation. In lobar pneumonia, in emphysematous blebs and in infarction, the pulmonic circuit bypasses the region and returns to the left atrium via the bronchial veins. The airless tissue of bronchogenic carcinoma and of bronchiectasis is also bypassed but secures an arterial blood supply via the bronchial artery. In mitral stenosis, both perfusion and ventilation are shifted to the upper portions of the congested lungs. On the other hand, with chronic obstructive lung disease, the reverse is usually the case and increased ventilation and perfusion occur in the lower lungs. When intravenous [133]xenon gas is used to measure lung clearance, the gas is washed out predominantly after one minute. When there is decreased perfusion, the clearance is only slightly delayed, but with chronic obstructive lung disease such as emphysema, asthma and chronic bronchitis with productive cough, there is a marked delay with wash-out exceeding two minutes. This is usually obvious clinically by the abnormal prolongation of expiration, which is frequently accompanied by expiratory wheezing. It is also confirmed when FEV_1 and VC are measured by spirometry. The normal FEV_1 is 80 percent of VC. With chronic airway obstruction, this ratio falls below 70 percent and may fall to 25 or 50 percent.

GAS TRANSPORT IN THE BLOOD

As part of the respiratory processes, mechanisms must be available for transport of oxygen from the pulmonary capillaries to the body's tissues and for carriage of CO_2 from the tissues to the lung. Oxygen transport is accomplished by two mechanisms: (1) physically dissolved in the plasma; or (2) chemically combined with hemoglobin as oxyhemoglobin. The amount of physically dissolved oxygen can be calculated if we know the partial pressure of the gas in the blood and its solubility in the plasma and red cells. Physiologically, this mode of oxygen transport is quantitatively unimportant. In some pathologic conditions, however, where the hemoglobin transport mechanisms are seriously deficient, it is possible to utilize this mode of transport more effectively by the use of hyperbaric oxygenation (exposure of the patient to environments of two or more atmospheres [1,420 mm. Hg] oxygen).

The major amount of oxygen carried from the pulmonary capillary to the peripheral tissues is chemically combined with hemoglobin. Each gram of hemoglobin can combine with 1.34 ml. of oxygen according to the equation:

$$Hb + 4O_2 \rightleftharpoons Hb\ O_8$$

The relationship between the physically dissolved oxygen and that chemically combined with hemoglobin is expressed by the oxyhemoglobin dissociation curve shown in Figure 2-3. This illustrates the importance of P_{O_2} as a determinant of oxyhemoglobin transport. In the pulmonary capillaries where the oxygen tension is high, chemical combination of oxygen with hemoglobin is virtually complete. When the blood moves to the peripheral tissues, however, and the oxygen tension is diminished, hemoglobin releases the oxygen that has been transported, making it available for oxidative reactions at the tissue level.

Although a solution of hemoglobin in water maintains its saturation with oxygen (at 90%) at a P_{O_2} of 40 mm. Hg nearly as well as it does at 100 mm. Hg (approximately 97%) in the blood, such a fall in P_{O_2} markedly depresses O_2 saturation, thus yielding oxygen to the tissues. The unloading of oxygen is enhanced by body temperature and by the presence of CO_2, which increases hydrogen ion concentration and depresses pH. This unloading or dissociation of oxygen by hemoglobin by increasing P_{CO_2} is known as the *Bohr* effect. Oxygenated hemoglobin becomes acid, which facilitates its action with CO_2 in releasing its oxygen (Fig. 2-4).

There are two separate types of human hemoglobin—adult (A) and fetal (F). Normally, fetal hemoglobin disappears within a few months after birth. The fetal hemoglobin has a different dissociation curve, enabling it to carry its oxygen at higher P_{CO_2} levels. The effect of other abnormal forms of hemoglobin such as in sickle cell anemia with hemoglobin S, is currently being investigated, but is not adequately established.

CARBON DIOXIDE TRANSPORT

Carbon dioxide transport is accomplished by a number of mechanisms. Approximately 5 percent of the CO_2 is physically dissolved in blood plasma and roughly 30 percent is in combination with hemoglobin in the form of carbaminohemoglobin. The remainder of the CO_2 transport occurs in the form of bicarbonate ion. As CO_2 enters the red cell from the plasma, it undergoes hydration to form carbonic acid which ionizes into hydrogen and bicarbonate ions. This reaction is catalyzed by the enzyme carbonic anhydrase in the red cell. Most of the bicarbonate formed then diffuses out into the plasma and is replaced in the red cell by the diffusion of chloride ions (chloride shift). Thus, carbon dioxide is carried in the form of bicarbonate ion, which is mainly produced in the red cell but transported in the plasma. When the blood returns to the pulmonary capillaries, the various reactions described above proceed in the opposite direction, resulting in CO_2 removal from blood to the alveolus.

Thus, the transport of carbon dioxide involves reactions which produce substances that alter the acidity and alkalinity of the blood (the pH). To avoid wide variations in blood pH, chemical buffering mechanisms are present in the blood and tissues, the most important of these being the proteins present in the plasma and the hemoglobin molecule of the red cell. An essential "physiologic" buffer is also provided by the ionization of the weak acid, H_2CO_3, to hydrogen and bicarbonate ions. According to the law of mass action, this ionization proceeds as follows:

$$pH = \frac{pK + \log HCO_3^-}{(CO_2) \ *} \text{Henderson-Hasselbalch equation}$$

The pK for blood is around 6.1 with this system; pH is controlled within narrow limits by varying the concentrations of bicarbonate and CO_2. If the pH of the blood becomes more acid because of loss of bicarbonate ion, the lungs, by hyperventilating and decreasing the CO_2 can return the HCO_3/CO_2 ratio to normal, raising the pH. Similarly, with severe obstructive pulmonary disease, and underventilation, accumulated CO_2 lowers pH. Such respiratory acidosis causes renal response. The kidney increases renal excretion of hydrogen ions and increases reabsorption of bicarbonate. A renal adjustment in the opposite direction occurs with alkalosis.

Carbonic anhydrase is inhibited by sulfonamides and also by the antienzyme acetozolamide (Diamox). High doses of this antienzyme may give rise to CO_2 retention and respiratory acidosis.

REGULATION OF RESPIRATION

The respiratory processes present a complex system which must be coordinated to assure normal blood oxygenation and CO_2 excretion. Breathing is largely an involuntary act, but one that can be greatly modified by volitional effort. The regulatory mechanisms which control the system include those related to nervous response and those responsive to changes in the blood gas tensions or pH. Normal cyclic respiratory activity results from the output of neurons in the medulla oblongata. These are "pacemakers" of the respiratory system. Areas higher in the brain stem are concerned with adjustments to the normal respiratory activity while cortical areas permit modifications such as breath-holding or voluntary hyperventilation.

Various reflexes originating in the lung and pulmonary vasculature have also been identified. Their quantitative importance in the control of normal

---

*CO_2 is used in the denominator rather than the acid H_2CO_3 because it is present in much larger amounts in the blood.

respiratory efforts remains uncertain. Mechanisms such as the cough reflex are of considerable importance in helping the lung rid itself of physical and chemical irritants. In addition, reflex mechanisms are important in helping to modify respiratory activity during swallowing or vomiting.

EFFECT OF BLOOD GASES ON RESPIRATION

The control of respiratory activity through changes in blood gas tensions and pH is accomplished by central and peripheral chemoreceptors. The central chemoreceptors are located in the medulla oblongata, but appear to be distinct from the medullary nerve centers. These chemical centers are mainly responsive to changes in the carbon dioxide tension and hydrogen ion concentration of the arterial blood and cerebrospinal fluid. If, for example, a patient with diabetes develops acidosis and increased hydrogen ion concentration of his blood, the central receptors act to increase ventilatory activity, blow off carbon dioxide and return blood pH toward normal. This form of hyperventilation is seen in patients with diabetic acidosis (Kussmaul breathing). Lowering of the P_{CO_2} or hydrogen ion concentration to subnormal levels will diminish ventilatory activity.

The central chemoreceptors are of great importance in the maintenance of normal ventilatory activity and in the body's response to abnormalities in the chemical constituents of the blood. Their activity can be modified in the presence of chronic obstructive pulmonary diseases such as emphysema. In severe emphysema, mechanical ventilatory activity is insufficient to rid the body of the CO_2 formed by the metabolic processes. As a consequence, the P_{CO_2} rises, producing a stimulus toward hyperventilation (in an attempt to blow off the excess CO_2). However, there is further CO_2 production from the overactive muscles of respiration and the diseased lungs must attempt to hyperventilate even more to blow off the CO_2. This is an inefficient mechanism. In such individuals, the chemoreceptors adapt so that excessive levels of carbon dioxide in the blood do not produce a persistent hyperventilation and respiration is then governed by diminished P_{O_2} levels.

Thus, with chronic respiratory acidosis, the medullary centers cease to respond effectively to increased P_{CO_2} and are governed by decreased arterial P_{O_2}. For this reason, the administration of oxygen tends to depress the respiratory center in severe asthmatic and emphysematous patients and is to be avoided if breathing can be enhanced by bronchial dilators. In individuals with pulmonary hemangioma and venous-arterial shunts, arterial oxygen saturation remains low and P_{CO_2} relatively high in spite of normal ventilatory physiology. Even the breathing of pure oxygen does not completely saturate the arterial blood and the P_{O_2} remains around 97 percent. Damage to the respiratory center itself may lead to a depressed tidal volume and absence of hyperventilation, despite P_{CO_2} elevation.

Hypoventilation of the lungs may result from degrees of respiratory paralysis or diseases of the respiratory muscle. It is usually caused by restricted ventilatory motion (from thoracic deformities or pleural effusion) or diseases decreasing the amount of lung tissue or causing loss of elastic recoil by fibrosis or congestion. Obstructive lesions in the airway may be a factor. The result is anoxemia (decreased P_{O_2}) and respiratory acidosis (increased P_{CO_2}). The diminished alveolar P_{O_2} reduces the percent of saturation of hemoglobin below 97.5. The retention of P_{CO_2} in the alveoli raises the arterial P_{CO_2} and causes a fall in the plasma pH. If the patient breathes oxygen in high concentration, alveolar P_{O_2} and arterial O_2 saturations rise but P_{CO_2} values in the alveoli and blood do not fall correspondingly. These relationships can be calculated on the O_2-CO_2 alveolar diagram of Rahn and Fenn (Fig. 2-5).

THE PERIPHERAL CHEMORECEPTORS

The peripheral chemoreceptors—the aortic and carotid bodies—respond in similar fashion to blood pH and P_{CO_2}. They are important in the body's defense against hypoxemia. Their role in stimulation of ventilation becomes important when the arterial oxygen tension decreases to about 50 mm. Hg.

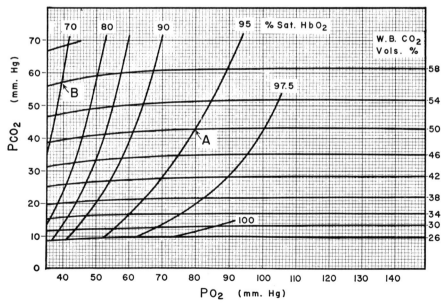

Fig. 2-5. Alveolar P_{O_2}-P_{CO_2}. At Point A, P_{O_2} of 80 and P_{CO_2} of 43 meet and a 95% O_2 saturation is indicated. At Point B, O_2 saturation of 70% and WBCO$_2$ of 58 volume percent meet and a P_{CO_2} of 57.5 mmHg and a P_{O_2} of 39.4 mmHg are indicated.

3

Classification and Major Features of Pulmonary Disease

Diseases of the lung or lower respiratory tract that are well defined both clinically and pathologically are classified into (A) ventilatory, (B) circulatory, and (C) parenchymal. *Ventilatory disturbances* involve the tracheobronchial airways, the most common being acute or chronic bronchitis, attacks of asthma and retained infected bronchial secretions—bronchiectasis. They may involve the pleura, chest wall or diaphragm and thus affect the bellows action of the thorax. *Circulatory disturbances* are caused by direct damage to the pulmonary vascular bed or restriction of its blood flow. The inhalation of noxious gases (steam, smoke and irritant war gases), rickettsial infections, emboli or severe hypoxia produce direct vascular impairment. Restricted pulmonary blood flow occurs with mitral or pulmonic valvular stenosis, with hypovolemic shock or with right ventricular failure. *Parenchymal diseases* are caused by changes at the alveolar level. They include all forms of pneumonitis (viral, bacterial, mycotic or parasitic), forms of pneumoconiosis resulting from inhaled irritant dusts such as silica, and so-called collagenous diseases of unknown etiology. Malignant disease may involve any category, some cancers originating in the bronchi, others in the alveoli or pleura and metastatic involvement occurring via the blood stream.

Acute respiratory diseases (particularly those ocurring in childhood) are *not readily classified* on this anatomic basis. The common "chest cold," producing catarrhal inflammation of the bronchi, bronchioles and at times, the alveoli, as well as a nasopharyngitis accompanied by sneezing, sore throat and cough is self limited, usually treated by home remedies and is rarely subjected to clinical analysis or pathologic study. The different types of adenoviruses that may act as etiologic agents and the high variability of the seasonal attacks defy anatomic classification.

TABLE 3-1. Variation of Signs and Functions in Cardiac and Respiratory Diseases

Determination	Cardiac Failure *	Cardiac Asthma	Emphysema	Bronchial Asthma	Pulmonary Fibrosis	Shock †
Cardiac Output	Minus	Minus	N (normal)	N	N	Minus
Venous Pressure	Plus	Plus	N to Plus	N	N	Minus
Circulation Time	Plus	Plus	N to Minus	N to Minus	N	Plus
Blood Volume	Plus	Plus	N to Plus	N	N to Plus	Minus
Arterial Pressure	Plus to Minus	Plus to Minus	N to Plus	N	N to Plus	Minus
Respiratory Rate	Plus	Plus	Plus	Plus	Plus	Plus
Pulmonary Rigidity	Plus	Plus	N	N	Plus	N
Intrapleural Pressure	Plus	Plus	Plus	Plus	Plus	?
Vital Capacity	Minus	Minus	Minus	Minus	Minus	N
Reserve Air	Minus	Minus	Severe Minus	Minus	Minus	N
Residual Air	Plus	Plus	Plus	Plus	N to Plus	N
Gaseous Mixing	Minus	Minus	Minus	Minus	Minus	N
BMR	Plus	Plus	N to Plus	Plus	N to Plus	Minus
Arterial P_{O_2}	N to Minus	Severe Minus	N to Minus	Minus	Minus	N to Minus
Alveolar P_{O_2}	Minus	Minus	Minus	Minus	Minus	N to Minus
Venous P_{O_2}	Minus	Minus	Minus	Minus	Minus	Minus
Tissue P_{O_2}	Minus	Minus	Minus	Minus	Minus	Minus
Arterial P_{CO_2}	Minus	N to Plus	Plus	Plus	N to Plus	Minus
Venous P_{CO_2}	N to Minus	Plus	Plus	Plus	Plus	Minus
Alveolar P_{CO_2}	Minus	N	Plus	Plus	N to Plus	Minus
Tissue P_{CO_2}	N	Plus	Plus	Plus	Plus	Plus
Arterial pH	N to Plus	N to Minus	N to Minus	Minus	Minus	Minus
Lacticemia	N to Plus	Plus	N to Plus	N to Plus	N to Plus	Plus
NaCl	Plus	N to Plus	N to Minus	Minus	Minus	Minus in most forms

* Congestive

† Acute cardiac failure

Classification of Lung Diseases

1. **Ventilatory**

   A. *Acute Asphyxia*
      Choking
      Drowning
      Smothering

   B. *Loss of Intrathoracic Pressure*
      Hydrothorax
      Pneumothorax
      Paralysis of diaphragm
      Flail chest

   C. *Constricted or Obstructed Airway*
      Foreign body
      Retained secretions
      Bronchitis
      Asthma
      Whooping cough
      Anatomical deformity
         produced by:
           Bronchial neoplasms
           Intrathoracic mass (goiter enlarged thymus or aneurysm)
      Emphysema (obstructive lung disease)

3. **Respiratory or Parenchymal**

   A. *Pneumonic Consolidation*
      Bacterial, viral, rickettsial, mycotic or parasitic infections
      Pulmonary tuberculosis

   B. *Pneumoconiosis*
      Silicosis
      Asbestosis
      Byssinosis

   C. *Alveolar-Capillary Block Syndromes*
      Sarcoidosis
      Hamman-Rich syndrome
      Wegener's granulomatosis
      Amyloidosis
      Goodpasture's syndrome
      Scleroderma
      Alveolar proteinosis
      Pulmonary hemosiderosis
      Diffuse alveolar carcinoma

   D. *Pulmonary Carcinoma*
      Primary infiltrating carcinomas
      Metastatic carcinoma or sarcoma

Ventilatory disturbances usually diminish vital capacity or timed vital capacity (FEV_1). In chronic cases, the end results may be over-expansion of the lung (emphysema) or collapse (atelectasis); the former the result of partial obstruction of the airway, the latter the result of complete obstruction or compression by changes in the pleural cavity. *Circulatory disturbances* often produce abnormalities of the blood gases (P_{O_2} and P_{CO_2}). Acute vascular obstruction, if not fatal, produces localized coagulation necrosis or infarction. Diffuse vascular narrowing often causes pulmonic hypertension and terminates in cor pulmonale. The findings and results of *parenchymal pulmonary involvement* depend upon the extent and duration of the changes. Most forms of pneumonitis whether patchy, lobar or diffuse, produce temporary changes both in ventilatory capacity and at times in the blood gases but usually resolve without permanent damage. However, if significant amounts of lung tissue are destroyed, the end result may be organization with fibrosis and scarring or patchy necrosis with cavitation.

Classification of Lung Diseases (Contd.)

2. **Circulatory**

   A. *Congestive Heart Failure*
      Left ventricular failure
      Infarction

   B. *Pulmonary Emboli*
      Phlebothrombosis
      Amniotic emboli
      Fat embolism

   C. *Injury and Leakage of*
         Capillary Bed
      Steam, smoke or war gases
      Rickettsial fevers
      Hypotonic intravenous
         infusion
      Severe anoxia
      Bacterial or endotoxin shock

   D. *Arteriovenous Shunt*
      Congenital angiomatous lesions
      Patent ductus arteriosus

   E. *Vascular Sclerosis with*
         Pulmonic Hypertension
      Scleroderma
      Other collagen diseases
      Fibrosing forms of pneumonitis

The different forms of pneumoconiosis produced by irritant dusts often produce diffuse irreversible scarring.

The symptoms noted by the patient include the common triad of dyspnea, cough and increased expectoration, at times with the spitting of blood or pus. Wheezing, cyanosis or clubbing of the fingers may be noted by the physician along with rales or diminished breath sounds determined by auscultation. Wheezing typifies ventilatory involvement, bubbly rales indicate vascular or cardiac disease with edema and fine rales or suppressed breath sounds accompany parenchymal disease. In present day practice, definitive diagnosis rarely is ventured without the aid of an x-ray film of the chest if severe symptoms persist for one to several weeks.

Fever and cough associated with sore throat or sneezing and mild cervical adenopathy are the commonest causes of acute illness in the United States and are usually referred to as acute respiratory disease (ARD) or as "cold or flu." Nasopharyngitis plus acute bronchitis are responsible for the symptoms and the causative organism is usually one of the adenovirus group of which more than 30 have been distinguished. The illness is usually self-limited and rarely subjected to diagnostic studies unless appearing in epidemic form. The extent to which the bronchial passages (as opposed to the respiratory alveoli) are involved varies but frank consolidation is rarely present. This common clinical condition when extending beyond the upper respiratory passages that are initially involved, constitutes an acute bronchitis rather than a pneumonitis. However, rales and roentgenographic evidence of pulmonary infiltration occur in about 10 percent of the cases, although dyspnea is rarely present.

MAJOR SYMPTOMS

Dyspnea in pulmonary disease is usually the result of reduced ventilatory capacity, which is known as *hypoventilation*. This refers to decreased gaseous exchange at the alveolar level often resulting in retained carbon dioxide (a blood level of 45 to 60 mm. Hg) or respiratory acidosis—findings which are usually present only after exertion or at times with exacerbations of respiratory infections. Lesser degrees of anoxemia are usually present (90 to 95 mm. Hg), although these may fall to lower levels. The respiratory center is stimulated by the retained CO_2 and increased hydrogen ion concentration in the blood. More rapid shallow breathing is often the outstanding feature in such chronic cases.

In acute respiratory failure such as massive pleural effusion or spontaneous or traumatic pneumothorax leading to massive collapse or with threatened suffocation such as choking or laryngeal spasm, oxygen saturation falls to low levels—50 to 75 mm. Hg. Respiratory excursions are increased in depth and the condition of *hyperventilation* exists, which reduces the level of CO_2 to 20 to 25 mm. Hg. In this situation, anoxemia is a stimulus to the respiratory center. With life-threatening degrees of suffocation, the markedly increased negative pressure in the thorax dilates the pulmonary capillary bed and some degree of pulmonary edema is usually present.

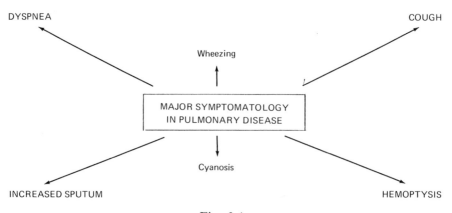

Fig. 3-1.

In chronic respiratory insufficiency which accompanies dyspnea in advanced emphysema or pulmonary fibrosis or status asthmaticus, the respiratory center is relatively insensitive to retained CO_2, which is stabilized by urinary excretion of hydrogen ions and retained bicarbonate. Injudicious administration of pure oxygen to such patients may induce coma.*

Patients with dyspnea usually experience orthopnea, which is an exaggeration of dyspnea in the reclining position. The mechanical work of ventilation is increased in recumbency because of increased airway resistance when the individual is lying flat. There is also some diminished lung compliance. In milder cases, the patient may complain of insomnia rather than orthopnea.

In patients with chronic respiratory deficiency with hypoventilation, the retention by the kidney of sodium ions to combat respiratory acidosis is usually accompanied by a corresponding loss of potassium. This must be considered when using diuretics to combat pulmonary edema which also lowers potassium. On the other hand, hyperventilation in normal subjects causes an increase in serum potassium and this increase may be marked if patients with elevated P_{CO_2} are hyperventilated to reduce the CO_2 value. In this instance, there is a renal excretion of sodium and retention of potassium. Voluntary hyperventilation for two minutes has been recommended by Rotsztain as a diagnostic test in respiratory insufficiency. Patients with severe chronic obstructive pulmonary disease can rarely reduce their P_{CO_2} values by more than 12 percent with hyperventilation, whereas in normal volunteers, this decrease averages 47 percent. If hyperventilation is used to lower high levels of CO_2, attempt should not be made to reduce this level beyond a moderate degree by this method.[9]

In America, the common cause of hypoventilation is referred to as obstructive lung disease. This includes asthma, emphysema and restriction of lung expansion or recoil by pleural effusion, pneumothorax, extreme obesity (Pickwickian syndrome), or loss of elasticity in chronic cardiac congestion or varying degrees of pulmonary fibrosis such as forms of pneumoconiosis. In England, the emphysematous patient is referred to as having chronic bronchitis, but the condition of chronic bronchitis per se does not restrict the airway.

Cheyne-Stokes Respiration or Periodic Breathing. In this form of abnormal breathing, a period of rapid deep breathing occurs for approximately one minute alternating with a similar period of shallow ineffectual breathing and apnea. The patient overventilates for a brief period with an alternate period of apnea. This abnormality occurs with cardiac decompensation or with severe anoxemia in patients who may be comatose with a delayed lung

---

* For patients in respiratory distress with cyanosis, the administration of 30 percent oxygen is recommended.

to brain circulation time.[46] The periods of hyperpnea are sufficient to keep the P_{CO_2} low and result in a higher level of alveolar ventilation than is required for the elimination of CO_2. A chronic case of Cheyne-Stokes respiration in a patient surviving coronary thrombosis and with narrowing of the lumen of the carotid artery has been reported by Bates and Christie.[9]

A number of respiratory poisons, including morphine and general anesthetics, produce this type of respiration through the depression of the respiratory center. *Biot's* respiration is a variant of periodic breathing in which alternate hyperpnea and apnea occur in abrupt attacks for irregular periods. It is usually seen with lesions of the medulla, especially in meningitis.

Kussmaul Breathing. In this type of breathing, inspirations are forced and regular, but expirations are unaffected. It was initially described in diabetic acidosis and may occur in the metabolic acidosis accompanying intestinal obstruction. This form of dyspnea has also been referred to as "air hunger" and results from direct stimulation of the respiratory center by the retention of hydrogen ions.

Cough is a protective reflex stimulated by irritation of the tracheobronchial tree or pleura. The afferent impulses arise at the endings of the vagal nerves in these tissues. Rarely, cough may be produced by diseases of the ear, stimulating the auricular branch of the vagus nerve (Arnold's nerve). The reflex consists of a brief and exaggerated inspiration, closure of the glottis for the first portion of a forceful expiration (increasing intrapulmonary pressure), and then a sudden opening of the glottis expelling any offending material in the air passages. The cough reflex is stimulated not only by diseases of the lower respiratory tract and pleura, but also by intrathoracic masses such as aortic aneurysm or substernal goiter compressing the trachea or involving the recurrent laryngeal nerve. Congestion of the airways in cardiac decompensation or the aspiration of fluids or foreign substances (including irritating gases) also stimulates cough.

A dry or nonproductive cough (often described as a "hacking" cough) is found with the common cold (upper respiratory infection associated with laryngitis, pharyngitis or tracheitis). A dry or brassy cough is also caused by pressure on the trachea in the presence of mediastinal tumors or aneurysms. Excessive smoking or irritant gases are additional causes. A productive cough with increased amounts of sputum occurs with bronchopulmonary infections such as pneumonia, tuberculosis, bronchiectasis or lung abscess. A profusely productive cough with foul smelling sputum occurs with bronchiectasis, lung abscess and pulmonary gangrene, when putrifying bacteria infect devitalized tissue. Pulmonary infarction may produce a productive cough and later may be complicated by lung abscess.

Paroxysmal coughing with repeated uncontrolled attacks at times termi-

MAJOR CAUSES OF COUGH

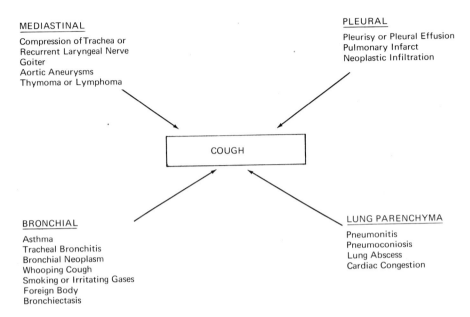

MEDIASTINAL

Compression of Trachea or
Recurrent Laryngeal Nerve
Goiter
Aortic Aneurysms
Thymoma or Lymphoma

PLEURAL

Pleurisy or Pleural Effusion
Pulmonary Infarct
Neoplastic Infiltration

COUGH

BRONCHIAL

Asthma
Tracheal Bronchitis
Bronchial Neoplasm
Whooping Cough
Smoking or Irritating Gases
Foreign Body
Bronchiectasis

LUNG PARENCHYMA

Pneumonitis
Pneumoconiosis
Lung Abscess
Cardiac Congestion

Fig. 3-2.

nating with vomiting, occurs with whooping cough and with primary or metastatic neoplasms involving the pleura or with similar involvement by miliary tuberculosis. Both pleural and pericardial effusion may be present. Advancing pulmonary lesions in tuberculosis or bronchogenic carcinoma or unresolved and organizing pneumonia may produce similar attacks. The paroxysms are usually worse at night after prolonged activity or exertion or talking.[98]

Cyanosis. Severe degrees of respiratory insufficiency are usually accompanied by cyanosis, which is a purplish discoloration most readily visible in the skin at the lobes of the ears, in the lips, or in the fingernail beds. The cyanosis is produced by hypoxia with reduction of oxyhemoglobin in the systemic capillaries. Cyanosis may also be of cardiac origin associated with severe degrees of either right or left ventricular failure or may occur with abnormal admixtures of arterial and venous blood in congenital heart disease. Chronic respiratory insufficiency is frequently accompanied by moderate polycythemia. This is true with right ventricular strain in patients with emphysema or status asthmaticus. The polycythemia is compensatory providing additional hemoglobin for the carriage of oxygen.

Causes of Cough

INFECTIONS OF RESPIRATORY PASSAGES, LUNGS, PLEURA
Unproductive
- Upper respiratory infections
  - Streptococcic pharyngitis
  - Diphtheria
- Early bronchial or pulmonary infections
  - Bronchitis
  - Pneumonia
  - Tuberculosis

Productive
- Fully developed or chronic bronchopulmonary infections
  - Bronchitis
  - Pneumonia
  - Tuberculosis
  - Whooping cough
  - Bronchiectasis
  - Pulmonary abscess
  - Mycotic pneumonia
  - Pleurisy
  - Unresolved pneumonia

CONGESTION OR FLUID IN LUNGS OR PLEURAL CAVITY
Productive
- Pulmonary infarction (embolism)
- Congestive heart failure (pulmonary congestion)
- Pulmonary edema with cardiac failure, drowning, irritant gases or massive collapse
- Pleurisy (with effusion) (pneumo-, hydro-, or pyothorax)

INTRATHORACIC NEOPLASM OR MASS
Usually Unproductive
- Substernal goiter
- Bronchogenic carcinoma or adenoma
- Mediastinal tuberculosis or lymphoma
- Esophageal diverticulum
- Aortic aneurysm
- Peri cardial effusion
- Pleural invasion by mammary carcinoma
- Metastatic malignancy

BRONCHIAL OBSTRUCTION OR IRRITATION OF RESPIRATORY PASSAGES OR PLEURA
Usually Unproductive
- Foreign body in air passages (swallowing the wrong way)
- Tonsillitis
- Pneumoconiosis
- Asthma
- Retropharyngeal abscess
- Injury (fractured rib, thoracentesis)

Causes of Cough (Contd.)

Irritant gases or dust, smoking
Nasal polyps
Postnasal drip

PSYCHOGENIC OR NEUROGENIC
Unproductive
Psychoneurosis or neurosis
Injury to recurrent laryngeal nerve in thyroidectomy or deep x-ray therapy

---

Hemoptysis. The coughing or spitting up of blood, when more than a trace is present in the sputum, suggests pulmonary tuberculosis, bronchogenic carcinoma, bronchiectasis or a suppurative pneumonitis with or without lung abscess. More rarely, hemoptysis occurs with pulmonary infarction or bouts of left ventricular failure. It may also complicate aortic aneurysm and pulmonary emboli in cases where these lesions are difficult to demonstrate in the roentgenogram. The pulmonary emboli may occur during parturition (amniotic embolism) or may be of venous origin in tall men after periods of long standing. In children, hemoptysis is sometimes seen with whooping cough. It also may occur in individuals with blood dyscrasias and a bleeding tendency.

Systemic Effects of Respiratory Insufficiency. In patients with chronic respiratory insufficiency or acute respiratory failure, cyanosis is accompanied by other findings caused by anoxemia or the retention of CO_2. Severe hypoxia affecting the vasomotor center of the medulla results in *systemic hypertension.* This was frequently seen in cases of bulbar poliomyelitis. The hypertension in these cases subsided when the patient was

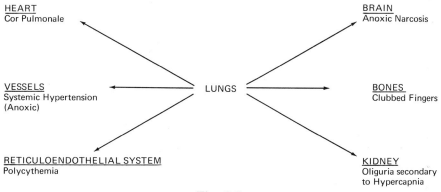

SYSTEMIC EFFECTS OF LUNG DISEASE

HEART
Cor Pulmonale

BRAIN
Anoxic Narcosis

VESSELS
Systemic Hypertension
(Anoxic)

LUNGS

BONES
Clubbed Fingers

RETICULOENDOTHELIAL SYSTEM
Polycythemia

KIDNEY
Oliguria secondary
to Hypercapnia

Fig. 3-3.

placed in a respirator and the anoxemia relieved. The occurrence of hypo-ventilation that is sufficiently severe to elevate the P_{CO_2} to 80 to 100 mm. Hg is accompanied by muscular twitching and mental confusion and may be followed by convulsions, coma and death. At autopsy there is lysis of cerebral neurons resulting from the hypoxia.

In patients with chronic respiratory insufficiency occurring with emphy-sema, status asthmaticus or progressive pulmonary fibrosis (pneumoconio-sis or postirradiation) there is compensatory *polycythemia* in which the increased number of erythrocytes compensates for the lack of oxyhemo-globin. In these patients, loss of the pulmonary capillary bed results in *pulmonic hypertension*. This leads to left ventricular strain and hyper-trophy and eventually, to right ventricular failure with hepatic engorgement and dependent edema.

Pulmonary Hypertrophic Osteoarthropathy. Clubbing of the distal ends of the fingers with rounding of the fingernails and periosteal new bone formation of the terminal phalanges occurs in patients with chronic hypoxia. These changes are common in cyanotic congenital heart disease and in bronchiectasis and also occur with bronchogenic carcinoma. In some patients, a periosteal thickening of the long bones of the extremities

TABLE 3-2. Etiologic Classification of Primary Diseases of the Lungs

Trauma	Penetrating chest wound
	Obstructing foreign bodies in trachea or bronchi
Burns, Radiation Injuries	Steam burns, irradiation pneumonitis and fibrosis
Toxic Injuries	Irritant gases (choline, phosgene, etc.)
	Irritant dusts (beryllium, silica, etc.)
Infections	Acute and chronic bronchitis
	Viral, rickettsial, bacterial, mycotic and parasitic pneumonitis
Hypersensitivity	Bronchial asthma
	Collagen pneumonitis
	Anaphylaxis
Aging	Senile emphysema
Congenital	Congenital atelectasis, hyalin membrane disease
	Pulmonary cysts
	Muscular cirrhosis
	Eventration of the diaphragm
	Diaphragmatic hernia
	Antitrypsin enzyme deficiency, cystic fibrosis
Neoplasia	Benign and malignant tumors

is visible in the roentgenogram accompanied by polyarthritis or arthralgia of the spine and joints of the extremities. Pathologically, the arthritic changes are accompanied by synovial thickening. The subperiosteal new bone formation is laid down around the normal cortex of the bone and may or may not fuse with it.[88] These changes have subsided following correction of congenital heart disease by open heart surgery, have been similarly benefitted by lobectomy in patients with bronchiectasis or carcinoma and may remit after vagotomy.

The osseous changes in the digits are the result of increased vascularity which has been demonstrated by increased skin temperature by infrared photography (thermography), by elevated digital pulse pressure and by postmortem arteriography.[51]

The systemic effects of pulmonary disease are mediated for the most part by changes in the chemical composition of blood in regard to P_{O_2}, P_{CO_2} and H^+. The cerebral effects of hypoxia, the occurrence of polycythemia and pulmonary osteoarthropathy are related to these changes. The structural distortions occurring with emphysema and with fibrosing pneumonitis obstruct the capillary circulation, hindering the passage of blood from the right to the left ventricle and ultimately may cause death from cardiac failure.

PULMONARY IMPAIRMENT SECONDARY TO PRIMARY DISEASE OF THE MAJOR ORGANS (PULMONARY CO-IMPAIRMENT)

Functional failure of major organs frequently spreads the burden of their affliction to the lungs. This is particularly true of left ventricular failure, which produces acute or chronic congestion of the lungs, at times with hydrothorax. Diseases of the central nervous system accompanied by coma and often the result of an overdose of barbiturates, narcotics (heroin) or alcohol, are major causes of aspiration pneumonia. More specific forms of asphyxia occur with neoplasms or infections of the central nervous system producing bulbar paralysis and impairment of the respiratory center of the medulla. Thrombi or solid material released into the systemic veins produces pulmonary emboli, at times with fatal right ventricular failure, so-called acute cor pulmonale. A special form of pulmonary embolism produces metastasis to the lungs and pleura with carcinoma or sarcoma primary in other organs.

Pleural effusion or hydrothorax is of varied origin. It may be produced by metastatic involvement of the pleura in malignant disease, but also occurs with benign tumors of the ovary (Meig's syndrome) and with ascites in hepatic cirrhosis. Hydrothorax also occurs in patients with edema or anasarca, in congestive heart failure or with renal failure and uremia.

The ventilatory capacity of the lung is reduced in patients with kyphoscoliosis, which deforms the thorax. This also occurs with extreme obesity in the so-called Pickwickian syndrome.[27]

Alpha-1 antitrypsin deficiency, believed to be an hereditary defect of the liver, and fibrocystic disease of the pancreas (also hereditary) both produce impairment of bronchial secretions resulting in infections and emphysema.

4

Diagnostic Procedures

In patients with the symptom triad of dyspnea, cough and sputum, age is important in determining the diagnostic possibilities. In children and teenagers, forms of pneumonitis and bronchial asthma predominate. In adults, chronic bronchitis, emphysema, congestive cardiac failure, tuberculosis and cancer are the common ailments. Children usually suffer acute or recurrent attacks of pulmonary disease; elderly adults are often chronic cases. If asthma appears for the first time after the age of 60 years, emphysema and right ventricular failure are the likely causes. Shortness of breath has many causes. It is found in heart diseases, anemia, obesity and with pleural effusion, which may complicate ovarian neoplasm or hepatic cirrhosis as well as heart or lung disease. Fever, leukocytosis and an elevated sedimentation rate occur with various forms of pneumonitis, but are also present with cancer of the lung. Auscultation and percussion are helpful in localizing the site of lung involvement, but acute or persistent symptoms warrant a roentgenogram or fluoroscopic examination of the chest.

RADIOGRAPHIC EXAMINATIONS

The major radiographic techniques for examination of the lungs include:

Fluoroscopy
X-ray films (A/P and lateral views at standard distance)
Bronchograms following Lipiodol injection into the trachea and bronchi
Angiopneumogram following injection of radiopaque material via catheter into the pulmonary artery
Tonograms
Pressure roentgenograms with Valsalva's maneuver
Radioisotopic examination (Lung scan)

43

Fluoroscopy. The ventilatory functions of the lungs can be observed under the fluoroscope by noting the range of motion of the two halves of the diaphragm during inspiration and expiration and the movement of the chest wall (alternate widening and narrowing of the intercostal spaces). The degree of aeration of the lung fields and opaque shadows also may be noted as well as the contour or pulsation of the mediastinal structures and the presence of effusions in the pleural cavities. In spite of its usefulness, this type of study is discouraged as a routine procedure because of the radiation hazards to the examiner.

Routine Chest Films. The anterior-posterior film of the chest is made at a standard distance following maximum inspiration while the diaphragm is held in this position. Lateral films are made with the same technique. These films depict:

1. The status of the thoracic cage including the ribs, pleura, the contours of the diaphragm and the airways of the upper respiratory tract as it enters the chest.

2. The size, contour and position of the mediastinal and hilar contents including the heart, aorta, lymph nodes and root of the bronchial tree.

3. The texture and degree of aeration of the lung parenchyma.

4. The size, shape and number, locations and density of pulmonary lesions including cavitation, fibrous markings and zones of consolidation.
Ideally, a notation should be made of all these features when the films are examined. Because of the importance of localization, the salient anatomical features of the chest must be recalled.

Normal Divisions of the Lung and Their Variations. The two main branches of the right bronchus supply the right upper lobe and the right middle and lower lobes. The left bronchus divides into three branches— the first two supply the left upper lobe and the third, the left lower lobe (Fig. 4-1). On the right, the upper, middle and lower lobes are separated by the two interlobar fissures. The major fissure separates the lower lobe anteriorly from the middle lobe and posteriorly from the upper. A minor fissure separates the middle lobe from the upper. On the left, a single major fissure (corresponding to the major fissure on the right) separates the upper and lower lobes. All five lobes are almost completely covered by the visceral pleura. Minor variations may occur in the form of accessory lobes. The most common is an azygos lobe (on the upper right), produced by an indentation surrounding the more direct course of the azygos vein. Small posterior or inferior accessory lobes may occur medially in either the right or left lung (Fig. 4-2). The density of an upper right azygos lobe may be mistaken for a neoplasm. Fissures are not visualized in the roentgenogram unless thickened by a previous pleuritis, although the minor

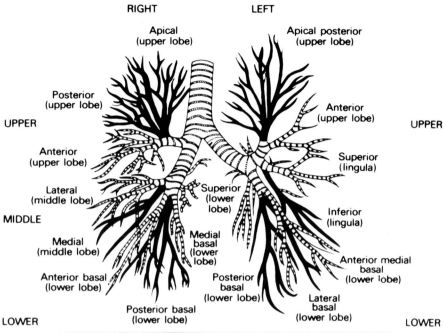

RIGHT   LEFT

Apical
(upper lobe)

Apical posterior
(upper lobe)

Posterior
(upper lobe)

Anterior
(upper lobe)

UPPER

UPPER

Anterior
(upper lobe)

Superior
(lingula)

Lateral
(middle lobe)

Superior
(lower
lobe)

Inferior
(lingula)

MIDDLE

Medial
basal
(lower
lobe)

Medial
(middle lobe)

Anterior medial
basal
(lower lobe)

Anterior basal
(lower lobe)

Posterior
basal
(lower lobe)

Lateral
basal
(lower lobe)

LOWER

Posterior basal
(lower lobe)

LOWER

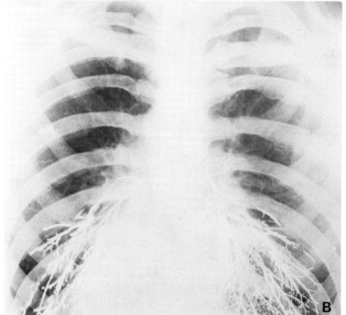

B

Fig. 4-1. (*Top*) Ramifications of the bronchial tree (Redrawn from Meschan, I.: Roentgen Signs in Clinical Practice. vol. 2. W. B. Saunders, Philadelphia). (*Bottom*) Normal bronchogram of lower lobes.

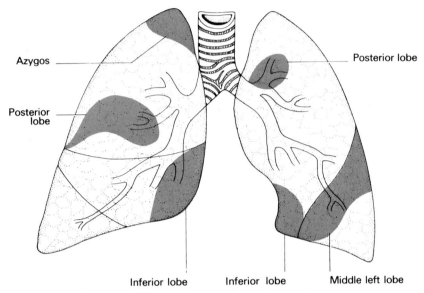

Azygos — Posterior lobe

Posterior lobe

Inferior lobe   Inferior lobe   Middle left lobe

Fig. 4-2. Occasional accessory lobes of the lungs.

fissure on the right (seen tangentially) may be discerned in the A-P view. Linear markings depicting the course of the arteries, veins and bronchi * (and their fibrous sheaths) radiate from the hilum and disappear in the midlung fields (Fig. 4-3). Their extent and density is increased by inflammatory changes in the bronchi or the inhalation of foreign material in pneumoconiosis. Bronchograms are needed if bronchiectasis is suspected and angiopneumograms when abnormalities of the vessels are under investigation.

Pleural changes visualized by the roentgenogram include:

1. Widening of the pleural space by pneumothorax, hydrothorax, chylothorax, hemothorax or purulent fluid (empyema);
2. Thickened bands of adhesions or calcified plaques;
3. Pleural nodulations caused by neoplasms, which may be confirmed by films made after an artificial pneumothorax.

Widening of the pleural space causes partial collapse of the ipsilateral lung and a shift of the mediastinum contralaterally. Pleural fluid casts a dense homogenous shadow. It may be free in the pleural space, unilaterally or bilaterally, or encapsulated within an interlobar space. Most frequently, fluid accumulates in the costodiaphragmatic angles where its presence must be confirmed by films at the *end of maximum inspiration* (Fig. 4-4). Mas-

---

* The normal bronchi are not visualized.

sive effusion is differentiated from massive collapse of the lung by the position of the mediastinal structures. Pleural effusion pushes these structures to the opposite side, massive collapse increases negative pressure and shifts the structures to the affected side.

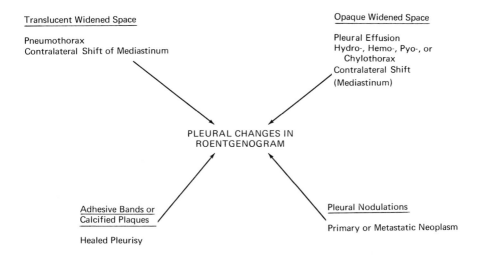

Translucent Widened Space

Pneumothorax
Contralateral Shift of Mediastinum

Opaque Widened Space

Pleural Effusion
Hydro-, Hemo-, Pyo-, or
     Chylothorax
Contralateral Shift
(Mediastinum)

PLEURAL CHANGES IN
ROENTGENOGRAM

Adhesive Bands or
Calcified Plaques

Healed Pleurisy

Pleural Nodulations

Primary or Metastatic Neoplasm

Abnormalities of the Diaphragm. The diaphragm arches over the abdominal contents. Its anterior attachments to the zyphoid and costal cartilages are higher than the posterior attachments about the first, second and third lumbar vertebrae. This downward, backward slope allows the liver and abdominal contents to obscure the posterior lower portions of the lungs in A/P roentgenograms. On quiet breathing, the excursions of the diaphragm are approximately 2 cm., increasing to 4 to 5 cm. with hyperventilation. Inequalities of excursion of the two halves of the diaphragm may be associated with diseases of the lungs, pleura, paralysis of the phrenic nerve or an intra-abdominal neoplasm. The diaphragm is pierced by the esophageal and aortic openings. This hiatus is the site of a sliding herniation of the stomach in approximately 3.5 percent of adults.[38] Detection requires upper gastrointestinal films following a barium swallow. Bleeding from esophageal ulceration may be caused by regurgitation of the herniated gastric contents. A bilaterally lowered diaphragm occurs in patients with an asthenic habitus, with emphysema and with chronic bronchial asthma. In such conditions, the heart shadow is centrally placed, elongated and has a "tear drop" contour. Elevation of the right diaphragm may be seen with hepatic cancer.

Mediastinal and Hilar Structures. The mediastinum contains the heart and the great vessels (including the aorta, pulmonary arteries and superior and inferior vena cavae). The region containing these structures (visual-

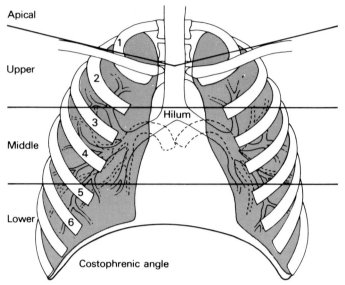

Fig. 4-3. Topography of posterior-anterior chest film showing linear marking radiating from hilum.

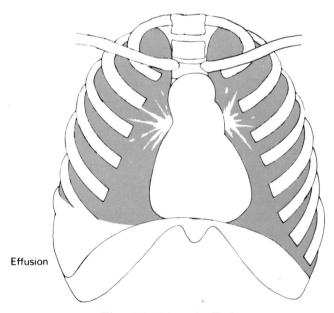

Fig. 4-4. Pleural effusion.

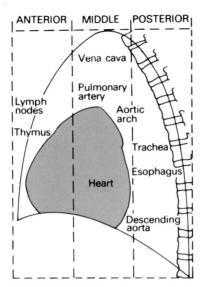

Fig. 4-5. Lateral view of the chest showing divisions of the mediastinum.

ized by lateral roentgenograms) is designated as the middle mediastinum (Fig. 4-5). The anterior mediastinum or retrosternal space is radiolucent. It contains the thymus or its remains, the anterior mediastinal lymph nodes and rarely, a substernal goiter. The posterior mediastinum contains the trachea, the bifurcation of the main bronchi, the esophagus and the arch, and the descending thoracic aorta. The phrenic nerves traverse the middle mediastinum and the vagi, the posterior mediastinum. The heart shadow is enlarged to the left in hypertension and in cases of congestive failure, aneurysms of the aortic arch are confirmed by pulsation under fluoroscopy.

The term hilum or "root" of the lung refers to structures between the medial surface of the lung and the mediastinum. The hilar structures are surrounded by pleura reflected from the lung surface. The hilus contains branches of the bronchi and pulmonic vessels and numerous lymph nodes. The pulmonary parenchyma is superimposed anteriorly so that the normal hilum is a semiaerated zone on either side of the mediastinum. This aerated space is frequently obliterated by pathologically enlarged lymph nodes and by bronchogenic neoplasms.

Widening of the mediastinal shadow or hilar masses require lateral views for accurate localization. Tumors or hyperplasia of the thymus, parathyroid adenomas, benign teratomas, and plunging goiters occupy the anterior mediastinum. Primary lymphomas or metastatic nodes (Fig. 4-6) involve the upper anterior or middle mediastinum. Esophageal diverticulae and neuromas (projecting from the vertebral region) occupy the posterior

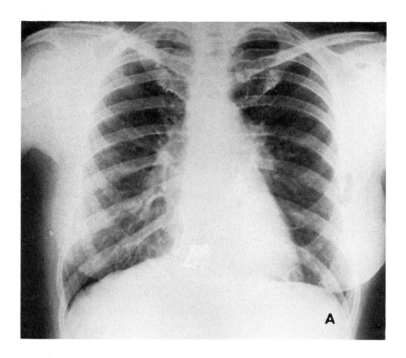

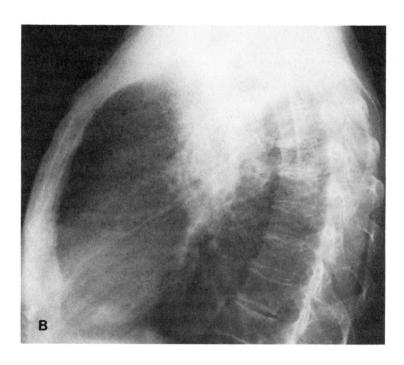

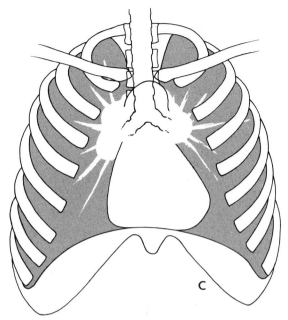

Fig. 4-6. (*A*) Hilar lymphadenopathy in a case of sarcoidosis. (*B*) Lateral view of hilar lymphadenopathy in a case of Hodgkins Disease. (*C*) Diagram, A-P view.

mediastinum. A superior sulcus tumor (bronchogenic carcinoma of an upper lobe), seen in lateral views, is in the upper portion of the posterior mediastinum. Aneurysms of the aortic arch are found in the upper middle mediastinum. In localizing these lesions, a barium swallow, outlining the esophagus, may be required. Radioiodine may be needed if a plunging goiter is suspected and clinical evidence of myasthenia gravis (with various eye signs) may aid in differentiating a thymic tumor. Bronchoscopic examination and biopsy are performed to confirm the presence of bronchogenic carcinoma.

LESIONS OF THE LUNG PARENCHYMA

The radiographic appearance of lesions of the pulmonary parenchyma can be divided into four major categories:
1. Zonal regions of increased density
2. Zonal regions of increased radiolucency with or without density
3. Nodular lesions, which may be solitary or multiple
4. Abnormal linear markings

Zonal Regions of Increased Density

The three common zonal densities in the roentgenogram are atelectasis, lobar pneumonia and pulmonary infarcts and at times, rapidly progressing tuberculosis and fungus infections.

Atelectasis. Pulmonary atelectasis refers to the collapse and loss of aeration in a segment or in an entire lung. It is caused by obstruction of a major air passage with resorption in the unventilated tissue or by the pressure of pleural effusion. The trachea is deflected toward the affected area. The atelectatic segment casts a dense shadow of diminished size. The opposite lung may show increased aeration.

When massive atelectasis of one lung follows bronchial obstruction with resorption of air, the affected lung shrinks in volume, shifting the mediastinal structures toward that side. The interspaces of the adjacent ribs are narrowed. However, if massive pleural effusion collapses the lung, the chest is expanded on the affected side with widening of the intercostal spaces. When the lung is consolidated by lobar pneumonia, there is no mediastinal shift and the two sides of the chest are of equal size.

Collapse of the right middle lobe by inflammatory disease such as tuberculosis or abscess or by neoplastic nodes, is termed the "middle lobe syndrome." However, the collapsed segment at times is in the lower portion

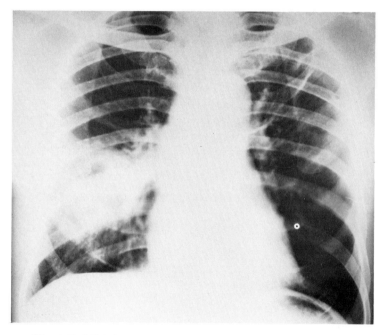

Fig. 4-7. Middle lobe syndrome in a case of lung abscess.

of the right upper lobe or in the upper portion of the right lower lobe. An esophageal traction diverticulum produced by mediastinal adhesions may accompany this process (Fig. 4-7).

Atelectasis of the newborn usually occurs in premature births. Complete expansion may require weeks (see hyaline membrane disease).

Lobar Pneumonia. Pneumococcic lobar pneumonia is characterized by rapid consolidation of a pulmonary lobe or contiguous lobes. (Chills, high fever, grunting respirations and marked leukocytosis are usually present). The zone of homogenous density affects an entire lobe or segment. The involved parenchyma does not decrease in volume. Hilar lymphadenopathy may be visualized. Zones of consolidation follow within hours and do not coincide with the clinical onset (Fig. 4-8).

Pulmonary infarction follows interruption of the blood supply (by embolism and thrombosis), which causes coagulative exudation in the affected segment. Cardiac decompensation with cardiomegaly and an overlying friction rub are usually present. A triangular or wedge-shaped zone of consolidation is visualized with its base toward the pleura. The zone of density occurs within several hours after the vascular occlusion and resolution requires several weeks (see Fig. 4-8).

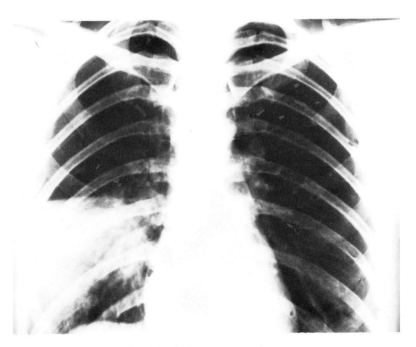

Fig. 4-8. Lobar pneumonia.

Increased Radiolucency

Abnormal radiolucent changes in the lung fields, exclusive of pneumothorax, are produced by: (1) Intrathoracic herniation of the stomach—hiatal hernia; (2) a cavity-producing lesion or cyst either in communication with a bronchus or infected by a gas-producing organism; (3) diffuse overventilation of the lungs (pulmonary emphysema) without blebs (most common form); bronchopleural fistulas with pneumatocele and pneumothorax (at times a complication of staphylococcal pneumonia).

Cysts, Pneumatoceles and Blebs. Cysts of the lung are often congenital. Thin-walled cysts with a flattened surface against the diaphragm or pleura are difficult to distinguish from encapsulated pneumothorax. The involved lung shows no markings. If the surrounding lung contains increased markings, a cavity secondary to abscess or necrotizing tuberculosis may be present (at times with a fluid level). Cavitation secondary to fungus infection such as torula or coccidiosis is referred to as a "fungus ball" by radiologists (Chap. 8). Hydatid cysts from echinococcus granulosis may have an air-containing crescent or, if ruptured, resemble a simple cyst.

Bullae and Blebs in Emphysema. A *bulla* is an encapsulated air sac within the lung produced by confluent air spaces following the rupture of alveolar septa. A *bleb* is a zone of lateral emphysema under the visceral

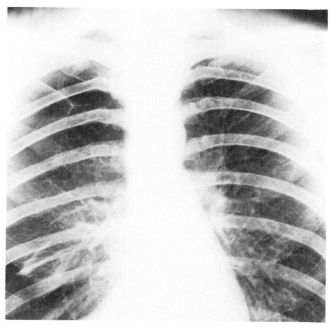

Fig. 4-9. Emphysema with bleb.

pleura. Air also may be forced into this position by severe coughing or laryngeal spasm (Fig. 4-9).

Emphysema. Diffuse increased radiolucence of both lungs occurs with emphysema. It is found in young individuals with a history of chronic asthma or develops in elderly adults. The expansion of the distal air spaces in this disease is irreversible. In the upper lobes of the lung, central lobular or obstructive emphysema results from dilatation of the respiratory bronchioles; in the lower lobes, periacinar or destructive emphysema results from widening of the alveolar air spaces and disintegration of their walls. The radiographic findings include increased radiolucency of both lungs, increased transverse diameter of the chest on lateral view, increased radiolucence of the paramediastinal tissues at the hilum and a central "tear drop" heart shadow. Vascular markings are diminished.

Pulmonic Nodular Density

Solitary nodular densities occurring in the lung fields include:

1. A congenital cyst with fluid (rare)
2. A benign tumor or hamartoma

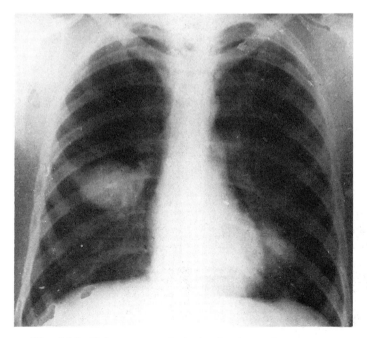

Fig. 4-10. Pulmonary metastasis of osteogenic sarcoma.

3. A healing tuberculoma or mycotic granuloma or a similar cavitating lesion with fluid
4. Pyogenic lung abscess with fluid level
5. Primary carcinoma of the lung
6. A solitary metastatic tumor (sarcoma or carcinoma) (Fig. 4-10).

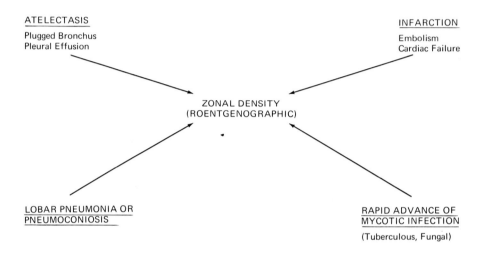

ATELECTASIS

Plugged Bronchus
Pleural Effusion

INFARCTION

Embolism
Cardiac Failure

ZONAL DENSITY
(ROENTGENOGRAPHIC)

LOBAR PNEUMONIA OR
PNEUMOCONIOSIS

RAPID ADVANCE OF
MYCOTIC INFECTION

(Tuberculous, Fungal)

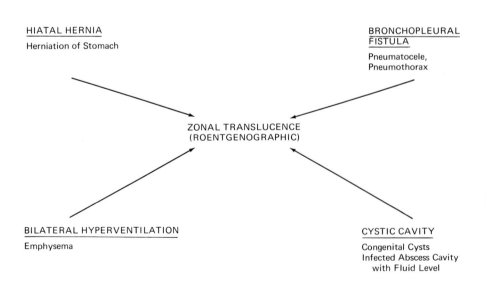

HIATAL HERNIA

Herniation of Stomach

BRONCHOPLEURAL
FISTULA

Pneumatocele,
Pneumothorax

ZONAL TRANSLUCENCE
(ROENTGENOGRAPHIC)

BILATERAL HYPERVENTILATION

Emphysema

CYSTIC CAVITY

Congenital Cysts
Infected Abscess Cavity
with Fluid Level

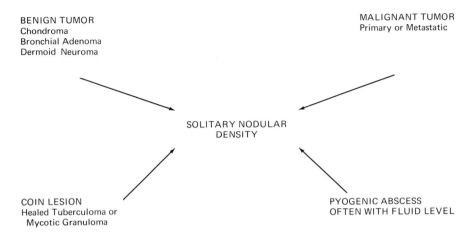

BENIGN TUMOR
Chondroma
Bronchial Adenoma
Dermoid Neuroma

MALIGNANT TUMOR
Primary or Metastatic

SOLITARY NODULAR
DENSITY

COIN LESION
Healed Tuberculoma or
Mycotic Granuloma

PYOGENIC ABSCESS
OFTEN WITH FLUID LEVEL

A visible fluid level in a circumscribed lesion indicates that a portion of its fluid or necrotic contents have been discharged via a bronchus. Although a pyogenic abscess, a tuberculosis cavity or a myotic granuloma is suggested, *malignant bronchogenic carcinoma* with necrotic tissue may give similar findings. In general, mycotic lesions are associated with visible enlargement of the mediastinal nodes. In the lower or outer lung fields, a healed tuberculoma may be distinguished from carcinoma only by biopsy. Tuberculomas retain a constant size on repeat films whereas bronchogenic carcinomas show progressive enlargement. Because of their size (5-cent to 25-cent piece) and contour, these are known as "coin lesions."

Multiple nodular densities, usually bilateral, include:
    A. Multiple discrete lesions
        1. Miliary tuberculosis
        2. Histoplasmosis
        3. Sarcoidosis (usually associated with enlarged hilar nodes)
        4. Metastatic carcinoma (often with lymphatic seeding)
        5. Pneumoconiosis including:
            Berylliosis
            Silicosis
            Asbestosis
            Anthrosilicosis
            Byssinosis (cotton dust)
            Bagassosis (sugar cane dust)
        6. Myeloid metaplasia (rare)
        7. Pulmonary alveolar carcinoma
        8. Loeffler's eosinophobe pneumonia
    B. Multiple nodules with infiltrating or irregular borders include:
        1. Mycotic granulomas

2. "Cottonball" pulmonary metastasis of carcinoma
3. Advanced forms of pneumoconiosis (Fig. 4-11)
4. Far advanced tuberculosis
5. All forms of bronchopneumonia (staphylococcal, streptococcal and atypical)
6. Pulmonary edema
7. Multiple abscesses with uremia.

The clinical history, laboratory examinations, culture of the sputum and biopsy aid in differential diagnosis.

Abnormal Increase of Linear Markings

Most lesions increasing the width or visibility of linear pulmonary margins involve the bronchi or major pulmonary vessels and extend outward from the hilum.

1. Chronic bronchitis associated with asthma or forms of pneumoconiosis producing increased peribronchial fibrosis.
2. Bronchiectasis with dilatation and abscess formation (limited usually to one lung and best visualized with the aid of the bronchogram)

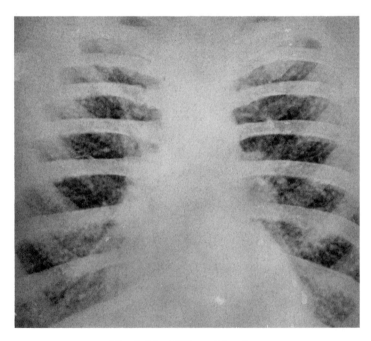

Fig. 4-11. Diffuse silicosis.

3. Hilar nodularity plus infiltrating markings bilaterally
   A. Collagen diseases (Wegener's granulomatosis, Goodpasture's syndrome, scleroderma, and systemic lupus erythematosus
   B. Forms of sarcoidosis
   C. Forms of pneumoconiosis

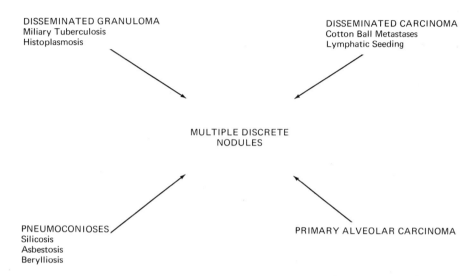

DISSEMINATED GRANULOMA
Miliary Tuberculosis
Histoplasmosis

DISSEMINATED CARCINOMA
Cotton Ball Metastases
Lymphatic Seeding

MULTIPLE DISCRETE NODULES

PNEUMOCONIOSES
Silicosis
Asbestosis
Berylliosis

PRIMARY ALVEOLAR CARCINOMA

SPECIAL RADIOLOGIC TECHNIQUES

Bronchography. Radiopaque materials injected into the trachea or a major bronchus for the roentgenographic visualization of the bronchial tree or one of its branches has been much improved since Lipiodol was first used in France in 1922. Materials such as propyliodone or Dionosil which are resorbed in three to four days, have made this a safe procedure. The patient is seated and the oropharynx anesthetized locally to abolish the gag reflex. A catheter is passed between the vocal cords and can be guided into the desired bronchus with the aid of the fluoroscope. This procedure is indicated for confirming the diagnosis of bronchiectasis and determining its distribution. It also permits the localization of obstructive lesions and is used to demonstrate bronchial compression by lesions in contiguous structures. It is particularly valuable in delineating massive atelectatic bronchiectasis (Chap. 4). Rapid tapering and narrowing of distal bronchi suggest asthmatic spasm, while more gradual tapering and peripheral bulge suggest chronic bronchitis.

Tomography or planigraphy is a technique for selectively exposing for x-ray film a predetermined layer of tissue to the exclusion of other depths.

The film and x-ray tube undergo reciprocal motion during the process. By this means, a layer of tissue from 0.5 to 1.0 cm. in thickness can be filmed at different depths in the lungs. Localizing a cavity or calcified plaque with definite demarcations may be thus achieved. Actually, this permits the outlining of a lesion when it has been obscured by superimposed structures. It is particularly advantageous in outlining the great vessels or the major bronchi when deformities are suspected from the routine film. When tomography is combined with scanning of the lung by intravenously administered isotopes, the more hazardous procedure of angiography may be avoided.

Lung Scanning. The lungs can be scanned with radioactive isotopes to delineate the distribution of pulmonary blood flow and also the distribution of gas in the alveoli. Pulmonary perfusion is depicted by scanning with radio-tagged microspheres that appear as transient emboli in the pulmonary capillaries. Either cameras or scanners are used for imaging. The diameters of the capillaries vary from 7 to 15 microns and microspheres vary in size from 5 to 100 microns. These particles remain in situ for 5 to 20 minutes and are then metabolized by macrophages of the reticuloendothelial system. The metabolic isotope technetium [99m] (aggregated with albumin or ferric hydroxide in aqueous suspension) is used * because of its short half-life (6 to 7 hours) and its penetrating gamma rays. A dose of two millicuries is given intravenously and measurements are registered over a period of 5 to 20 minutes.[91A] Scans registering pulmonary perfusion are used to demonstrate: (1) thromboembolism; (2) neoplasms and inflammatory lesions obstructing pulmonary airways; (3) vascular changes in emphysema; and, (4) vascular abnormalities in congenital cardiac disease or hemangiomas causing A/V shunting. (Fig. 4-12 A&B)

Radioactive gas (Xenon[133]) can be used to measure regional ventilation and lung volume (it can also be used to study regional vascular perfusion). Measurements must be made within seconds after administration of the gas. The scintillation camera depicts the distribution of the gas during a period of 5 to 30 seconds and accumulated counts are registered. For determining regional ventilation the gas can be inhaled, but for the determination of perfusion ventilation ratios it is administered intravenously.

Angiography of the Pulmonary Vessels. Pulmonary arterial pattern and flow can be demonstrated by injecting radiopaque fluid through a catheter, inserted via an arm vein into the right atrium, right ventricle or main pulmonary artery. Although the procedure is not without risk, it permits

---

* Aggregated albumin labeled with Iodine[131] is also used.

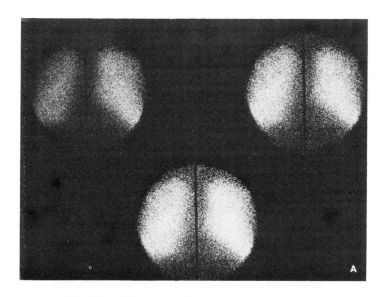

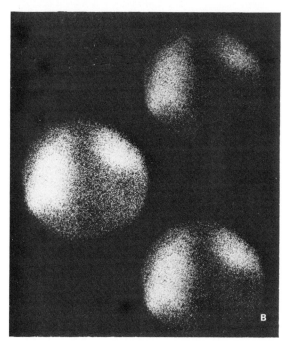

Fig. 4-12. (*A*) Normal lung scan. (*B*) Lung scan showing embolus
and infarction in left lower lobe.

definitive diagnosis and location of arteriovenous fistulas, emboli and congenital anomalies of the major vessels. Simpler diagnostic techniques are preferred to this hazardous procedure in most cases of pulmonary disease. Since the introduction of "perfusion lung scan" with radioactive microspheres, this form of radionucleotide study is preferred for the evaluation of patients suspected of thromboembolic disease (Fig. 4-13 A&B).

OTHER DIAGNOSTIC TECHNIQUES

Diagnostic Bronchoscopy. This specialized technique is used to confirm the presence of benign or malignant bronchial neoplasms or to determine the cause of zonal atelectasis or bronchiectasis that may result from obstructing bronchogenic tumor or foreign body, a tuberculous granuloma or extrinsic stenosis. With suspected abscess, the bronchial orifice draining the exudate may be localized by this means and material obtained for culture. The most frequent indication for the use of the bronchoscope is to obtain biopsy material in the presence of a bronchial neoplasm.

Bronchial catheterization and brushing to obtain exfoliated cellular material for microscopic diagnosis has been employed recently to substitute for bronchoscopy.[92]

Patients selected for bronchoscopy or bronchial catheterization are those with abnormal chest x-ray films in which the lesion appears to impinge or occlude a major bronchus or its branches. Atypical tuberculosis and bronchiectasis as well as mycotic infections have been confirmed by bronchial catheterization.

Bronchospirometry. (VENTILATORY CAPACITY AND LUNG VOLUME). Nodular or destructive pulmonary lesions that are localized or patchy in distribution rarely produce significant changes in ventilatory capacity. Such lesions caused by tuberculosis, mycotic infections or malignant disease may disseminate fatally without inflicting respiratory failure. In such cases, spirometry (although diagnostically unimportant) is useful in following the clinical course or in evaluating the risk of radical surgery such as pneumonectomy. These measurements are important in the diagnosis of unexplained dyspnea, cyanosis or respiratory acidosis. However, the clinical usefulness is handicapped by the absence of simplified instruments for determining the numerous measurements recommended by specialists.

Vital Capacity and FEV₁. Two functional tests are available to the clinician. One measures airway obstruction or decreased elastic recoil of the lungs expressed as degrees of expiratory slowing (expiratory slowing refers to diminished flow rate of expired air in liters/second). FEV_1

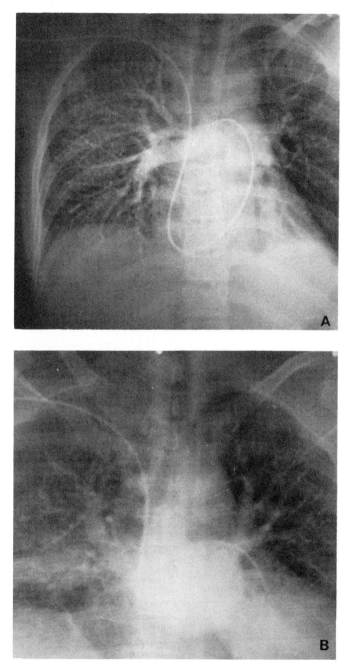

Fig. 4-13. (*A*) Normal angiogram. (*B*) Angiogram showing pulmonary infarct.

(forced expiratory volume in one second) can be performed on a simple vital capacity machine with the signals of "blow" and "stop at the end of one second, determined by a stop watch. FEV_1 can then be related to vital capacity (FEV_1/VC), performed on the same machine. FEV_1/VC in percentage determines the degree of expiratory impairment, which may result from airway obstruction (in asthma, emphysema or chronic bronchitis), loss of lung elastic recoil (in cardiac congestion or diffuse infiltrative disease) or a combination of both. The normal individual exhales 83 percent of his vital capacity in one second. The FEV_1 times 30 approximates maximum breathing capacity ("indirect maximum breathing capacity"). When the reduction in FEV_1 is due to pulmonary fibrosis or reduced volume of total lung capacity, the vital capacity is lowered more severely than the flow rate. The ratio appears normal but vital capacity is reduced. With airway obstruction, the reverse is true and an FEV_1/VC ratio below 70 percent is diagnostic of an obstructive disorder of the airways, Most patients with pulmonary disease have a noticeable prolongation of expiration.

In patients with infiltrative disease such as silicosis, asbestosis, sarcoidosis, Hamman-Rich syndrome, scleroderma and other collagen diseases, mild expiratory slowing ($FEV_1 = 1.5$ instead of normal $2.0+$ liters/second) represents an early stage of the disease. In adult patients with emphysema or chronic bronchitis, a similar finding is favorable for survival of five or more years if there is no cardiac decompensation. With FEV_1 of 1.0 to 0.75 liters/second, chronic hypercapnia (respiratory acidosis) and right ventricular strain are present and pulmonic hypertension is usually present.

Residual Volume and Total Lung Capacity. The residual volume (or residual air) is the volume remaining at the end of maximum expiration that is exchanged only by diffusion and cannot be measured directly by the spirometer. *Residual volume plus vital capacity gives the total lung capacity.* In normal adults, residual air averages 1.2 liters and with vital capacity of 4 to 5 liters, total lung capacity is between 5 and 6 liters. If the clinician suspects that total lung volume is increased by emphysema and blebs or reduced by fibrosing disease, the residual volume must be measured for confirmation.

Measurement of residual volume is based on washing out the N_2 from the lungs after forced expiration. Since the residual air is 80 percent N_2, the amount of nitrogen determined will represent 80 percent of the residual volume. "Wash out" is performed by having the patient breathe pure O_2 for 7 minutes and collecting the expired gas in the spirometer.

Residual volume is increased beyond the normal adult value of 1.2 liters in patients with airway obstruction in asthma, emphysema and in forms of chronic bronchitis with peribronchial fibrosis. It represents pulmonary hyperinflation. Thus, when FEV_1 is diminished, residual volume is usually increased. With prolongation and difficulty in expiration, intrapleural pressure is increased because active muscular contraction of expiratory muscles decreases the volume of the thoracic cage faster than air is expelled. The further expiratory handicap may be induced since positive "tissue pressure" may exceed intraluminal pressure in the bronchioles and tend to narrow them during expiration.

Reduction of Total Volume. Since total lung capacity can be calculated when vital capacity and residual volume are known, a ratio is obtained by dividing residual volume by total lung capacity and expressing this in percentage. RV/TLC=20 percent as an average in normal adults. In infiltrative diseases of the lung such as pneumoconiosis or sarcoidosis, restriction of total volume is accompanied by increased residual volume (loss of elastic recoil). In such patients, RV/TLC may be increased to 40 to 50 percent.[25]

Total lung volume can be estimated from x-rays obtained at the end of maximum inspiration and measurement of the anterior-posterior diameter of the chest by means of calipers. The area of the lung determined by planimetry is multiplied by the external diameter. This gives a volume which is usually 200 to 300 percent of that determined by methods for washing out nitrogen and measuring the nitrogen volume. To obtain the actual lung volume, a formula is applied based upon empirical relationship of this value.[8] Increased lung volumes with expansion of total lung capacity is judged by increased radiolucence in the roentgenogram. If vital capacity and total lung capacity are known, the residual volume, which is the amount of air that cannot be expelled on expiration, can be calculated. The residual volume of air normally increases in the years beyond 50 as the vital capacity decreases. Hyperventilation in diseases with airway obstruction usually have a similar effect—timed vital capacity is diminished and residual volume increased. This is true of emphysema and bronchial asthma and in many cases of chronic bronchitis with overinflation. Where facilities for spirometry are unavailable, the clinician, by means of the roentgenogram, chest diameter and vital capacity, can confirm his diagnosis of ventilatory dysfunction.

Restricted Ventilatory Capacity (Diminished TLC *)
   Radiation fibrosis
   Kyphoscoliosis
   Marked obesity (Pickwickian syndrome)
   Chronic congestion with mitral stenosis

---

* TLC=Total lung capacity

Left ventricular failure

Massive pleural effusion

Advanced infiltrative disease (sarcoidosis, scleroderma, Hamman-Rich syndrome, diffuse lymphogenous metastases, diffuse alveolar cell carcinoma of the lung, forms of pneumoconiosis)

Expanded Ventilatory Capacity (Increased TLC)

Emphysema

Pulmonary cysts

Pulmonary bullae

Forms of bronchitis with overinflation

Ventilatory Obstruction (Reduced Airway) (FEV_1 Decreased)

Chronic bronchitis

Bronchial asthma

Emphysema

Infiltrative pulmonary disease (miliary tuberculosis, pneumoconiosis, collagen diseases), sarcoidosis, radiation fibrosis)

Pulmonary fibrosis—healing phase of infiltrative disease

Hamman-Rich syndrome

TABLE 4-1. Diagnostic Criteria in Chronic Lung Disease with Airway Obstruction

	Spasmodic or Allergic Asthma	Asthma With Overinflation	Emphysema	Bronchitis With Overinflation	Chronic Bronchitis
$\dfrac{FEV}{VC}$	—	—	—	—	N or —
$\dfrac{RV}{TLC}$	N	+	++	+	N
Age	5 to 35		55 to 75		45-65
Sputum	After attack		Scanty mucoid		Copious purulent
P_{CO_2} (arterial)	++	+	N	+	+
P_{O_2} (arterial)	——	—	—	—	—
Chest x-ray	N		Radiolucent		Fibrotic

$++$ = Increase

$--$ = Decrease

N = Normal

Increased Reserve Volume (RV Increased)
Status asthmaticus
Emphysema
Bronchitis with overinflation
Advanced infiltrative disease (sarcoidosis, pneumoconiosis, collagen disease)
RV = Reserve volume
FEV_1 = Forced expiratory volume/one second

Blood Gases

In cases of acute respiratory embarrassment such as massive collapse of a lung, extensive bilateral pneumonitis, severe status asthmaticus and in the advanced stages of chronic emphysema or pneumoconiosis where there is cyanosis and threatened carbon dioxide narcosis, determination of P_{O_2} and P_{CO_2} blood levels is indicated to measure the degree of anoxemia and hypercapnia. Acute pulmonary edema following the inhalation of noxious gases or in the presence of left ventricular failure should be similarly evaluated. These blood gases can be measured electrometrically. While arterial sampling has been preferred in the past, the microanalytical technique using capillary blood from a previously warmed finger tip is suitable (Chap. 2).

The changes in the arterial gas tensions produced by failing alveolar ventilation (assuming normal distribution of perfusion and ventilation and normal respiratory quotient) are tabulated below.

The electrode system for gas analysis determines P_{O_2} by an electrode with a constant polarizing voltage of 0.6 volts at which the current generated by oxygen is directly proportional to the oxygen tension diffusing to the reactive surface of the electrode. The current produced is a result

TABLE 4.2 Change in Blood Gases with Diminished Alveolar Ventilation

Alveolar Ventilation (L./min.)		Arterial			
		P_{O_2} (mm. Hg)	O_2Hb (%)	P_{CO_2} (mm. Hg)	pH (if no change in HCO_3)
5.0	Normal	100	95.7	40	7.40
4.0		82	93.7	50	7.32
3.0		68	87.0	75 *	7.20
2.0		30	40.0	105 *	7.05

* Range of impending CO_2 narcosis.

of the reduction of oxygen at the electrode, which proceeds in accordance with the reaction:

$$O_2 + H_2O + 4e^- \text{ gives } 4OH^-$$

Each molecule of oxygen reacts with four electrons and this flow of electrons is the measurement recorded in terms of P_{O_2}. To make the P_{O_2} electrode specifically sensitive for oxygen, it is covered by a plastic membrane permeable to gas. The electrons reacting at the cathode are supplied by the oxidation of silver at the anode reacting with chlorine.

The measurement of P_{CO_2} potentiometrically is an adaptation of the electrode method of measuring pH. A combination of pH glass and reference electrode is in contact with a solution behind a gas-permeable membrane. As carbon dioxide diffuses across the membrane, hydration of CO_2 in the electrolyte water produces carbonic acid causing a change in hydrogen ion activity.

$$CO_2 + H_2O \rightleftharpoons H_2CO_3 \rightleftharpoons H^+ + HCO_3^-$$

The pH electrode senses the change in CO_2 concentration as changes in the pH electrode, developing a voltage exponentially related to P_{CO_2}. A ten-fold increase in P_{CO_2} is equivalent to a decrease of approximately one pH unit.

In this system of gas analysis, pH is measured directly.

In the body, the carbonic acid bicarbonate buffer system has two regulators. The concentration of CO_2 (which gives carbonic acid when hydrated) is controlled by respiration; the base bicarbonate is mainly controlled by the kidneys, the blood pH being determined by the ratio of the two. In venous plasma, the ratio of bicarbonate to acid is 20:1, giving a pH of 7.4. The absolute concentration of either factor is irrelevant since the ratio is the dominant factor. If the P_{CO_2} in mm/Hg is determined, multiplying by 0.03 gives HCO_3^- in millimoles/liter.

If H_2CO_3 is known in millimoles/liter, multiplying by 33 gives P_{CO_2} in mm. Hg.

The CO_2 concentration by itself cannot be translated into pH, but with pH, it is useful.

Oxygen Saturation. Changes in P_{O_2} reflect changes in blood oxygenation but the amount of oxygen carried is not related linearly to P_{O_2} but is defined by the oxyhemoglobin dissociation curve. At high levels of P_{O_2}, this saturation varies little and is between 90 and 97 percent (Fig. 2-4). These relationships are changed in heavy smokers who may have about 10 percent COHb in their blood. On gram of hemoglobin carries 1.39 ml. O_2. If the concentration of oxyhemoglobin is known, multiplying hemoglobin concentration in grams percent by percent of saturation by 1.39 gives O_2

content in volume percent, which equals about 17 volumes $O_2/100$ ml. blood.

The composition of alveolar air and, in turn, arterial P_{O_2} and P_{CO_2} vary both with total alveolar ventilation and with the patient's tissue metabolism. Increased metabolism raises O_2 consumed and lowers venous P_{O_2}. At the same time, increased CO_2 is produced raising P_{CO_2} in the venous return to the lungs.

Sputum Staining and Culture

When sputum is available, special methods and stains for acid fast bacilli are valuable diagnostic aids. A diagnosis of active tuberculosis requires demonstration of the causative organism. If these are not revealed in successive examinations of the sputum, gastric washings for organisms are indicated. Another technique is to obtain bronchial washings by means of the bronchoscope for the demonstration of organisms or tumor cells, when bronchogenic carcinoma is suspected. Such examinations may be augmented by culturing fungi, pneumococci or Friedländer's bacillus in cases of pneumonitis. Fortunately, because of the use of antibiotics, the typing of pneumococci is no longer performed routinely in cases of lobar pneumonia, but cultures to disclose staphylococcus are used to determine sensitivity to antibiotics.

The special diagnostic tests performed on bronchial secretions obtained as sputum or by other methods include the following:

1. Sputum from bronchial asthma for identification of Curschmann's spirals (Fig. 4-14) and Charcot-Leyden crystals and eosinophiles;

2. Sputum with acid staining for tubercle bacilli;

3. Sputum stained with Perl's stain for iron to demonstrate hemosiderin in the macrophages in mitral stenosis;

4. Sputum stained with periodic acid Schiff (PAS) for microscopic examination for mycotic infections,[60] followed by culture on Saboraud's media;

5. Culture of sputum followed by test for antibiotic sensitivity in cases of staphylococcic, pneumococcic or streptococcic pneumonia;

6. Gastric washings with the use of a stomach tube with centrifuging and staining of sediment for acid-fast bacilli (and Papanicolaou smear for bronchogenic carcinoma);

7. The use of a bronchoscope and bronchial washings for microscopic specimens for diagnosis of bronchial carcinoma.

Diagnostic Therapeutic Trial

Chronic heart failure with pulmonary congestion producing dyspnea, cough and expectoration may be indistinguishable in the roentgenogram

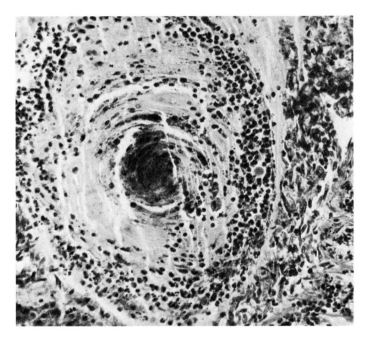

Fig. 4-14. Curschmann's spiral in bronchial asthma. (×150)

from forms of fibrosing interstitial pneumonitis or organizing forms of bronchial pneumonia. The differential diagnosis in such cases is aided by instituting treatment—digitalis and diuretics for congestive heart failure. Absence of improvement in the roentgenogram and clinical findings is in favor of primary pulmonary disease.

In elderly adults, status asthmaticus or recurrent asthmatic attacks precipitated on recumbency is usually associated with emphysema and right ventricular failure. In allergic bronchitis, response is obtained with bronchial dilators such as Isuprel and intravenous aminophylline and avoidance of pollens, dusts and danders. On the other hand, emphysematous cardiacs (so-called cardiac asthma) respond to digitalization, although "leaf preparations" of digitalis must be avoided because a number of these patients previously treated are sensitive to them.

Valsalva Maneuver. In patients with emphysema or interstitial fibrosis, measuring systemic blood pressure during the valsalva maneuver (forced expiration against a closed glottis) can be used to indicate the presence of pulmonic hypertension (Chap. 6).

Exploratory Thoracotomy and Transpleural Biopsy. When bronchogenic carcinoma is suspected from the roentgenogram and if the lesion is peripheral and difficult to distinguish from the "coin lesion" of a healed tuberculoma, a definitive pathologic diagnosis is in order. If this cannot be made from bronchial biopsy or from cells obtained from pleural effusion through thoracentesis, exploratory thoracotomy is indicated. Needle biopsy through the intact chest wall under local anesthesia is frequently undertaken but if the lesion is operable, neoplastic cells may be implanted in the chest wall in the needle track. When pleural effusion is present, the tapped fluid should be centrifuged and sectioned in order to determine whether or not malignant cells are present. In similar cases where a spread of malignant disease is suspected, a needle biopsy that can core or punch out a bit of thickened pleura can be used to obtain tissue for pathologic examination.

Skin Testing

Bacterial and fungal antigens are commercially available for the diagnosis of forms of pulmonary infection. These include purified tuberculin protein and antigens of histoplasmosis, coccidioidomycosis and blastomycosis. A negative battery of such skin tests may suggest a diagnosis of sarcoidosis. In some mycotic infections, the pulmonary symptoms are produced by hypersensitivity to the fungus and the patient may have severe asthmatic attacks. This has been demonstrated for aspergillosis and mucormycosis. In such cases, skin testing may be diagnostic.

Serologic Tests

Only a few serologic tests are of value in lung disease, but the cold agglutination test is important in mycoplasma pneumonia and serologic tests are available for the more common mycotic infections.

5

Diseases Affecting Ventilation

Normal respiration requires an unimpeded flow of air in and out of the tracheobronchial tree in response to the excursions of the chest wall and diaphragm and the elastic recoil of the lung tissues. If air cannot gain free access to a single portion of the lung, the residual air is absorbed and the nonaerated tissue collapses. This condition is known as *obstructive atelectasis*. If the excursions of the lung are restricted or immobilized by fluid or air in the pleura or by paralysis of the diaphragm, *compression atelectasis* results. (Congenital atelectasis, a separate form, is discussed separately). Inhaled air can be trapped in the lung and cause over-expansion in the tissue where it is retained. This is known as *emphysema*. Because inspiration is an active muscular effort that is readily increased, whereas expiration is chiefly a passive recoil, partial or a valvelike obstruction in a major bronchus or spasmodic bronchial constriction, which occurs in asthmatics, can lead to such pulmonary inflation. In diseases of the pulmonary parenchyma, air can escape from a branch of the bronchial tree and be trapped in the surrounding tissues. This is known as *interstitial emphysema*. The entrapped air may infiltrate into the soft tissues of the neck or thorax. With advancing age, the pulmonary tissues lose their elastic recoil (diminished compliance) and this may be a factor in emphysema in the aged. In addition, there may be changes in the bony thorax, such as scoliokyphosis, which results in such overstretching. In general, emphysematous changes in the lung are more poorly understood than the conditions that produce atelectasis.

Ventilatory disturbances do not result in lung volume changes only. A reciprocal relation exists between ventilation and the pulmonary circulation. With congestion of the pulmonary circulation in cardiac failure, increased pulmonary rigidity (or loss of compliance) decreases vital capacity and dyspnea is the main symptom. On the other hand in chronic emphysema, when the alveolar walls rupture and fibrose, the pulmonary circulation is impared and right ventricular failure eventuates.

In circulatory collapse following severe trauma or hypovolemic shock, pulmonary edema and fat emboli lead to hyalin membrane formation, leukocytic exudation and eventually, alveolar destruction and fibrosis— so-called "shock lung syndrome." [49] On the other hand, acute asphyxia from smothering or choking leads to anoxic leakage of the capillary bed and pulmonary edema. These are discussed in the chapter under circulatory disturbances.

LESIONS OF THE CHEST WALL AND DIAPHRAGM
(Ineffective Enclosure of Respiratory Organs)

Wounds of the Chest Wall. Penetrating or crushing injuries to the chest embarrass respiratory movements. *Open or sucking wounds* are caused by penetrating injuries which establish a communication through the wall between the exterior and the lungs and pleural spaces. If air passes freely through the wound in either direction, a compression pneumothorax is avoided. However, if a slitlike wound in the pleura acts as a valve permitting ingress but not egress of air, then increasing amounts of entrapped air compress the lung on the affected side (tension or pressure pneumothorax). With *pneumothorax,* percussion yields a typical hyperresonanance and breath sounds are distant or absent. In cases of pressure pneumothorax, the trachea is shifted to the uninvolved side and dyspnea is marked. Shock frequently supervenes in pressure pneumothorax due to hypoxia and impaired cardiac filling. (Fig. 5-1A & B)

Removal of the trapped air is imperative. This is accomplished by repeated aspiration with a syringe or by the insertion of a rubber tube anteriorly through an intercostal space. The exterior end is then placed in a bottle with a water seal system or an improvised one-way valve made with the finger of a rubber glove, tieing the proximal end about the rubber tube and cutting the other end to provide flaps. If pneumothorax in severe chest injuries fails to be relieved by this method, a laceration in the trachea or major bronchus (requiring surgical intervention) may be present.

Closed wounds are those produced by crush injuries to the chest wall, which drive the end of a fractured rib through the pleura to lacerate the lung. Air and/or blood leak through from the bronchi and vessels of the lacerated lung into the pleural space to produce hemothorax, pneumothorax, or both. The patient suffers restricted respirations and ineffectual cough. Reflex bronchospasm and increased bronchial secretions result. Thus, infections (empyema) and compression of the lung (atelec-

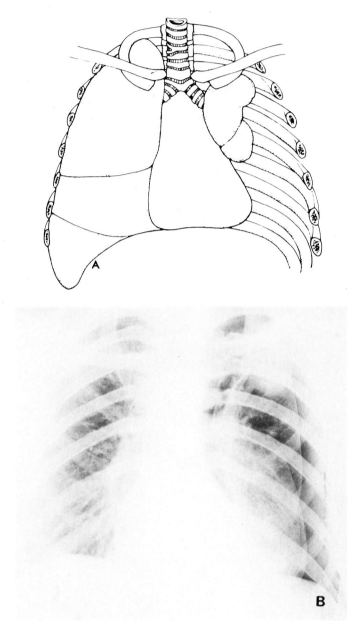

Fig. 5-1. (*A*) Pneumothorax with collapse of left lung. (*B*) Partial
left pneumothorax.

tasis) supervene unless treatment is promptly instituted. The aspiration of blood by thoracentesis is indicated, but a clotted hemothorax requires surgical removal of the clot and surgical collapse of the overlying chest wall.

Flail Chest. This is a serious defect of the chest wall resulting from trauma in which several ribs are fractured. The chest wall is sucked in by negative pressure on inspiration but expands with elastic recoil of the chest on expiration, giving rise to "paradoxical" motion. If a large area is affected, ventilation is impaired and the mediastinal contents are shifted to the affected side by negative pressure. Cardiac filling may be impeded.

Diaphragmatic Paralysis. Impairment of ventilation follows paralysis of the *phrenic nerve.* This may result from deliberate surgical resection of the nerve in the therapy of tuberculosis, compression of the nerve by tumor, or inadvertently during the removal of a cervical rib for relief of a scalenus-anticus syndrome. The effect of crushing the nerve persists for about six months before the phrenic nerve regains its function but in 5 percent of the cases, permanent diaphragmatic paralysis results. Because the phrenic nerve passes along the lateral aspect of the mediastinum anterior to the pulmonary hilus, it may be damaged by mediastinal neoplasms. The paralyzed diaphragm is elevated and loses its downward movement, undergoing passive paradoxical motion, as described in flail chest. In most cases, paralysis is compensated for by the use of accessory muscles of respiration. Weakening of the cough reflex on the affected side may result in inspissated secretions and atelectasis in the poorly ventilated lower lobes and chronic infection. Paralysis of the left nerve may be accompanied by vomiting and acute gastric distention. Such symptoms are transient and last only a few days.

Eventration of the Diaphragm. In a number of cases (both congenital and acquired), the diaphragm may be immobile on one side. The acquired form in adults is of unknown etiology and in infants, is an unexplained congenital anomaly. Surgical repair is indicated in the infant when symptoms include dyspnea, vomiting and gastric distention.

Similar distress occurs with infantile diaphragmatic hernia with an intrathoracic stomach. In adults, diaphragmatic hernia produces symptoms of less severity but similar in type. These include postprandial pain and dyspnea, vomiting and episodes of cardiac arrhythmia.

Dayman and Manning [28] have grouped all of these extrinsic causes of respiratory embarrassment together under the term "incomplete closure" as causes of pulmonary atelectasis. (Ineffective enclosure is a more expressive term.) The lung, when affected by a flail chest, a paralyzed diaphragm, or a flat, mechanically ineffective diaphragm (eventration) is *hypoventilated* and tends to undergo *paradoxical ventilation,* being expanded by elastic recoil of the normal pulmonary structures and compressed by intrathoracic negative pressure while the other lung is being normally expanded. Under these conditions, the injured lung invites cross-ventilation with the more vigorous normal lung, which may lead to infection and bronchiectasis when bronchial secretions follow the stream of pulmonary air flow. Similar complications may follow a large collapsed thorocotomy incision, the action of a cuirass respirator in poliomyelitis and a flat, mechanically ineffective diaphragm in advanced emphysema. The ineffective or flaccid lung during cough is prone to cross-ventilation, retaining inspissated secretions and acting as reservoir for infections.

ATELECTASIS

Congenital Atelectasis. Although there are some observations which suggest that respiratory movements may occur in utero, normal infants begin life with pulmonary atelectasis, which is combatted by crying and forcible respirations at birth. If the infant has been stillborn, this can be confirmed at necropsy by the presence of atelectasis or the failure of lung expansion. This is congenital atelectasis. In infants who survive but a few days, foci of incomplete expansion or atelectasis persist (Chap. 11).

Hyaline Membrane Disease (Resorption Atelectasis). A major cause of atelectasis in the newborn is the formation of a hyaline membrane on the alveolar walls. Obstruction of the bronchioles by aspirated mucus, desquamated epithelium, vernix caseosa or amniotic fluid may be present. The lungs have a deep purple color, resembling the liver in consistency and do not float in water. Microscopically, the capillary bed is congested, the smaller bronchioles contain inspissated material and the surrounding lung tissue has a glandular appearance with numerous cells trapped in the interstices between the alveoli. This condition is found in 2.4 percent of live births and is more common in premature infants.[58] Hypoxia producing plasma leakage from the anoxic capillaries is a contributing factor but the underlying cause is functional immaturity of the lung with surfactant deficiency. The membrane contains cellular debris, plasma protein and fibrin in various stages of polymerization. It covers the bronchioles, alveolar ducts and the alveoli, leaving the epithelial lining beneath intact but stimulates phagocytic activity by macrophages and neutrophils. The membrane and subjacent alveolar walls are ruptured by small hemorrhages. The hyaline is produced by the clotting of leaking plasma enmeshing the cellular debris present in the newborn. This condition is discussed in Chapter 11 under the respiratory distress syndrome of the newborn.

Obstructive and Compression Atelectasis. Plugging or constriction of a major bronchial airway is followed by reabsorption of the stagnant alveolar air with collapse of the parenchyma supplied by the bronchus. The negative pressure of inspiration draws blood into the affected lobe and pulls the mediastinal structures toward the collapsed tissue. When air, pleural effusion or hemothorax exerts (Fig. 5-2) pressure from the pleura on the underlying lung (in the conditions previously discussed), the parenchyma is collapsed by pressure, the affected tissue is dry and bloodless and the mediastinal contents are pushed away from the compressed tissue. In both forms of atelectasis, the collapsed pulmonary tissue is nonfunctioning and tends to undergo fibrosis. Inspissated secretions in the unused airway may become infected and lead to bronchiectasis.

Obstructive atelectasis may result from a retained foreign body (Fig. 5-3) or inspissated secretions in unconscious patients undergoing general anesthesia or those with respiratory paralysis, immobilizing the diaphragm. A mediastinal tumor may compress the bronchus from without or a benign bronchial adenoma may obstruct it from within. Abolition of the cough reflex during and following major abdominal surgery may be complicated by retained secretions and *"massive postoperative collapse."* Reabsorption of air is followed by chest pains, cyanosis, tachycardia, dyspnea and fever. These symptoms appear 24 to 48 hours after the operation. PCO_2 may be maintained at normal levels by hyperventilation of

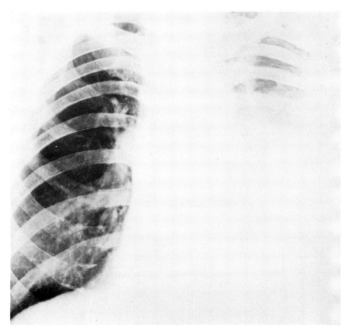

Fig. 5-2. Massive pulmonary effusion.

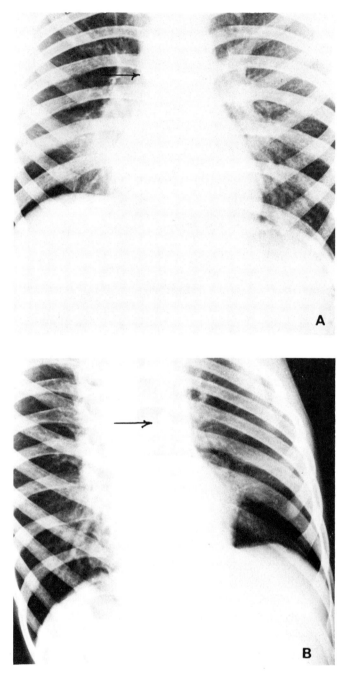

Fig. 5-3. Bronchial foreign body. (*A*) A-P view. (*B*) Oblique view.

the uninvolved lung, but shunting of blood from airless tissue lowers PO_2. Postoperative atelectasis may be prevented by aspiration of secretions during the operation and by encouraging coughing and deep breathing postoperatively and by turning the patient from side to side. Early ambulation is highly effective. In the presence of this postoperative complication, suction through a catheter introduced into the bronchus is indicated if attempts to induce coughing are ineffective. Atelectasis developing without surgical operation often requires bronchoscopy both for diagnosis and treatment. Rotation or sudden movement of the patient (once massive atelectasis has occurred) is hazardous because traction on the great vessels during mediastinal shift may produce sudden death through cardiac arrest.

Compression Atelectasis with Pneumothorax, Hydrothorax or Hemothorax. When a lung is collapsed by pneumothorax, hemothorax or hydrothorax, the collapsed parenchyma (as previously noted) is dry, practically airless and its volume is reduced. The mediastinal contents are pushed to the opposite side of the chest. In hydrothorax, the effusion may result from cardiac decompensation, cirrhosis with ascites, advanced renal disease or from pleural metastases or infection. Chylothorax follows rupture of the thoracic duct or its compression by cancer. Pneumothorax may be secondary to chest wounds as described above, but also occurs spontaneously.

The syndrome of spontaneous pneumothorax consists of the appearance of air or air and blood successively into the pleural cavity followed by atelectasis. The air gains entrance from the lung to the pleural cavity from lesions in the subpleural alveoli. The nature of the initial lesion varies.[95] Healed scars of pulmonary tuberculosis, congenital defects or rupture of old adhesions or emphysematous blebs connect the aerated lung tissue to the pleura. Coughing or forced expiration against a closed glottis permits the alveolar air to gain entrance to the pleural space. It is believed that the initial air usually penetrates into the mediastinum and subsequently ruptures from the mediastinum into the pleural cavity. The blood leaking into the pneumothorax in patients with pre-existing pulmonary disease fails to clot because of its previous defibrination by the whipping action of the heart and lungs. If the blood clots after its withdrawal, recent or continuing hemorrhage is suggested. The difference between spontaneous pneumothorax and hemopneumothorax is a torn pleural vessel, which is usually part of an adhesion. The mortality of massive pulmonary collapse is relatively high in postoperative cases. It is low with simple pleural effusions or hydrothorax and fatalities occur in less than 15 percent of cases of spontaneous pneumothorax.

Middle Lobe Syndrome. The middle lobe syndrome refers to atelectasis of the right middle lobe * secondary to lymphadenopathy, tumor or pneumonitis that compresses a main stem bronchus. The patients suffer cough, recurrent respiratory infections, wheezing, hemoptysis and chest pain. Roentgenograms reveal lymphadenopathy or a mediastinal mass and a triangular shadow of atelectasis. Biopsy is necessary to determine the cause of the obstruction (Fig. 4-7).

Hyperventilation. The effects of acute atelectasis or massive collapse of a single lung is hyperventilation. The tidal volume and total ventilation in the remaining functioning lung is immediately increased. There is a prompt fall in arterial oxygen saturation that is considered responsible for the sudden hyperventilation.[78] In this hyperventilation in the contralateral lung after massive collapse of its fellow, there is both a fall in arterial oxygen tension and a fall in arterial P_{CO_2}, the latter a characteristic result of both voluntary and involuntary hyperventilation. Moreover, on exercise there may be a further fall in P_{CO_2}, but oxygen saturation remains below normal indicating that the hyperventilation cannot successfully combat all of the low arterial oxygen saturation. This compensatory hyperventilation does not occur if the remaining lung is diseased. However with a normal remaining lung following hemothorax or pneumothorax, the blood gases may be nearly normal at rest. In patients who have had a pneumonectomy, this compensatory expansion of the lung at the end of one year does not restore vital capacity, but does permit approximately normal function with exercise. After ten years in adults, the remaining lung tends to be less efficient. The emphysema responsible for this is a separate factor of aging and is not the result of hyperventilation in the opinion of Bates and Christie.[9]

INFECTIOUS DISEASES

Bronchiectasis. Bronchiectasis is a progressive and advanced stage of bronchial infection secondary to pre-existing bronchopulmonary disease, which produces atelectasis. The etiologic factor may be congenital bronchial stricture, causing saccular or cylindrical dilatation. Sources of infection may be a severe chronic sinusitis with postnasal drainage or the weakened bronchial wall (enclosed in atelectatic pulmonary parenchyma) becomes secondarily infected because it fails to maintain its viability through the loss of respiratory movements. The bronchiectasis may be secondary to fibrosing or healing pulmonary tuberculosis or to enlarged tuberculous nodes in children, which compress a major bronchus or to hereditary fibrocystic disease of the pancreas, which increases the viscosity of secretions.

---

* In some instances, an upper segment of the right lower lobe is involved.

Tumors, a foreign body or inspissated secretions may obstruct the drainage of the atelectatic tissues which become secondarily infected. The affected bronchi (Fig. 5-4) lose their ciliated epithelium, which is replaced by metaplastic squamous cells. The bronchial wall ulcerates and is infiltrated by leukocytes and scar tissue. Abscessed cavities form in dilated outpouchings. Bronchiectasis involving the peripheral bronchi is most frequent in the left lower lobe. These patients have a chronic cough, dyspnea, and copious amounts of foul-smelling sputum, aggravated in the mornings by accumulation during sleep. (At times, an excess amount of sputum is not present.) Hemoptysis and asthmatic wheezing are frequent manifestations. The diagnosis is confirmed by Dionosil injection, a radiopaque medium which outlines the cavities and bronchial dilatation in the bronchograms. When the bronchi are dilated along a major segment, cylindrical bronchiectasis is present; if multiple outpouchings occur, the condition is saccular (Fig. 5-4). Whether one or multiple lobes are involved or whether the condition is unilateral or bilateral is important in determining the advisability of surgery. Bronchoscopic examination is also required to determine the type and possible etiology of the bronchial obstruction.

The gross appearance of a sectioned lung is characteristic. Tortuous dilated pus-containing bronchi penetrate and ramify through the collapsed diseased lung. The bronchial cavities are lined by inflamed thickened mucosa coated by pus (Fig. 5-4). Saccular bronchiectatic cavities may measure several centimeters in diameter and if complicating tuberculosis, the walls are caseated.

In the granulation tissue in the infected bronchial walls, dilated blood vessels provide anastomoses between the bronchial artery and branches of the pulmonary artery, giving rise to arterial shunts between the two circulations. These are similar to A-V shunts in the systemic circulation and may give rise to left ventricular hypertrophy, and varying degrees of pulmonic hypertension. Bronchiectasis is most successfully treated by resection of the involved lobe or segment. Prolonged antibiotic therapy produces uncertain results because of failure of the antibiotic to reach into the thickened pus-containing walls of the dilated bronchi. The extent and duration of the disease determines the success of medical treatment. Incipient or bilateral disease is in favor of this approach. Postural drainage with the head lowered and the patient made comfortable should be used twice daily. Maintenance of the fluid intake to approximately 3,000 ml per day aids in keeping the secretions fluid. The use of potassium iodide or chymar pancreatic enzymes is of doubtful value in diminishing the tenacity of the secretions. The choice of antibiotics depends upon the predominant organism and its sensitivity.

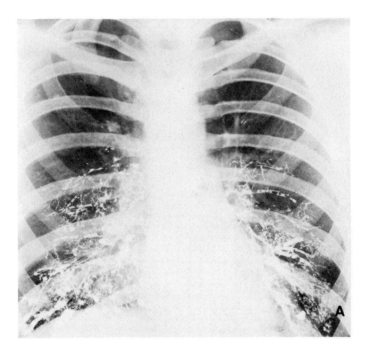

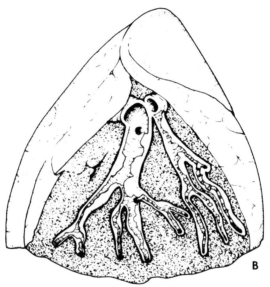

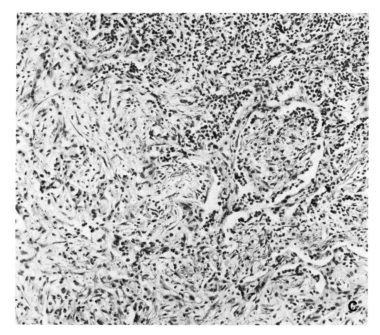

Fig. 5-4. Bronchiectiasis. (*A*) Bronchogram. (*B*) Gross specimen. (Drawing) (*C*) Micropathology. (×100)

Two special forms of congenital bronchiectasis occur. In one of these, the misshaped bronchi extend nearly to the pleura and appear to exist in lung tissue that has never developed normal alveolar tissue. Only one lobe or a single lung is involved. The cause is supposed to be an abnormal position of the left duct of Cuvier as it enters the sinus venosus, since the lower left lobe of the lung is usually affected. Other congenital anomalies may be at fault.

The other form of infantile bronchiectasis occurs in the hereditary disease cystic fibrosis or mucoviscidosis. In this condition, thick, viscous mucus plugs the bronchi and leads to bronchiectasis through secondary infection. There is a diffuse squamous cell metaplasia in the lining of the bronchi. The children rarely survive many weeks.

Pertussis. Whooping cough is an infection of the lower respiratory tract or broncheolitis, produced by the gram negative bacillus *Bordetella pertussis*. The disease is transmitted by droplet infection, the organism multiplying rapidly in the respiratory mucus membranes. The disease begins with a catarrhal stage with sneezing and a mild progressive cough 10 to 14 days after exposure. At the end of this time, necrosis of bronchial epithelium and an infiltration of leukocytes involves the bronchial tree

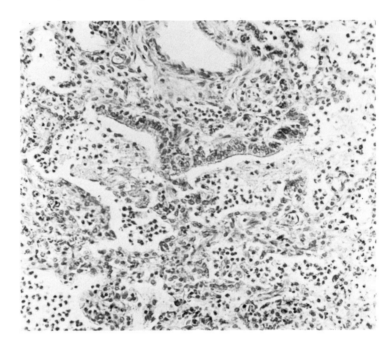

Fig. 5-5. Photomicrograph of the lung in pertussis. (×150)

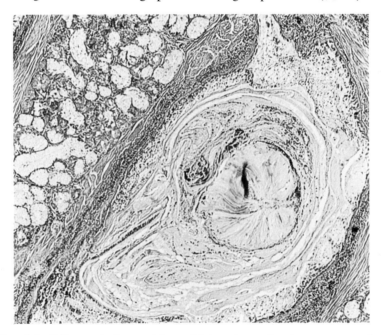

Fig. 5-6. Micropathology of bronchial asthma showing mucous plug.
(×150)

forming an inflammatory rim about the small bronchi and bronchioles described as a peribroncheolitis (Fig. 5-5). Suppurative lesions may appear in the surrounding parenchyma, but usually only edema and hemorrhage are found in this region.

The severe clinical features of the disease are produced by obstruction of the lower airways by mucus plugs, causing varying degrees of anoxia, respiratory acidosis and at times hypoxic convulsions. The cough or "whoop," which gives the disease its name and usually persists for two or three weeks, is characterized by paroxysms which end in a forced inspiration or whoop. The paroxysm in children frequently ends in vomiting. A characteristic leukocytosis (up to 30,000) with a predominance of lymphocytes is nearly always present.

The disease has been largely controlled by a course of immunization of children beginning at the age of three months. The vaccination is usually given as a combination with diphtheria and tetanus toxoids as a multiple antigen. Booster injections are given at one- to two-year intervals during childhood. Once the disease is contracted, chloramphenicol or tetracyclines are of moderate value. Rabbit antiserum is more effective. An attack of the disease confers a permanent immunity.

Acute Laryngotracheobronchitis. This is a disease usually of infants and children from which a group of parainfluenza viruses have been isolated. It is an upper respiratory infection usually with fever and a characteristic cough or croup due to the associated laryngeal edema. Approximately two-thirds of these patients have a so-called croup syndrome with inspiratory stridor accompanied by retraction of the rib cage. There is a variable degree of bronchial obstruction with inspiratory wheezes and the disease may extend to produce bronchopneumonia with marked dyspnea and rales over the lower chest. On x-ray examination, the patients with the complication of bronchopneumonia show a localized peribronchiolar infiltration involving a single or multiple lobes of the lung. A leukocytosis may be present.

In children, the tendency for the disease to involve the upper respiratory tract including the nose, pharynx and larynx may lead to death from laryngeal obstruction without clinical signs to warn of the seriousness of the illness. This is one of the major causes of "crib deaths." The involvement of the trachea and the bronchi by airway obstruction may be caused by the accumulation of inspissated tenacious mucus. Suction aspiration may be indicated and at times, tracheostomy.

ALLERGIC DISEASE

Allergic or Spasmodic Bronchial Asthma. Bronchial asthma is a functional constriction of the bronchioles caused by spasm of their muscular walls in response to inhaled antigens such as dusts, pollens, danders or secretions from upper respiratory infections in patients who are sensitized or allergic to such antigens. The disease usually has its onset in childhood or in early maturity and may be preceded by several years of seasonal hayfever. In children, chronic allergic rhinitis (with the formation of nasal polyps) or eczema may be present and in young adults, seasonal pollinosis is the most common factor.

During attacks, spasm of the bronchial musculature is accompanied by prolonged expiratory wheezes or by both expiratory and inspiratory wheezes with severe spasms. There is increased vascularity and hypersecretion in the bronchial mucosa. In prolonged attacks and in chronic cases known as status asthmaticus, inspissated secretions form obstructing plugs in the bronchioles. When these are coughed up at the end of an attack, they form small white twisted plugs in the sputum, known as Curschmann's spirals. An exudation of plasma cells, lymphocytes and eosinophiles infiltrate the bronchial wall and may be found in the sputum together with Charcot-Leyden crystals that are formed from the granules or nuclei of disintegrated eosinophils. In young individuals (particularly in children), there is a leukocytosis and relative lymphocytosis and eosinophilia. Rarely, death may occur in an acute attack from inspissated secretions in otherwise healthy individuals; more often, elderly asthmatics die because of the complications of chronic emphysema and right ventricular failure.

In the lungs of chronic asthmatics studied at autopsy, the small bronchioles (Fig. 5-6) show inspissated secretion with the characteristics described above for the sputum. The epithelial lining cells of the bronchioles contain one to two or more layers of tall columnar epithelium. The bronchial musculature is hypertrophied and the bronchial cartilages eroded. The bronchial epithelium rests upon a thickened hyalinized membrane.

An infiltrate of plasma cells and lymphocytes forming gamma IgE antibody surrounds the bronchial mucus glands and has been identified in the bronchial lymph nodes and also in tonsils and adenoids removed from asthmatic patients. The concentration of this antibody, also known as *reagin,* is higher in nasal and bronchial secretions than in the blood stream where it is also found in asthmatics. The union of this antibody with antigens (such as pollens, house dusts and animal danders) is responsible for the attacks. Tissue mast cells underlying the respiratory mucosa and PMN leukocytes contain the antibodies of the IgE class on their surface and are thus sensitized to contact with the antigens. Upon union, granules within the sensitized cells are released. These contain histamine, a slow reacting substance known as an anaphylaxis antigen (SRS-A), and substances known as *kinins* causing increased secretory activity of bronchial glands, bronchoconstriction with vasodilatation and edema in the bronchial walls. There is no cell destruction and serum complement is not involved.

The immunoglobulin, known as IgE, is a gamma-1 glycoprotein with a molecular weight of 200,000. In normal serum, its concentration is between 100 and 700 μg. per milliliter and in asthmatics, has been found to average as high as 2600 μg. This antibody is also known as a skin sensitizing antibody, since it is capable of transferring a positive skin reaction to an antigen if serum from the allergic individual is injected subcutaneously into a normal person (P/K reaction).* The presence of high serum titers of IgE are not peculiar to asthmatics; they have been found in pulmonary hemosiderosis, severe liver disease and in rare cases of multiple myeloma. The atopic individuals who are subject to respiratory allergies have an inherited permeability of their respiratory mucus membrane to the inhalants to which they react. Other peculiarities of the asthmatic consist of hyper-response to acetylcholine and to histamine given by inhalation. Another peculiarity of the asthmatic, according to Szentivanyi,[91b] is a deficiency of beta-adrenergic response. The alpha receptors, which produce broncho-constriction in response to norepinephrine, are relatively unopposed by the beta receptors, which respond to epinephrine. The beta receptors apparently are lacking in sufficient adenylcyclase, an enzyme responsible for hormonal sensitivity. In support of this theory is the finding that urinary levels of cyclic AMP† do not increase in asthmatics in response to epinephrine whereas a prompt rise occurs in normal individuals.[64a]

Adults with asthmatic attacks may have intrinsic asthma that is unrelated to the immunologic mechanisms described above. These patients are not hypersensitive to most allergens, but bronchial irritants such as acetylcholine or histamine (when inhaled) produce attacks. Pathologically, these patients also have hypertrophy of bronchomucus glands and thickening of the bronchial basement membrane. A number of these patients seem to have developed emphysema prior to and not after their attacks.[45]

In chronic bronchial asthma, upper respiratory infections may cause recurrent attacks. Psychogenic stimuli also may act as precipitants particularly in children. In adults, the addiction to sympathomimetic sprays may produce attacks on withdrawal. During severe episodes (because of

---

* P/K reaction: passive-transfer test of Prausnitz and Küstner.

† It is now believed that hormones act at the surface of their target cells by releasing adenylcyclase, which catalyzes the transformation of adenosine triphosphate (ATP) to cyclic AMP (adenosine 3'5' = monophosphate). The cyclic AMP accelerates the intracellular response, the synthesis requiring the enzyme phosphodiesterase. This type of intracellular response is required when tissues respond to epinephrine or to other catecholamines. (Butcher, R. W.: Role of cyclic AMP in hormone actions, New England J. M. *279:*1378, 1968).

hypoxia) the respiratory center is under the control of the oxygen content in the blood. Suppression of this center by the injudicious use of morphine may result in fatal asphyxia. Asthmatics who have been controlled on relatively high doses of steroids suffer from adrenal suppression. With an attack of pneumonitis (particularly in children), a fatal infection may ensue unless the hospital staff is aware of the previous cortisone therapy and the dosage increased during the infection.

Elderly asthmatics with emphysema and chronic dyspnea suffer from right ventricular strain and are often benefitted by digitalis therapy. These patients have a moderate polycythemia and the role of the circulation in precipitating night attacks can be demonstrated by placing them in the supine position without elevation of the head. This provokes an immediate attack, and adrenalin should be available for injection.

Patients with intermittent attacks of asthma of moderate severity rarely show abnormalities of arterial P_{O_2} or P_{CO_2} between attacks. During attacks, oxygen saturation is usually below 93 percent (average 89%) and arterial CO_2 tension averages 43 mm. Hg.[101] The maximum breathing capacity approximates 30 L./min., as compared to 65 L. per min. when the patients were free of asthma. Pulmonary arterial pressure increases during asthmatic attacks, averaging 52/24 mm. Hg. Williams and Zohman[101] attributed this pulmonic hypertension to increased alveolar pressure produced by the asthmatic airway obstruction. However, cor pulmonale rarely develops in patients with intermittent attacks unless there are repeated episodes of status asthmaticus. In this chronic condition, there is regional asphyxia produced by the widespread plugging of bronchioles by mucoid secretions. During status asthmaticus, the respirations may increase to 30 to 40 per minute with a corresponding pulse rate of 140 to 150 per minute. The expiratory excursions are increased with definite "pulling or labored" respirations. An increased P_{CO_2} between 80 and 90 may occur and the pH may reach 7.2 to 7.1. With relief from the attack, the values rapidly return to normal and the chest clears of rales.

Death occurring during a bronchial asthma attack is due to suffocation. Bronchospasm, plugs of tenacious secretion in the bronchioles and edema of the bronchial walls combine to obliterate the peripheral airways.[26] Fatalities in asthmatic patients may occur between attacks from right ventricular failure or from pneumonia due to chronic overdosage of cortisone therapy, which lowers immune response.

Asthmatic attacks in children or young adults (without preceding hayfever), occurring as a result of exposure to animal danders, eiderdown pillows, household dusts or foods, may be relieved by preventing exposure to the provocative antigen or by desensitization if the antigen can be demonstrated by skin testing. This type of therapy is effective in the early stages of the disease. Patients with a history of attacks for several years duration and with seasonal exacerbations caused by pollinosis, usually have crossed sensitizations to multiple substances and only a minority respond to desensitization.

Asthmatic attacks are controlled by a variety of methods, including sympathomimetic amines used as inhalant sprays, injections of adrenalin, or the chronic administration of cortisone therapy. Intravenous injections of aminophylline are effective during attacks. None of these methods of control is completely satisfactory. In a number of patients with chronic or recurrent attacks, quinoline therapy over a period of months may result in an arrest of the condition for periods of two or more years.[45] Following discontinuation of this therapy, however, the patient can redevelop his allergy. In elderly adults who do not have a history of asthma prior to the age of 60 years, attacks of wheezing and dyspnea with inspiratory and expiratory rales is usually a manifestation of emphysema or right ventricular failure. The latter are *cardiac asthmatics* and respond to digitalis therapy. Purified digitoxin or other synthetic products are preferable to digitalis leaf, since a number of asthmatics are sensitive to digitalis. A number of these patients are also sensitive to salicylates.

EMPHYSEMA

Pulmonary Emphysema. Emphysema is a chronic impairment of normal ventilatory capacity in the lungs of men and women usually beyond the age of 50 years, characterized by dyspnea and cough with overinflation of the pulmonary parenchyma. Pathologically, the air sacs and alveoli distal to the terminal bronchioles are increased in size by dilatation and destruction of their walls. In some forms, the dilatation appears to involve selectively the terminal bronchioles (centrilobular emphysema); in other cases, the alveoli of entire lobes are dilated (panlobular emphysema); and in many cases, both types of change are present in the overinflated lungs. The underlying cause is peripheral airway obstruction leading to trapping of inspired air during passive recoil of expirations [20] (Fig. 5-7). In most cases, the anterior-posterior diameter of the chest is increased and vital capacity and FEV_1 are decreased. Residual air is correspondingly increased. Abnormally prolonged enforced expiration following a maximum inspiration is characteristic. Chronic bronchitis or attacks of pneumonitis and irritant inhalants (including excessive smoking) are thought to play a role in the centrilobular form of the disease.[93] In both types of emphysema, the vasculature of the capillary bed is diminished, leading to pulmonary hypertension and, ultimately, to cor pulmonale.[48]

Emphysema may be observed in childhood in patients suffering from

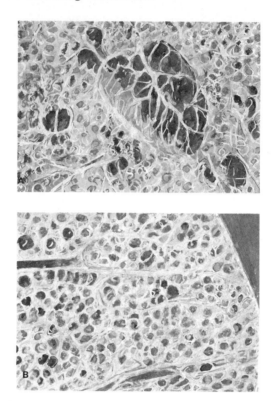

Fig. 5-7. Forms of emphysema. (*A*) Centrilobular. (*B*) Diffuse panacinar.

repeated asthmatic attacks. Distortion of the chest wall with kyphosis and bowing of the sternum is usually present.

The clinical diagnosis of emphysema is substantiated radiologically by increased translucence in the x-ray film and increased narrowing of the pulmonary arteries distal to the large hilar vessels (Fig. 5-8A & B). Bronchograms reveal splaying or widening of the angles of the major bronchi in the region of the hilum and frequently, difficulty in filling the peripheral bronchi of smaller caliber. The clinical diagnosis is considered substantiated if measurement of residual air is increased beyond the normal of 30 percent of total lung capacity. When residual volume is increased beyond the normal 30 percent to 45 percent of total volume, the emphysema is moderate; when increased to 45 to 55 percent, severe emphysema is present. Arterial oxygen saturation is diminished, falling from the normal 97 percent to a value of 90 percent or less. P_{CO_2} values range from 47 to 60 mm. Hg and blood pH from 7.39 to 7.35. Beerel and Vance [11] found

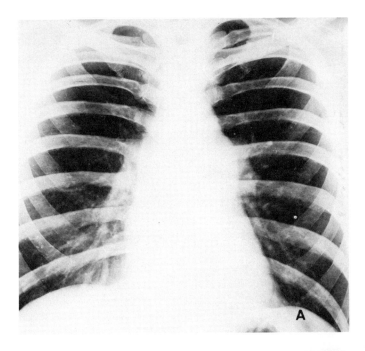

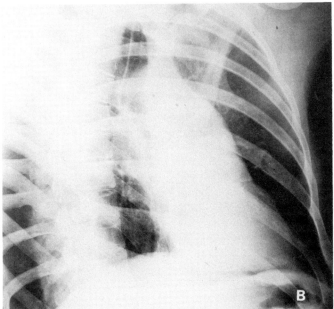

Fig. 5-8. Roentgenograms of emphysema. (*A*) A-P view. (*B*) Lateral view.

that these values were similar if the determination was made on blood obtained from the brachial artery or from blood obtained at the fingertip that had been adequately warmed. A moderate polycythemia is usually present and pulmonary artery pressure is increased, rising with diminished arterial oxygen saturation.

Whereas the normal blood pressure in the pulmonary circuit is about 25/10 mm. Hg, Ebert and his co-workers [33] found in 24 patients that the pulmonary systolic pressure was raised to 50-72 mm. Hg, and the diastolic to approximately 22 mm. Hg. In autopsy studies, Hicken et al.[48] could not correlate the weight of the right ventricle with the degree of pulmonary emphysema in patients with the panacinar form. Right ventricular hypertrophy however, was correlated with centrilobular emphysema in 75 percent of the cases.

Once the disease is well established in adults, the systemic blood pressure also may be elevated (circa 160/95) and the Valsalva maneuver causes a drop in pulse pressure, indicating there is difficulty (in the pulmonic circuit) in passing blood from the right to the left side of the heart.[44] The exact cause of this increased pulmonic vascular resistance is not established. Some observors believe there is elongation and narrowing of the precapillary arteries that are stretched over the dilated alveoli; others find increased muscular thickening in the arterial walls with narrowing of their lumens.

The pathogenesis of emphysema is varied and the ultimate mechanism of increased airway resistance that causes the dilatation and rupture of the air sacs is unknown. Chronic bronchitis, including bronchiolitis in heavy smokers and in patients who have had multiple severe attacks of pneumonitis, is thought to play a role, but the increased prevalence of chronic bronchitis may be secondary to the emphysema in many cases. Inspissated bronchial secretions that act as a check valve to expiration appear to be important in patients suffering from status asthmaticus. Constriction of these airways secondary to fibrosis occurs in miner's asthma, following exposure to silica compounds, asbestos and other lung irritants. If the bronchioles are plugged or disappear, the persisting alveoli may receive air (via the pores of Kohn) from the adjacent acini, which remains trapped during expiration. This is known as the "air pool" theory. On the other hand, infiltration of the lungs by irritant dusts with disappearance of their blood supply may cause atrophy of the muscular and elastic walls of the respiratory bronchioles causing their distention and eventual disruption of adjacent alveoli.[86]

Hereditary Factors. Two forms of emphysema arising on an hereditary basis are known. In patients with fibrocystic disease of the pancreas inherited as a recessive trait, the development of emphysema complicates chronic pulmonary infections. This may be related to the discovery of a factor in their serum that inhibits the action of respiratory cilia and which can be demonstrated in explants on rabbit tracheal mucosa. In patients with hereditary alpha 1-antitrypsin deficiency (also inherited as a recessive trait), emphysema with dyspnea on exertion appears as a primary disease usually below the age of 40. There is usually no history of infection and roentgenograms of the chest show hyperventilation of the lower lungs with diminished vascular markings. The dyspneic state is accompanied by only moderate hypoxemia and normal P_{CO_2}. Cardiac complications are rare, but cor pulmonale develops terminally in the presence of infection. Only a few develop polycythemia. Of 33 patients, homozygous for alpha$_1$-antitrypsin deficiency, Eriksson [36] found 23 with emphysema (chronic obstructive bronchopulmonary disease). All of the males over the age of 40 years had this disease. He suggested that the primary antienzyme defect was in the liver and the pulmonary damage was due to lysing enzymes from leukocytes responding to subclinical respiratory infections that were unopposed by antitrypsin. Recent evidence indicates that the enzyme is formed in the liver in these patients but fails to escape into the serum. (Vordon *et al.*)[45B] The lytic damage, however, has not been demonstrated microscopically and only one of the patients was studied at autopsy. This patient had panacinar emphysema. However, emphysema has been produced experimentally in dogs by administering the proteolytic enzyme papain.[73] Damage in these dogs was localized in the region of the bronchioles.

Course of Disease. In the early stages of emphysema, the patient usually complains only of dyspnea on exertion with or without a moderate cough and the diagnosis is made by prolonged expiration (on maximum inspiration and expiration) or diminished FEV_1. Bronchial dilators in the form of ephedrine or theophyllline and antibiotics at the onset of respiratory infections are satisfactory forms of treatment. However, despite initial improvement in symptoms, there is continuous slow decline in ventilatory function with FEV_1 decreasing 75 ml./year (which is two to three times the normal rate with aging).[18] This is accompanied by obliteration of capillaries by increased fibrosis diminishing perfusions (Fig. 5-9). When FEV_1 is in the range of 1.5 liters, cardiac complications are not severe or may be absent, but with FEV_1 in the range of 1 liter, less than 50 percent of the patients will survive for 5 years.

At this stage, there is accompanying hypercapnia or cor pulmonale. In this advanced stage of the disease, the patients are improved on digitalis therapy and the intermittent use of cortisone or antibiotics for episodes of severe dyspnea with cough during bouts of respiratory infection. In a review of 229 cases of emphysema, approximately 15 percent had attacks of bronchial asthma and more than 40 percent had evidence of left ven-

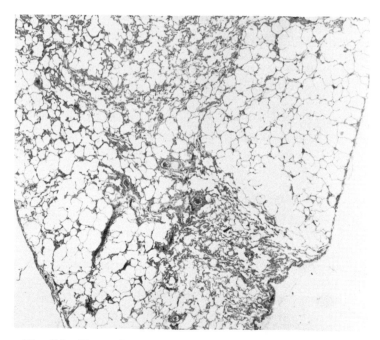

Fig. 5-9. Photomicrograph of panacinar emphysema. (×25)

tricular hypertrophy at autopsy as well as EKG evidence, either with normal systemic blood pressure or with moderate elevation. Baum et al [10] have recently confirmed these findings by cardiac catheterization, finding left ventricular dysfunction in the majority of 15 cases studied. Left ventricular hypertrophy was found whether or not right sided heart failure was present. Among the possible causes of this left ventricular strain are broncho-pulmonary vascular anastomoses and impairment of coronary outflow secondary to increased right atrial pressure since intrathoracic negative pressure is diminished or lost in chronic emphysema. Regardless of cause, many patients with emphysema die of pulmonic hypertension and right ventricular failure without developing severe respiratory deficiency.

Elderly patients with advanced emphysema and varying degrees of cardiac decompensation are frequently admitted to the hospital with acute respiratory infections which precipitate respiratory acidosis. A similar acidosis with respiratory failure may occur in such individuals following major surgery. The chronic hypercapnia and respiratory acidosis fits the nomogram reproduced in Fig. 2-5, indicating the amount of sodium bicarbonate or THAM-E required to offset the accumulation of hydrogen ions. The retention of CO_2 leads to mental confusion, which may be followed by CO_2 narcosis. Oxygen therapy may be required. When oxygen is indicated in such patients with emphysema, the mortality rate is high. Such attacks are less frequent in patients who have been previously digitalized.

Transplantation of a lung in patients with advanced emphysema has resulted in failure with one exception. A major reason is the vascular resistance in the remaining emphysematous lung in which hyperinflation and further hypoperfusion is precipitated. A more drastic operation has recently been reported in which the heart and both lungs were transplanted into a patient who survived only a few days.[89]

Bronchiolar Emphysema or Muscular Cirrhosis of the Lung. In this rare form of emphysema, both the terminal bronchioles and alveoli show arrested development. The number of alveolar ducts is fewer and enter into single or less elaborate aggregates of alveoli with thickened walls that appear to be an extension of collagen and elastic fibers proliferating from the bronchioles. At times, cystic expansion of emphysematous changes appear to be derived directly from the bronchioles, suggesting that the emphysematous changes are superimposed upon a poorly developed or arrested form of lung structure. The gross appearance of the lung is characteristic. The surface is uneven, noncrepitant and doughy, resembling the finely nodular surface of the liver in Laennec's cirrhosis. The condition is always bilateral, but most patients survive into adult life despite progressive dyspnea and chronic cough. One fatal case has been reported in an infant.[84] In the 12 cases reported through 1957, hypertrophy of the muscular coats of the respiratory bronchioles with a diminished number of dependent alveoli was the outstanding feature. Grossly, this condition resembles the honey-combed lung of scleroderma (systemic sclerosis) and also the congenital cystic lymphangiectasia of the lung.

Chemical Bronchitis and Acute Emphysema. Acute destruction of the epithelial lining of the bronchi with desquamated cells and edema fluid filling the small bronchioles was frequently observed in fatal cases of gas poisoning in World War I. (Winternitz).[104] Nonfatal cases of chemical bronchitis with broncheolitis and acute emphysematous changes (over inflation) occur in firemen overcome by smoke and among chemists working with fuming nitric acid, ammonia, or other irritant gases.

The patients suffer fever and cough and dyspnea on exertion. If a history of exposure is not obtained in cases where the degree of poisoning is nonfatal but repeated, the condition is often mistaken for influenza. The distinctive clinical feature is the occurrence of both systemic and pulmonic hypertension. The systemic pressure may rise to 220/120 and persist for a week or more after exposure. In fatal cases, such as occur with steam or chemical poisoning, the bronchial epithelium is necrotic or desquamated, the muscle walls of the bronchioles disintegrate and there is an outpouring of fibrin, red blood cells and leukocytes into the alveolar spaces. In chronic cases, pulmonary hypertension and the associated systemic hypertension is thought to result from the vasoconstriction and the shunting of blood away from the nonaerated tissue. Patients recovering from the acute episode may subsequently die of right ventricular failure secondary to progressive pulmonary fibrosis.

CHRONIC BRONCHITIS IN THE AGED

Chronic bronchitis in the aged with increased productive cough and with exacerbations of fever, wheezing and dyspnea commonly complicates emphysema and is more common during the winter months in temperate climates. Fog and dampness exacerbate the condition by apparently increasing the bronchial secretions. In England, during the winter months, the incidence has been estimated between 130 and 140/1,000, varying with the sex and being more common in men. The peak of age incidence is between 60 and 75 years. When complicated by bronchopneumonia, it is the leading cause of death among respiratory diseases. Pathologically, proliferation of the mucus glands and edema of the bronchial walls with minimal amounts of lymphoid exudate identify the condition. There is an associated emphysema and occasional alveoli which are collapsed by inspissated exudate. Patches of bronchial erosion may alternate with the areas of mucus gland hyperplasia (Fig. 5-10A and B).

Chronic bronchitis is usually a complication of other diseases such as chronic congestive heart failure, recurrent attacks of asthma and advanced emphysema. Industrial dusts or gases and excessive cigarette smoking are contributing causes. Its relation to fatal bronchopneumonia in the aged during the winter months is frequent in geriatric institutions, but few bacterial studies have been made to elucidate the nature of the infectious organisms. These are apparently similar to those carried in the upper respiratory tract in ordinary individuals and include pneumococcus, staphylococcus, streptococcus and hemophylus influenza. The flora in these patients with chronic bronchitis often remains the same during acute exacerbations although infection by pneumococci often is responsible for the severe acute exacerbations. Increased cough and purulent sputum accompany these exacerbations, which may be reduced in frequency during the winter months in northern climates by the prophylactic use of broad spectrum antibiotics (tetracycline or chloromycetin). This is not justified except in the elderly in which the condition is complicated by cardiac decompensation.

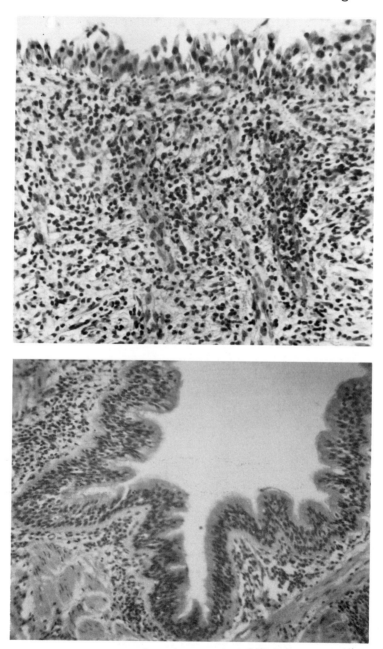

Fig. 5-10. (*Top*) Photomicrograph of acute bronchitis. (*Bottom*)
Photomicrograph of chronic bronchitis. (×150)

BRONCHIAL ADENOMA

Cough, hemoptysis and nonasthmatic wheezing are frequent symptoms of bronchial adenoma. The adenoma is usually visualized by means of bronchoscopy and confirmed by biopsy. Recurrent, unresolved pneumonia in a single lobe, atelectasis or localized bronchiectasis may complicate these tumors. Hemoptysis may occur five to eight years (or more) prior to the discovery of the tumor. Usually, the tumor is obscured in the roentgenogram by atelectasis or pneumonia. The cytology of bronchial washings is usually unrewarding. Rarely, the tumor may complicate tuberculosis.[14] (Chapter 12)

6

Pulmonary Circulatory Disease

There are four major conditions which affect the perfusion capacity of the lungs; two of these have their origin in the vascular system, the other two are dependent upon changes originating in the pulmonary parenchyma. The primary vascular abnormalities are: (1) those affecting the general circulation or cardiac output and (2) those involving the local pulmonary vasculature. The changes in the pulmonary parenchyma that affect perfusion are: (1) Zones of nonaeration due to such conditions as atelectasis, a bleb or at times, an infarct or a pneumonic zone of consolidation or neoplasm. Blood is usually shunted away from such a zone. (2) Chronic obstructive lung disease (usually emphysema), which results in vasoconstriction or pulmonic hypertension.

ACUTE PULMONARY EDEMA

Vascular leakage with flooding of the alveoli is a life-threatening emergency. It may be precipitated by an increase of hydrostatic pressure within the pulmonary capillaries; by fall in the protein concentration of the plasma with loss of capillary osmotic pressure or by damage to the capillary walls which increase their permeability.

A rise in pulmonary capillary hydrostatic pressure may occur acutely with attacks of left ventricular failure. The resultant pulmonary congestion and edema causes bubbly rales, dyspnea, cough with frothy sputum and cyanosis. There is an elevation of P_{CO_2} and a fall in P_{O_2}, which in severe cases requires oxygen therapy to tide the patient over an impending fatality. The most common causes of left ventricular failure with elevated pulmonary venous pressure are long-standing systemic hypertension, mitral stenosis and aortic stenosis. The sudden elevation of pulmonary venous pressure produces vasostasis in the capillary bed of the lungs. The elevated hydrostatic pressure and the effect of hypoxia on the capillary wall (which promotes leakage) combine to extravasate fluid into the pulmonary alveolar spaces.

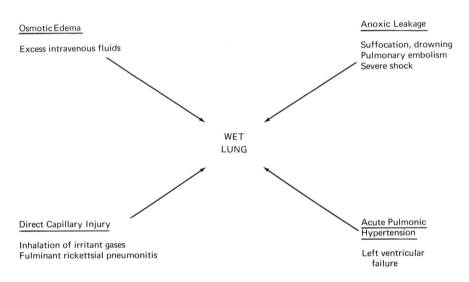

MAJOR CAUSES OF ACUTE PULMONARY CONGESTION & EDEMA
(WET LUNG)

Osmotic Edema

Excess intravenous fluids

Anoxic Leakage

Suffocation, drowning
Pulmonary embolism
Severe shock

WET
LUNG

Direct Capillary Injury

Inhalation of irritant gases
Fulminant rickettsial pneumonitis

Acute Pulmonic
Hypertension

Left ventricular
failure

The pulmonary edema associated with attacks of left ventricular failure can often be combatted with digitalis or drugs that combat auricular fibrillation or cardiac arrhythmias, and with diuretics. Oxygen, of course, is required in severe cases. Phlebotomy may be life saving. In subacute cases, rotating tourniquets may be applied to the extremities at the time or just before a phlebotomy of 500 ml. of blood. Aminophylline intravenously diminishes bronchial constriction and augments cardiac contractility. Intravenous diuretics such as furosemide or ethacrynic acid are given.

The pulmonary edema that occurs in uremia or with acute renal failure in shock is a complicated disorder. The loss of electrolytes and at times, serum albumin lowers plasma osmotic pressure. At the same time, cardiac impairment, through the retention of potassium or nitrogenous wastes, elevates venous hydrostatic pressure in the pulmonary venous circulation. At times, severe degrees of hypertension contribute to the cardiac failure.

Pulmonary edema may follow the rapid intravenous administration of hypotonic solutions. The rapid addition of such fluids to the circulation lowers the osmotic pressure within the pulmonary capillaries resulting in leakage and edema.

Capillary Injury With Pulmonary Edema. Direct injury to the capillary walls resulting from the inhalation of noxious gases produces edema or wet lung. Extensive experience with this form of pulmonary edema resulted from the use of poisonous gases during World War I. Similar capillary injuries may result from the inhalation of smoke, live steam, fuming nitric acid or ammonia. If hypertonic saline infusions are given to combat such edema, the patient's condition becomes worse because the intravenous fluids aid in maintaining hydrostatic pressure and capillary leakage. The preferable treatment is restriction of fluids and the administration of diuretics to reduce blood volume. In these cases of chemically induced pulmonary edema, the exudation of plasma from the damaged capillaries seals off the diffusion surface of the alveoli and limits diffusion. The inhalation of pure oxygen is required to combat anoxia and hypercapnia. An extracorporeal oxygenator if available, may be life saving.[49]

Anoxia With Capillary Leakage. While chronic hypoxia causes pulmonary vasoconstriction and nonaerated portions of the lungs may be bypassed, this is not true for severe acute hypoxia. Acute hypoxia damages the pulmonary capillary bed and causes leakage of edema fluid. Such hypoxic leakage occurs in exertion at high altitude, during diminished cardiac output in post-traumatic shock and with acute left ventricular failure. Similar leakage occurs with suffocation and in drowning if laryngeal spasm seals the airways. There is also capillary leakage with massive pulmonary embolism (so-called acute cor pulmonale). In suffocation, congestion and edema in the lungs is increased by violent respiratory efforts which increase negative intrathoracic pressure and suck more blood into the pulmonic circuit.

With nonfatal degrees of gas poisoning such as the inhalation of smoke by firemen or more dilute chemical fumes that may affect chemists working with a faulty hood, there is severe bronchial spasm and excess bronchial secretion from the irritated lining membranes. The result is an acute form of emphysema accompanied by both intrapulmonic and systemic hypertension. How much of this is due to the reponse of the vasomotor and respiratory centers in the medulla is not known. Some of these patients have been misdiagnosed as forms of acute viral pneumonitis, but the elevated blood pressure is the key to the diagnosis. However, antibiotics are indicated to prevent secondary bacterial infection and pneumonia.

Capillary and arteriolar rupture with intrapulmonic hemorrhages may follow blast injuries in warfare. The blast wave compresses the chest and residual alveolar air. There is then sudden release as the blast wave passes and this release of compressed air in the rapidly expanding alveoli ruptures their walls and their capillaries.

The pulmonary capillaries are injured by exposure to irradiation, particularly in therapeutic dosage given for carcinoma of the breast or bronchogenic carcinoma. A leakage in the capillary bed and destruction of the respiratory epithelial lining of the bronchi in the earlier phase, predisposes to pneumonitis. Postirradiation pneumonia usually occurs at the end of two to three weeks, shortly after the completion of the therapeutic course of irradiation. The late effects (produced by healing) are pulmonary fibrosis, which results largely from vascular sclerosis.

Edema and thickening of the alveolar septums and the walls of the arterioles with capillary exudation occurs in rickettsial fevers. Thrombosis of capillaries and arterioles is more frequently seen in Rocky Mountain spotted fever and Old World typhus; hemorrhagic exudate and pericapillary infiltrate is more pronounced in scrub typhus. Frank pulmonary edema does not occur unless large amounts of intravenous fluids are administered at the height of the rickettsial pneumonitis.

Pulmonic Vessels in Shock (Shock Lung Syndrome). Post-traumatic shock is accompanied by peripheral vasoconstriction in the systemic circuit, thus in theory conserving blood for vital organs. However, in posthemorrhagic and traumatic shock, there is a similar vasoconstriction in the pulmonic circuit which may cause fatal hypoxia. Arterial oxygen tensions below 50 mm. Hg have been recorded.[49] In laboratory animals, the pulmonic vasoconstriction adjusts this vascular bed to the greatly reduced central blood volume. However, edema, hemorrhage and necrosis of the alveolar walls may result from this pulmonic ischemia, augmenting the decreased arterial oxygen saturation.[102] In shocked laboratory animals who have been rendered hypovolemic, reinfusion of the withdrawn blood has failed to alleviate the pulmonic vasoconstriction. The original experiments performed on dogs were repeated on primates (baboons) in whom there was a reversal of vascular changes upon resuscitation.[15] In clinical post-traumatic shock, both fat and air emboli in the pulmonic circuit complicate the picture. However, when the patients have been maintained by extracorporeal oxygenation for several days, recovery has occurred.

PULMONARY CONGESTION WITH CHRONIC CARDIAC DECOMPENSATION

Long-standing pulmonary congestion with elevated pulmonary venous pressure is common with mitral stenosis and severe degrees of mitral insufficiency which are usually of rheumatic origin. The alterations in the lungs which produces a rusty appearance and rigid texture are known as "brown induration." Microscopically, the alveoli contain numerous hemosiderin-laden macrophages (heart failure cells), which may be coughed up in the sputum. The arteriolar and capillary walls are thickened by deposits of fibrin and fibrous tissue and their lumens are distended with red cells. At times, iron liberated from macrophages may accumulate in the internal elastic lamellae of the arteries (pulmonary hemosiderosis). Small thrombi and hemorrhages may occur in the tortuous vessels. When the capillary pressure in congestive heart failure rises above 30 mm. Hg the excess over osmotic pressure produces varying degrees of pulmonary edema. However, a moderate excess of hydrostatic pressure can occur without significant edema because of the increased rate of fluid drainage by the pulmonary lymphatics, which return the leakage to the venous circulation.

Right Pleural Effusion. Pleural effusion in the right chest is often a source of increased dyspnea and of insomnia in cardiac decompensation. The pulmonary capillary bed is greater on the right than on the left, but the lymphatic plexus is smaller on the right. Thus, with anoxic and capillary leakage, fluid has an increased tendency to accumulate in the pleural space. Once an appreciable amount has accumulated, the lymphatics are compressed in the adjacent pleura and the effusion tends to persist.

Cardiac Asthma. Patients with longstanding right ventricular strain secondary to left ventricular failure or to emphysema suffer orthopnea. In some of these individuals, the assumption of the reclining position leads to attacks of bronchiolar constriction and asthmatic wheezes. In such patients, this reflex response occurs within seconds as blood from the distended veins reaches the right heart on reclining. This may be a paraendocrine response secondary to serotonin release by the argentaffine cells in the lungs.

PULMONARY EMBOLISM

Fatal Thromboembolism. A variety of emboli are carried by the venous system to the right side of the heart and thence to the pulmonary capillaries, where they may interrupt the circulation to varying degrees. The most common type of embolus is thromboembolism that arises from detached fragments of thrombi which have formed in the right auricular appendage or, more frequently, in the veins of the lower extremities. Propogating thrombi producing massive pulmonary embolism usually form in the veins of the calf in debilitated patients after prolonged bed rest or in the larger veins of the leg or pelvis following abdominal operations. The tail of the thrombus elongates by eddy currents fed into the main channel and a prolonged segment, following its detachment, passes through the right atrium and right ventricle and lodges most often at the bifurcation of the pulmonary artery where it forms a "saddle thrombus." Blockage of over 65 percent of the pulmonary circulation results in acute right ventricular failure and death within minutes (acute cor pulmonale). The stagnating blood in the blocked pulmonary vasculature leaks from the anoxic capillaries and the lungs at autopsy ooze edema fluid and red blood cells on sectioning (Fig. 6-1).

Nonfatal Thromboembolism. Obstruction of a single branch of the pulmonary artery by thromboembolism is not fatal except where there is preceding coronary insufficiency or cardiac decompensation with mitral stenosis. Obstruction of minor branches when the circulation is slowed by cardiac decompensation results in *pulmonary infarction* (Fig. 6-2). The tissue affected by the circulatory block undergoes coagulation. At necropsy, a triangular zone of tissue has a firm raised "stuffed" feeling and is airless and dry on sectioning. The overlying pleura is covered by fibrinous exudate. Clinically, a pulmonary infarct is manifested by a zone of consolidation, a pleural fraction rub, pain on deep breathing, fever and hemoptysis. If the patient is a known cardiac, particularly one with mitral stenosis, the diagnosis is relatively easy.

Diagnosis. In patients not in congestive cardiac failure, the triad of hemoptysis pleural friction rub and a pre-existing thrombophlebitis was formerly considered presumptive evidence of pulmonary embolism. However, with diagnosis aided by radionuclide scanning (scintigraphy) the

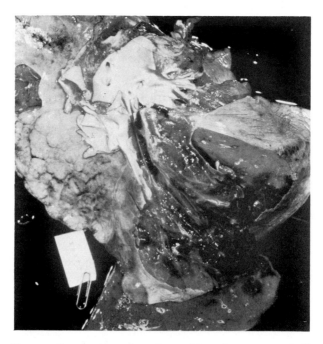

Fig. 6-1. Propagating venous thrombus with pulmonary embolism and infarction.

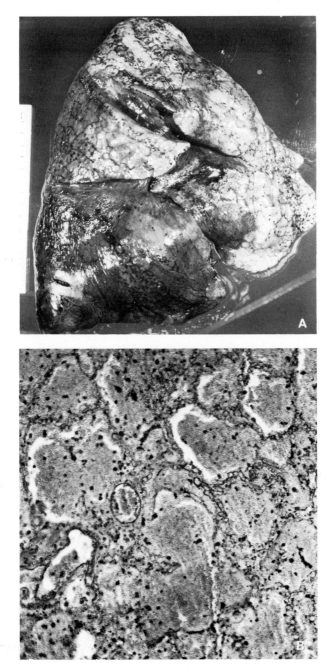

Fig. 6-2. Massive pulmonary infarct. (*A*) Gross specimen. (*B*)
Photomicrograph. (×150)

majority of the patients have nonspecific symptoms. These include dyspnea (86%), cough (70%), followed by pleural pain (58%) and finally, hemoptysis (38%).[81] A frequent physical finding is accentuation of the pulmonary secondary sound and a respiratory rate greater than 20 per minute with tachycardia greater than 100 per minute and a low grade fever (101°F.). The electrocardiogram may show disturbances of rhythm with paroxysmal atrial fibrillation or flutter and either atrial or ventricular ectopic beats and a rightward shift of the QRS axis. T-wave inversions of the right precordial leads indicative of right ventricular strain are important when present. Lung scans are particularly helpful, but cannot be interpreted without radiographic films to rule out other pathology. The final diagnosis may require angiography, which depicts the anatomic defect in the plugged vessel but this is not without risk. Intravenous heparin is used in the acute phase of the disease followed by anticoagulant therapy by mouth (coumarin derivatives).

Other Varieties of Pulmonary Embolism. In divers, gas embolism results from the sudden release from atmospheric compression, which permits nitrogen to bubble out of solution from the blood. Fatal pulmonary embolism may result; in other instances more widespread involvement occurs in the venous system and the central nervous system also suffers. In aviators, this is known as altitude sickness.

During the London blitz, pulmonary thromboembolism (at times fatal) resulted from prolonged pressure in the veins of the calf or lower leg muscles in tall men, particularly air wardens who stood for long periods. This has been referred to as the "long, thin man syndrome."

The intravenous injection by drug addicts of drugs in tablet form containing talc and other fillers results in widespread obstruction of the pulmonary vascular bed with the formation of granulomas in the vessel walls. Pulmonary hypertension and right ventricular failure may result.

Bone marrow and fat gain entrance into the circulation following severe injuries in which there are fractures of the major bones and damage to the soft tissues (Fig. 6-3). Bone marrow at times with small bone spicules may be found in the small pulmonary vessels in patients dying from the severity of the injury without significant pulmonary symptoms. Fatal fat embolisms result from the large amount of fatty tissues liberated by trauma. The amount of fat and its ready emulsification are important. Grossly, the lungs are congested and edematous and the oily embolic material oozes from the cut surface of the lungs. The kidney and the brain may be involved by the emboli passing through the pulmonary capillaries into the systemic circulation.

Trophoblast Embolism. Small emboli of trophoblastic tissue often occur during pregnancy and are found at autopsy in women dying during preg-

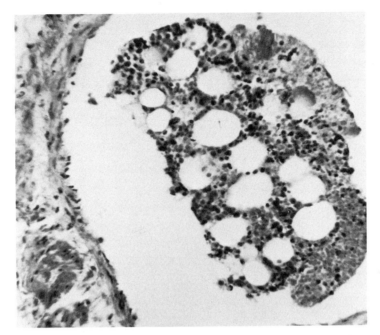

Fig. 6-3. Bone marrow embolus following fracture. (×100)

nancy or shortly after parturition of other causes. They have been reported in 43.6 percent of obstetrical deaths.[6]

Amniotic Fluid Embolism. This serious and usually fatal complication of childbirth which occurs either during or shortly after delivery, is accompanied by severe dyspnea, tachycardia cyanosis and vascular collapse (Fig. 6-4). Death may follow in minutes, hours or days. At autopsy, the lungs are heavy, congested and edematous. Microscopically, the pulmonary arterioles and capillaries contain droplets of mucinous amiotic fluid which can be demonstrated by PAS staining. In addition, fetal debris carried in the fluid may include bits of fetal skin, meconium, lanugo hairs and trophoblasts. The venous infusion of amniotic fluid is favored by violent uterine contractions in the presence of vascular rupture in cases of partial detachment of the placenta, cervical tears or rupture of the myometrium. The incidence of amniotic fluid emboli is unknown, since in nonfatal cases, the reversible shock experienced by the patients is usually attributed to postpartum hemorrhage. In surviving patients, intravascular coagulation lowers fibrinogen and results in hemorrhages. This and other coagulative defects result from thromboplastin from the fetus entering the maternal circulation.

Parasitic Emboli. Extensive parasitic emboli are most common as a result of infestation with the various forms of schistosoma organism.

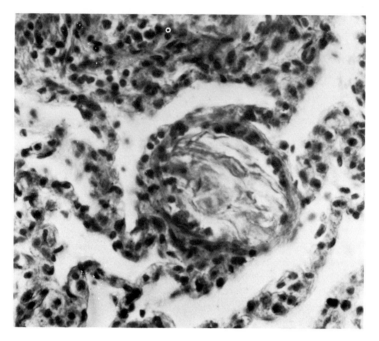

Fig. 6-4. Amniotic fluid embolus. (×200)

Numerous ova are carried by the bloodstream to the lungs, usually in cases where there is extensive hepatic involvement. The ova within the pulmonary arterioles produce fibrinoid necrosis of the vessel walls and a perivascular granulomatous reaction. Subsequent scarring obliterates the vascular lumen. Larger arteries may undergo thrombosis. The pulmonary involvement may result in hypertension of the lesser circulation, right ventricular hypertrophy and failure.[68]

Tumor Emboli. Multiple pulmonary foci of metastatic cancer are common in the advanced stages of malignant disease and are usually referred to as "seeding." The roentgenogram may resemble that of miliary tuberculosis. Chronic cough and dyspnea are the usual symptoms. In exceptional cases, the progressively severe pulmonic hypertension and right ventricular hypertrophy may lead to death from cor pulmonale when the primary tumor has gone undetected.[90]

CHRONIC PULMONARY HYPERTENSION

Pressure in the pulmonary arteries normally varies between 20/10 to 25/15 mm. Hg. A systolic pressure between 40 and 69 mm. Hg is considered moderate hypertension and over 70 mm. Hg is considered severe.

The increased pressure is said to arise *arterially* when it is the result of increased cardiac output. Venous hypertension refers to that caused by increased resistance to exit pressure via the pulmonic veins.

Arterial hypertension occurs from congenital atrial or ventricular septal defects which permit shunting of blood from the left to the right ventricle, increasing blood flow from the right ventricle. A similar boosting action from the force of the left ventricle occurs in cases with a patent ductus arteriosus or in cases of bronchiectasis in which arteriovenous shunts are formed between the bronchial artery and pulmonic veins.

Venous pulmonic hypertension is produced by mitral stenosis or severe mitral insufficiency, which elevates pressure in the pulmonic capillaries. This provokes compensatory right ventricular hypertrophy with increased output.

MAJOR CAUSES OF PULMONARY HYPERTENSION

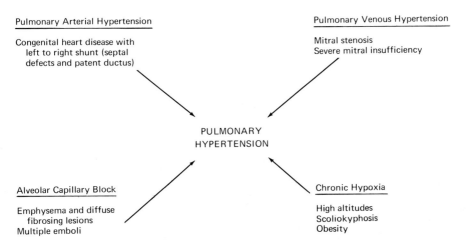

Either form of sustained pulmonic hypertension causes medial hypertrophy and fibrosis of the pulmonary arteries which withstand the effects of increased pressure. Such mural thickening diminishes the lumen of the vessels and serves to aggravate the hypertension. Ultimately, right ventricular failure results. In some cases of pulmonic hypertension, with congenital heart disease, there is intravascular fibrin precipitation, endothelial proliferation and thrombotic occlusion of the small vessels.[53]

A third form of pulmonic hypertension originates at the capillary level in emphysema, pneumoconiosis and other lesions which produce diffuse fibrosis and obliteration of capillary vessels. In such cases, the alveolar capillaries are first more tortuous then compressed and finally obliterated.

There is an associated loss of alveolar septa extending hypoxia to surrounding regions with additional loss of capillaries. Such widespread post-hypertensive changes eventually extend to the larger pulmonary arteries whose walls are thickened and fibrosed. In diffuse pulmonary schistosomiasis and lymphatic spread of pulmonary metastases, there may be hypertension of the capillary type.

Unexplained forms of pulmonic hypertension occur. A few cases termed idiopathic appear to be familial.[87] Forms secondary to pulmonic hypoxia occur in kyphoscoliotics ("heart failure of hunch-backs") and also in short, adipose individuals with shallow breathing—the "Pickwickian syndrome." A mountain form occurs in natives living at high altitudes in the Andes, who hyperventilate because of low oxygen pressure. According to Naeye,[69] these hypoxic forms act directly on the musculature of the pulmonary arteries.

In patients beyond the age of 50 who have suffered with emphysema, obesity with lax abdominal muscles and kyphoscoliosis over a period of years, the author has found that the pulmonic hypertension is associated with moderate to severe systemic hypertension with blood pressures in the region of 165/95.[44]

Attempts have been made to estimate the degree of change in the pulmonic capillary bed and the degree of hypoxia required to produce pulmonic hypertension. An approximate 50 percent reduction in the capillary bed or a drop in arterial saturation approaching 80 mm. Hg, was associated with pulmonic hypertension in uranium miners.[66] The two factors of reduced capillary network and respiratory hypoxia may act or interact as cause and/or effect. Apparently, either may come first. Thus, cor pulmonale and hypertension may occur early in emphysema without concomitant vascular changes. The role of reduced perfusion can now be more readily estimated by scanning with radioactive materials.[22] (See Chapter 3.) The role of hypoxia in producing vasoconstriction has been demonstrated in human volunteers by administering 5 percent oxygen by catheter to the main bronchus of one lung while the other is under normal ventilation. Diffuse vasoconstriction occurs in vessels of all sizes.[41]

As noted in Chapter 4, pulmonic hypertension can be demonstrated by taking the patient's pulse pressure before and again during the Valsalva maneuver. Compression of the inferior vena cava against the liver during this maneuver limits return blood flow to the right ventricle. If pulmonic hypertension is present, there is further difficulty in blood flow from right to left and the pulse pressure drops and may actually disappear through elevation of the diastolic pressure.[44]

There is no adequate treatment for pulmonic hypertension. Digitalis therapy to support the right ventricular contractions may greatly extend the patient's capacity for activity. This, plus bronchial dilators of the theophylline type produce symptomatic relief.

PULMONARY VASCULAR SHUNTS

The double blood supply of the lungs has numerous points of junction in the capillary bed of the bronchi and bronchioles. The blood supply to the tracheobronchial passages is from the left ventricle via the bronchial arteries while venous blood from the right ventricle, via the pulmonary artery, passes through the capillary bed of the alveoli. On its return from the tracheobronchial passages via the bronchial veins to the superior vena cava, a small portion of this blood passes via anastomoses to the major pulmonary veins joining that which originated from the pulmonary artery. Because of this connection, under pathologic conditions about one-third of the blood proceeding from the pulmonary artery may by-pass the alveolar capillaries entirely and return via the bronchial veins. This abnormal shunting is precipitated by zones of nonaerated pulmonary tissue. This is possible because such nonaerated zones produce local vasoconstriction in the pulmonic circuit through hypoxia.[41] This shunting occurs in cases of lobar pneumonia and atelectasis where an entire lobe is nonaerated. This conservation of blood flow prevents the rise of P_{CO_2}, which occurs when nonventilated tissue is perfused by the pulmonary capillaries. However, if the shunts are large due to arteriovenous aneurysms, the oxygenation of blood is prevented by by-passing large zones of aerated tissue. In patients who suffer multiple pulmonary emboli, severe degrees of hypoxia are prevented by shunting.

The opposite type of reflex also exists in the lungs, but its mode of action has not been explained. If zones of pulmonary tissue fail to receive a blood supply (which, coming from the pulmonary vein, is high in CO_2 concentration) the alveolar air continues to have a low concentration of CO_2. This low concentration of alveolar CO_2 stimulates bronchiolar and bronchial constriction.[91a] It is probable that attacks of cardiac asthma are precipitated by failure of the right ventricle to perfuse the alveoli in the midlung fields.

Pulmonary Hemangiomas and Arteriovenous Fistulas. Angiomatous lesions of the lungs are rare and may complicate hereditary vascular lesions such as Osler-Rendu-Weber disease or Lindau-Hipple disease. Only the larger cavernous lesions cause disturbances of the pulmonary blood flow. However, the arterial channels may progressively enlarge over the years and cause the shunting of the deoxygenated pulmonary arterial blood into the systemic circulation via an arteriovenous fistula. If sufficient blood is thus shunted from large pulmonary vessels to the systemic circulation, oxygen desaturation results. If more than 30 percent of the pulmonary blood flow is thus shunted, cyanosis will result and there is a secondary polycythemia and increased blood volume. In these rare cases, cyanosis is not accompanied by diminution of vital capacity or other lung volumes and the lesion can be disclosed by scanning the lungs by radio-tagged microspherules (Chap. 3).

Resection of these growths is indicated; sudden hemothorax may eventuate in untreated cases. Although right ventricular hypertrophy is rare, it may occur.[87]

ENDOTHELIAL DAMAGE

Rickettsial and Hemorrhagic Pneumonitis. Rickettsial infection, transmitted by the bite of insects, produces spotted fever, so-called because of the hemorrhagic lesions in the skin. Old World typhus, transmitted by the body louse, is the best known form, but pulmonary symptoms are transient and not severe with this infection. The rickettsial diseases with varying degrees of pneumonitis are Rocky Mountain spotted fever (caused by *Rickettsia rickettsii*), scrub typhus (caused by *Rickettsia tsutsugamushi*) and Q fever (caused by *Rickettsia burneti*). The pneumonitis produced by Q fever is accompanied by fever, cough and chest pains and signs of consolidation or infiltration in the roentgenogram, resembling atypical pneumonia. It is the least severe of the three and usually followed by complete recovery. Pathologically, it produces an exudate in the bronchioles and alveoli with numerous eosinophilic granulocytes.

Severe pneumonitis with damage to the blood vessels occurs with Rocky Mountain spotted fever and with scrub typhus (Fig. 6-5). In these two diseases, the rickettsia parasitize the endothelial cells, causing thrombosis or rupture with extravasation of red blood cells in the small vessels and capillaries of the lung. There is little or no alveolar exudate. The dilatation and damage to the vascular bed of the lungs is responsible for the term hemorrhagic pneumonitis. The cough is nonproductive and hemoptysis is rare. A superimposed bacterial bronchopneumonia may be present in fatal cases.

The patient's serum in Rocky Mountain spotted fever and in scrub typhus carries agglutinin against proteus-X strains of bacteria, which is known as the Weil-Felix reaction. This diagnostic test is usually positive after the second week. The American wood tick is responsible for Rocky Mountain spotted fever and infected ticks are now widespread throughout most of the United States. The itch mite responsible for the transmission of scrub typhus is a trombiculid mite in which the larva or chigger parasitizes vertebrate hosts is endemic in Japan and in parts of Southeast Asia.

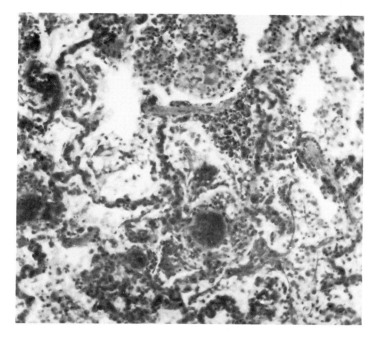

Fig. 6-5. Scrub typhus with hemorrhagic pneumonitis. (×150)

Rickettsia burneti, the agent responsible for Q fever, is transmitted to livestock by ticks but man is an incidental host and is not infected by the tick but by inhalation of infected dust or drinking raw milk from animals that bear the rickettsial organism.

Rickettsial fevers are treated by chloromycetin or tetracycline derivatives.

7

Infections of the Lower Respiratory Tract

The mortality of pulmonary infections has been markedly reduced by antibiotic therapy for pneumonia and isoniazid for tuberculosis. However, bacterial pneumonitis still complicates many systemic and pulmonary diseases and viral pneumonitis is still a leading form of illness in the United States. The report of the Committee of Diagnostic Standards in Respiratory Disease of the American Thoracic Society lists 33 bacteria, 14 viruses, 19 fungi and 19 parasites causing infectious reactions in the lower respiratory tract.[24]

Specific antibiotic therapy requires the identification of the causative organism. Nevertheless, the type of involvement depicted in the roentgenogram and the pathologic findings are still used to define different types of pneumonitis. *Lobar pneumonia* refers to diffuse consolidation of one or several lobes by infection (usually the pneumococcus or rarely, *Klebsiella pneumoniae*). *Lobular or bronchopneumonia* refers to patchy consolidation and may be of bacterial or mycotic origin. *Staphylococcus aureus* or hemolytic streptococci are common causes. *Interstitial pneumonitis* is caused by perivascular exudate of moderate degree, usually of viral or undetermined origin but also produced by rickettsial disease (Table 7-1 and Fig. 7-1). *Necrotizing or cavitary pneumonitis* refers to patchy destruction of the pulmonary parenchyma and is characteristic of tuberculosis and of fungus infections other than histoplasmosis. It also occurs in plague. The necrotizing forms of pneumonitis, if not rapidly progressive, are preceded by a granulomatous inflammation or tubercle formation (Fig. 7-2). *Organizing pneumonia* is a form of permanent scarring that may follow any type of pneumonitis, but is rare in viral or influenzal infections. *Lung abscess* is also a complication of pneumonitis, but may be secondary to a pulmonary infarct or penetrating wounds of the chest wall or a foreign body in the bronchus (Fig. 7-3).

TABLE 7-1. Forms of Pneumonitis

ANATOMIC TYPE	ETIOLOGIC AGENTS	PATHOLOGY
Lobar	Pneumococcus 99% *Klebsiella pneumoniae* 1%	Pyogenic and fibrinous exudate in alveoli
Patchy, Lobular or Bronchopneumonia	Hemolytic streptococcus Group A *Staphylococcus aureus*	Pyogenic and fibrinous exudate chiefly in bronchioles
Interstitial or Infiltrative	Influenza virus A, B, C *Mycoplasma pneumoniae*	Monocytic interstitial infiltrate with edema
Necrotizing or Cavitary	*Mycobacterium tuberculosis* *Francisella tularensis* *Pasteurella pestis* Systemic mycoses (coccidioidomycosis, torulosis, histoplasmosis, etc.)	Granulomatous exu- date or hemorrhagic or caseous necrosis

PNEUMOCOCCIC LOBAR PNEUMONIA

Lobar pneumonia is an infection of the lower respiratory tract spreading diffusely through one or more lobes, characterized by an acute onset with high fever, chest pains, varying degrees of cough, dyspnea, cyanosis, a frothy bloody sputum and frequently, abdominal distention and herpes

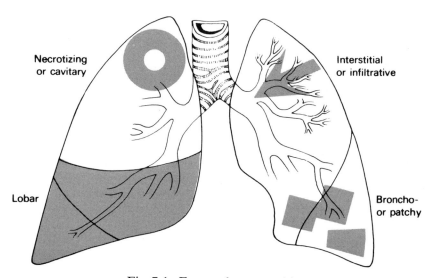

Fig. 7-1. Forms of pneumonitis.

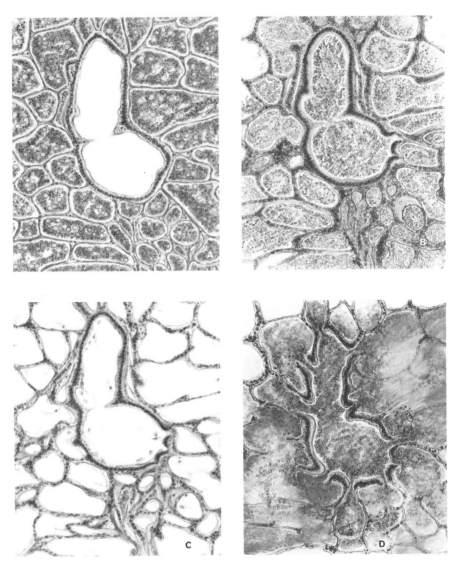

Fig. 7-2. Micropathology of various forms of pneumonitis. (*A*) Lobar pneumonia. (*B*) Lobular or bronchopneumonia. (*C*) Interstitial (viral) pneumonia. (*D*) Necrotizing pneumonia. (Drawn ×100)

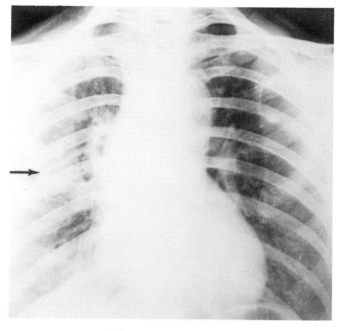

Fig. 7-3. Lung abscesses.

about the mouth. There is also a marked leukocytosis. Rales and friction rubs may be heard over the involved tissue because of the exudate and fibrin extending into the alveoli and deposited on the pleural surfaces. In over 90 percent of the cases, one of the 32 types of pathogenic pneumococci is responsible for the disease. The fulminant onset of pneumonia in adults is thought to result through a hypersensitivity reaction to prior exposure to the pneumococcus. A viral respiratory infection immediately preceding the attack is often a precipitating cause, since strains of the pneumococci can be cultured from the nasopharynx of 50 percent of the normal population during the spring and winter months when the disease is prevalent. Recent studies suggest that an enzyme (neuraminidase) elaborated by the pneumococcus may account for the shocklike state in fatal cases since no bacterial toxin has been demonstrated. Fatalities from the disease are lowest in children, increasing progressively after the age of 40 years. Recovery from the infection confers no lasting immunity, since humoral antibodies disappear rapidly during convalescence. In fact, there seems to be an increased susceptibility to subsequent attacks because of a persistent hypersensitivity response to the organism. The antigens of the bacillus, in addition to a hemolysin and a purpuric factor, include a specific "aggressin" derived from the so-called 'C' factor in the capsule, which facilitates invasiveness. It is to this antigen that immunizing antibody is formed in man and in experimental animals and from which an antisera was formerly devised for use in treatment before the advent of penicillin.

Roentgenograms made several hours after the onset of acute symptoms show a hazy zone of consolidation affecting an entire lobe or pulmonary segment. The zone of density is homogenous, the hilar lymph nodes are more prominent and the shadows of the pulmonary arteries are distended and straightened by hyperemia accompanying the inflammatory state (Fig. 7-4).

The pathologic changes through which the infection evolves have been well documented because of the former frequency and high rate of fatality of the disease. Four successive stages are recognized: (1) In the first 4 to 12 hours, in a wet stage, known as *engorgement,* fluid pours into the alveoli from the dilated leaking vascular bed. (2) In the next 48 hours, a fibropurulent stage (*red hepatization*) occurs in which red blood cells, polymorphonuclear leukocytes and fibrin fill the alveoli that harbor the proliferating pneumococci. (3) From the third to the eighth day, a further purulent stage is reached (*gray hepatization*), in which the leukocytes and fibrin consolidate the involved tissue. (4) On the seventh to the eleventh day, the final or *resorptive* stage is reached in which the exudate is lysed and resorbed by macrophages—a process of resolution through which the normal structure of the tissue is restored. During this stage, the patient often passes through a crisis in which both the fever and blood pressure fall, and a shocklike state may occur. Immunity occurring in this stage is in part serologic and in part cytologic due to action of the macrophages. Gradual subsidence of fever with resolution is known as lysis. If sufficient necrosis has occurred in the infected tissue, organization by an ingrowth of new blood vessels and by fibroblasts may produce permanent scarring or pulmonary fibrosis. In patients with delayed immunity and spreading infection, there is a spread of pneumococcic infection, which may give rise to the complications of empyema, lung abscess, pericarditis, endocarditis, septic arthritis, osteomyelitis, otitis media and meningitis or brain abscess.

Large numbers of pneumococci are present in the sputum, usually coughed up throughout the course of the patient's pneumonia. These can be readily identified by the Neufeld "quellung" response in which the capsule of the organism swells in the presence of homologous antisera mixed with the sputum rendering them readily visible microscopically.

Penicillin remains the drug of choice, since the pneumococcus rarely develops a resistance to this antibiotic. If in doubt, broad spectrum tetracycline drugs should be used and the sputum cultured for staphylococci, which may be penicillin-resistant.

In most cases of lobar pneumonia caused by the pneumococcus, the

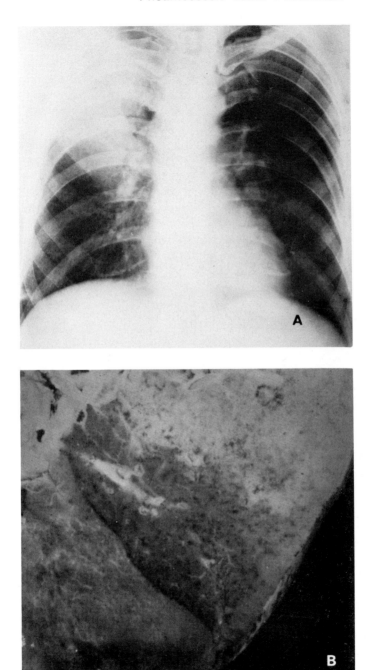

Fig. 7-4. Lobar pneumonia. (*A*) Roentgenogram. (*B*) Gross specimen.

lungs are restored to normal following resolution whether the infection subsides by crisis or lysis or is aborted by antibiotic treatment. Although the temperature subsides within hours with effective antibiotic therapy, resolution and the return of the lungs to normal requires several days. In severe cases in which the pneumococcus can be cultured from the bloodstream, the danger of complications is increased and prognosis must be more guarded.

Vital capacity and functional residual capacity are limited in both lobar and bronchial pneumonia and the rigidity of the lung (loss of compliance) is much increased, which explains the rapid shallow respirations that are present in the disease. However, neither the sudden reduction in lung compliance nor the mechanism of adjusting the respiratory depth and rate to lung rigidity has been explained. Oxygen uptake is reduced by the pneumonitis. In cases of lobar pneumonia, right heart catheterization has revealed no significant change in pulmonary arterial pressure.[3]

STAPHYLOCOCCIC PNEUMONIA

Staphylococcic pneumonia is often a complication of measles or whooping cough in children and may appear in infants under one year of age. It is also frequent in children with cystic fibrosis. Staphylococcic pneumonia in adults may be preceded by viral influenza and is one of the major causes of fatality in influenza epidemics. A patchy bronchopneumonia is the rule, producing secondary cavitary abscesses which may result in pneumothorax or empyema (Fig. 7-5). The onset is usually acute with high fever, a pink purulent sputum and varying degrees of cyanosis. Many strains of *Staphylococcus aureus* producing pneumonic involvement elaborate penicillinase, an enzyme rendering them resistant to the effect of penicillin.

Although when penicillin was first introduced nearly 90 percent of *S. aureus* were sensitive to this antibiotic, now more than 80 percent of the strains responsible for serious hospital-acquired staphylococcal disease are penicillin-resistant and it is estimated that 20 to 40 percent of the general population is similarly resistant.[67]

In hospital practice, the danger of spread in medical and surgical wards and in the newborn nursery may stem from direct contact with infected individuals, airborne dissemination or contact with clothing. The most susceptible individuals are those who have undergone major operative procedures, those with previous corticosteroid therapy with suppressed adrenals, those with diabetes or those with blood dyscrasias producing suppression of red or white blood cells or those with agammaglobulinemia.

The *Staphylococcus aureus* is a typical pyogenic or pus-producing

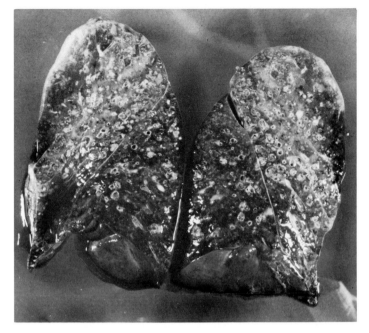

Fig. 7-5. Staphylococcic pneumonia, gross specimen.

organism and has, in addition, a coagulative factor which precipitates fibrin and a necrotizing toxin (necrosin). The actions of these two toxins tend to produce localized abscess formation in the involved pulmonary tissue with a central necrotic core and an outer rim of organizing tissues. In children, a spherical air-containing cyst (pneumatocele) may be found in the roentgenogram. In these young individuals as noted, the disease may complicate measles, whooping cough or cystic fibrosis. Rupture into the bronchi or pleura are frequent modes of extension and are responsible for a high percentage of fatalities.

Treatment is with the new semisynthetic penicillin derivatives, which are resistant to the bacterial enzyme, penicillinase. Some of the strains of staphylococci are resistant to methicillin by a mechanism other than penicillinase production and a combination of antibiotics may be required.

NECROTIZING BACTERIAL PNEUMONIAS

Tuberculosis, plague and tularemia may produce a necrotizing pneumonia that at times is rapidly progressive and fatal. In pulmonary tuberculosis, the initial lesion is usually a monocytic exudate evolving to tubercle formation, which is partially a healing response and partially a reaction to destroyed lung tissue.[65] However, in the chronic progressive form of the disease the lesion progresses to liquefaction necrosis and, at times, to secondary suppuration.[19] Before the use of streptomycin, pneumonic plague was frequently fatal in its initial stage of serosanguinous exudation flooding the alveolar spaces. In tularemia, pleuropulmonic involvement with pleural effusion occurs only in about 50 percent of the cases.[29]

Plague, also known as the pest or black death, is an acute febrile disease in which there is lymphadenopathy with bacteremia or septicemia and diffuse hemorrhages into the skin and mucosal surfaces. The disease is caused by the gram-negative bacillus *Pasteurella pestis*. A fatal form of pneumonia occurs during epidemics.

The rat is the host or reservoir for *P. pestis*. The rat flea becomes infected by taking blood from the plague-infected rat. These bacilli multiply in the midgut of the flea and massive infection blocks the esophagus and pharynx. When the flea takes its next blood meal, bacilli are regurgitated into the skin or capillaries of the new mammalian host via the insect's proboscis.

The plague bacillus secretes a gelatinous envelope which is heat labile and from which a highly toxic protein fraction can be isolated. The somatic antigen of the cell body is heat stable and water insoluble.

Where the infection produces septicemia, a fatal secondary pneumonia may occur. This pneumonic infection then may be transmitted from person to person by droplet infection. The incubation period is short, usually less than three days. The course is fulminant and death may occur within hours after the first symptoms of chills, high fever and marked leukocytosis. A positive blood culture may be obtained in these patients and bacilli may be recovered from the sputum.

The findings in the lungs at autopsy are characterized by necrosis of blood vessels and a serosanguinous exudate (Fig. 7-6). The necrotic zones of pulmonary involvement are surrounded by this exudate and infiltrated by granulocytes. Later, monocytes replace the polymorphonuclear leukocytes. Experimental studies [39] of pneumonic plague in monkeys indicate that edema or serous exudate in response to the toxic action of the bacillus occurs within 70 hours after infection. Inflammatory exudation and necrotic lesions are later manifestations.

The mortality of pneumonic plague, formerly irremedial, has been reduced to about 10 percent by streptomycin therapy. Within 10 to 12 hours after beginning treatment, the bacilli disappear from the sputum and the risk of spreading the disease to the attending staff or other individuals is much reduced. If resistance develops to streptomycin after 48 hours after attendant relapse, chloramphenicol is substituted. In spite of the effectiveness of antibiotic therapy, death may occur from toxemia. Im-

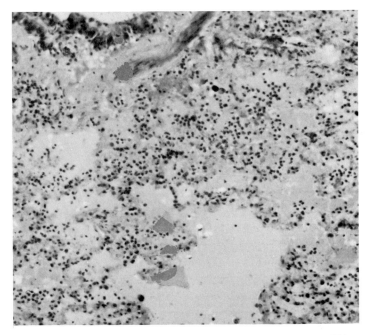

Fig. 7-6. Photomicrograph of pneumonic plague. (×150)

munity is not absolute in patients who recover. When professional personnel or the military are exposed to infection in regions in which the disease is endemic, sulfonamide is taken routinely as a preventive measure.

Tularemia. Tularemic infection is usually acquired from handling or eating infected rabbits or from the bite of blood-sucking flies or ticks, which transmit the causative organism, *Pasteurella* (or *Fransicella*) *tularense*. The incubation period is several days to one week, and, in fulminant cases characterized by involvement of the reticuloendothelial system and ulcerating lymphadenitis, death may occur within 4 to 12 days. In some cases, a diffuse primary pneumonitis with pleural effusion occurs in the absence of a generalized lymphadenitis, apparently from organisms gaining entrance via the respiratory tract. In the cases with generalized lymphadenitis, pneumonic involvement has been estimated [13] as 20 percent. The initial symptoms are a febrile influenzalike attack with high temperature and leukocytosis. The organisms can be isolated from the sputum, the pharynx or gastric washings and identified by fluorescent antibody staining technique. Agglutinins also appear in the patient's serum, but not until after the sixth day of the illness (Fig. 7-7).

Tularemic pneumonia is often accompanied by pleural effusion and, at times, by hydropneumothorax because of the rapidly progressing necrotic

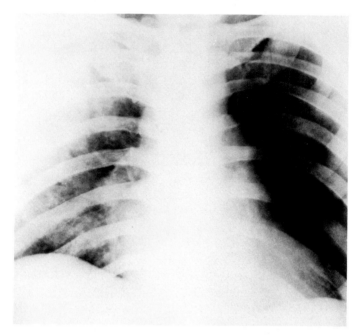

Fig. 7-7. Bronchopneumonia in a case of tularemia.

lesions. The tissue necrosis and the adjacent histiocytic infiltrate usually affects both lungs at their bases, accompanied by hilar lymphadenopathy. These are visualized in the roentgenogram as zones of increased density which have infiltrating borders and tend to become confluent; the intervening nonconsolidated tissue has a hazy appearance. The upper portions of the lung may escape involvement.

Streptomycin is the antibiotic of choice, but other broad spectrum antibiotics such as tetracycline or chloramphenicol also are effective. Vaccination against the disease with killed organisms is relatively ineffective, although the disease itself produces lasting immunity. The use of an avirulent vaccine is used to control tularemia in the Soviet Union, but has not been widely used in America.[94]

Pulmonary Brucellosis. This is a generalized systemic infection in which domestic animals (cattle, hogs and goats) act as a reservoir for the human disease. The brucella organism primarily affects the reticuloendothelial system and produces a subacute or chronic fever with characteristic undulations extending over months or years. Regional lymphadenopathy, splenomegaly and attacks of abdominal pain (because of mesenteric adenitis) are usually present. Other features of the disease may be pulmonary involvement, hepatomegaly and arthralgia.

The bronchopulmonary symptoms of brucellosis (unless the disease has been previously diagnosed) simulate viral pneumonitis except for the more frequent occurrence of serofibrinous pleurisy and hilar lymphadenopathy (Fig. 7-8). Rarely, there may be a miliary type of bronchopneumonia. The disease is most commonly seen in patients from rural or farming districts, and a history of drinking unpasteurized milk may be obtained. Agglutinating antibodies may be present in the patient's serum, but isolation of the cultures from blood or marrow puncture is more reliable. Tetracycline or streptomycin is an effective form of antibiotic therapy.

Secondary and Terminal Bronchopneumonias. Bacterial bronchopneumonia often occurs secondarily to other diseases of the lungs, particularly to forms of viral pneumonitis (such as Influenza A and B), to bronchitis, bronchiectasis, bronchogenic carcinoma and severe chest wall injuries. In debilitated individuals, it often occurs as a terminal event and it is also a postoperative hazard in the elderly. The common offending organisms are hemolytic streptococci, *Staphylococcus aureus, and Hemophilus influenzae.* More rarely, the pneumococcus or the *Klebsiella pneumoniae* (Friedländer's bacillus) appears as a secondary invader. *Hemophilus influenzae* pneumonia tends to produce a purulent bronchiolitis and to remain confined to the bronchial tree. It is particularly common in children. *Staphylococcus aureus* is prone to produce abscess formation and may be complicated by

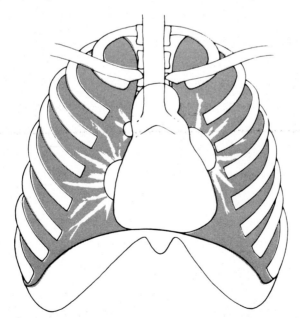

Fig. 7-8. Brucellosis bronchopneumonia. (Schinz, H. R. *et al.:* Roentgen-Diagnostics. vol. 3. Grune and Stratton, New York)

pneumothorax, as previously noted. Streptococcal pneumonia is often associated with empyema. Pneumonia produced by Klebsiella produces a thick, tenacious mucoid exudate. This organism may also cause a chronic pneumonitis with abscess formation accompanied by fibrotic healing. At times, mixed infections may occur with two of these organisms cultured from the diseased lungs in fatal cases.

The infections are treated with the broad spectrum antibiotics such as the tetracycline derivatives. In chronic Friedländer's bacillus infections, which at times follow lobar pneumonia, sulfadiazine and streptomycin have proved effective.

Aspiration Pneumonia. Aspiration pneumonia is caused by the inhalation of gastric contents or infected material from the pharynx. It is commonly associated with repeated vomiting, particularly in patients with an absent or weakened cough reflex during unconsciousness such as occurs with acute alcoholism, barbiturate poisoning, drug addiction or general anesthesia. The aspiration of noninfected gastric acid juice produces edema and hemorrhage within the alveoli followed by polymorphonuclear leukocytic exudate with transient consolidation which usually resolves. However, the gastric contents contain putrefactive organisms such as *Borrelia vincenti* and pneumonia or abscess may result. The necrotic foci of pneumonitis at their periphery may contain anaerobic streptococci. Obstruction of the smaller bronchi and bronchioles is believed to be essential to the infectious process.

The sequence of pneumonic changes in fatal cases of narcotic poisoning have been detailed by Siegel.[85A] (Siegel, H.: Human Pathology, 3:55, 1972).[85A] In cases of fatal narcosis, dying within 3 to 12 hours after overdosage, the lungs are voluminous and heavy with the dependent portions edematous and hemorrhagic, the anterior portions emphysematous. Erythrocytes and edema fluid distend many alveoli with mononuclear cells scattered through the alveolar walls. Foci of partial atelectasis alternate with acute zones of emphysema, caused by entrapped air.

If death occurs 12 to 24 hours after overdosage, zones of lobular pneumonia (some confluent) extend in patchy fashion adjacent to the zone of plugged bronchioles containing inspissated gastric debris. The alveolar exudate is predominated by polymorphs. With death occurring after 24 to 48 hours, the picture is that of confluent lobular pneumonia and rarely, small abscesses appear at the site of aspirated material. While this form of aspiration pneumonia has recently been referred to as "narcotic lungs," the picture is identical in cases of alcohol and barbiturate overdosage.

Influenza A and B. Influenza is an acute interstitial pneumonitis caused by types A or B influenza virus or variants (a type C virus is rare). Pandemic spreads of influenza viral infections are probably caused by a virulent variant. The incubation period is one or two days, and in recovered cases the specific antibody appears in the blood with maximal titers in the second or third week and disappearance in 6 to 12 months.

Clinical features include headache, nasopharyngitis, fever and chest pains with fine rales at the lung bases. Nasal congestion, sore throat, persistent headaches, fever, a dry cough, muscular aches and weakness indicate respiratory infection without defining its nature, which is presumed from the prevalence of similar cases in epidemics. Serologic diagnosis may be confirmed in convalescent cases by the capacity of the patient's serum to inhibit the ability of the cultured influenza virus to agglutinate red blood cells (hemagglutination inhibition test).

The influenza virus parasitizes and kills respiratory ciliated epithelium, producing patchy ulcerations which heal in four to five days by squamous cell metaplasia. These cells are derived from the basal cell layer of the lining. Within the alveolar septa of the pulmonary parenchyma, infection causes vascular dilatation, a monocytic exudate and a leakage of red blood cells and fibrin. A hyaline membrane may adhere to the wall of the alveolar ducts (Fig. 7-9). Winternitz, on the basis of his studies in the pandemic of Influenza in World War I, classified [103] the disease as an acute tracheobronchitis associated with secondary involvement of the pulmonary paren-

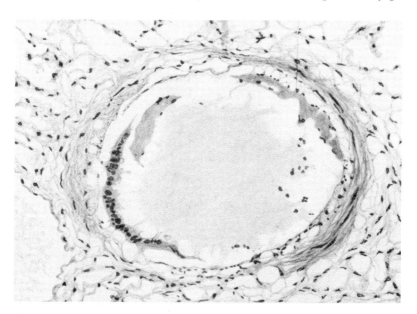

Fig .7-9. Early lesion of the bronchiole in influenzal pneumonia. (Winternitz, M. C. *et al.:* The Pathology of Influenza, Yale Univ. Press, New Haven)

chyma. Roentgenograms of the lungs rarely show consolidation unless there is secondary bacterial infection. This occurs usually in elderly individuals or those who have been chronically ill. More rarely, a fatal patchy or diffuse pneumonitis may be attributed to the virus.[60a]

The pathologic pulmonary changes found in fatal cases of influenza are usually complicated by secondary bacterial infection or by a pre-existing cardiac decompensation such as occurs with mitral stenosis or by an advanced stage of pregnancy, which also may be responsible for pulmonary congestion. The vascular leakage, producing pulmonary edema may be the result of multiple factors and may not be attributable to viral injury entirely. Interstitial myocarditis of a focal nature is described in a number of fatal cases and a form of fatal myocarditis (Fiedler's myocarditis) is sometimes referred to as postinfluenzal myocarditis. The relationship to the influenza virus A or B is not established and only rarely has the virus been recovered from pericardial fluid.

There is no specific therapy for influenza and treatment in uncomplicated cases is palliative and symptomatic. The degree of immunity produced by prior attacks or by vaccination with the virus is variable. The majority of young individuals may suffer reinfection within a period of four months. After a widespread outbreak of influenza, a low incidence of infection to the same virus in the affected community may be observed for several years. The majority of cases in America are caused by influenza types A and B; an additional type C apparently produces only mild upper respiratory disease. To date, there is no evidence of cross immunization between influenza A and B.

The experience of the USPHS and the Armed Forces Epidemiological Board with formalin-inactivated virus A and B grown in chick embryos and obtained from allantoic fluid has been extensive over the past decade. Many thousands of persons have been inoculated with both aqueous and mineral oil suspensions, the aqueous solution being administered subcutaneously and the mineral oil suspension intramuscularly. Both local and systemic reactions follow the injection and hypersensitivity responses to the fowl protein may occur. These authorities consider protection to be adequate in 75 percent of those vaccinated but there is no protection given to a variety of other upper respiratory diseases. Another disadvantage is the appearance of epidemics in response to strains different from A and B. To date, six types have been isolated in epidemics in the USA since 1930 (types: Swine-A, A, A', Asian, B, and C). An additional handicap in the use of these vaccines has been lack of standardization in their biological strength.

Atypical Primary Pneumonia. This is an infectious respiratory disease, usually mild and self-limited, with clinical features resembling the interstitial pneumonitis caused by influenza A or B virus. The causative organism is usually *Mycoplasma pneumoniae,* which was isolated from one of the rarely fatal cases by Eaton *et al.*[32] and originally designated as the Eaton agent. The serum of infected patients contains a factor which will agglutinate group O human erythrocytes in the cold, usually not manifested in high titers until the third week after onset of the infection. The infectious agent, now known as a form of mycoplasma, resembles the pleuropneumonialike organisms (PPLO)* in its variable configuration (at times referred to as the coccobacillus), its lack of a rigid cell wall and its capacity to grow in a cell-free environment. The organism is difficult to cultivate and grows in small colonies in the presence of ascitic fluid or other forms of enriched media. Diagnosis can now be confirmed by growth of the organism transferred by means of pharyngeal swab or from sputum to appropriate artificial media or cultivated in chick embryos. The organism persists in many patients in spite of the development of high levels of antibody following convalescence.

The clinical features resemble influenza infection, with throat irritation, cough, headache, malaise, anorexia and fever. Headache and cough are prominent. The incubation period is more prolonged than influenza and is usually one to three weeks. Unlike influenza, roentgenograms of the chest reveal infiltration spreading out from the hilum with decreased density toward the periphery, the shadows extending in irregular fashion (Fig. 7-10A). The infiltration in the roentgenogram precedes the onset of severe symptoms and is more than would be expected from the fine or sticky rales and lack of evidence of consolidation. The roentgenographic signs may be transitory or may persist after the disappearance of fever and undergo slow resolution during the next several weeks. The pathologic changes are not certain because of the rarity of fatal cases. In those reported, the lungs are congested and partially hemorrhagic, with small focal lesions resembling miliary granulomata with varying zones of consolidation and, at times, atelectasis or emphysema in isolated portions of the parenchyma. The bronchitis and broncheolitis may be severe with a characteristic tenacious exudate. This tenacious exudate is one of the reasons for the persistent cough. The bronchial mucosa is inflamed and ulcerated in small

---

* Three groups of PPLO organisms are currently recognized: (1) L-forms of known bacteria which lose their cell wall under adverse conditions such as exposure to penicillin, but may revert to ordinary form with continued subculture. (2) Permanent pleuropneumonia organisms without cell walls, producing a variety of pleuropneumonia infections in domestic animals and recoverable from nonvenereal inflammation of the genitourinary tract in man. (3) The *Mycoplasma pneumoniae,* resembling the other forms but differing from them in its nutritional requirements and in the character of cold hemagglutinins associated with the immune bodies which it provokes in patients with atypical pneumonia.

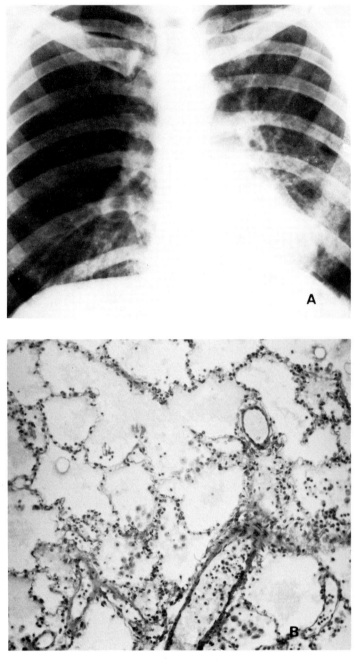

Fig. 7-10. Primary atypical pneumonia. (*A*) Roentgenogram. (*B*) Photomicrograph of lung tissue. (×150)

foci. Microscopically, there is a characteristic interstitial pneumonitis with a mononuclear cell infiltrate (Fig. 7-10B). However, there is, in addition, a broncheolitis in which the lumina of the bronchioles contain inspissated material and numerous polymorphonuclear leukocytes and fibrin. Some observers believe that acute myocarditis and hemorrhagic encephalitis may occur in fatal cases. There is always a lymphadenitis and the spleen may show acute follicular hyperplasia.

Fortunately, the disease responds to tetracycline antibiotics, which is the treatment of choice in interstitial pneumonitis in the absence of specific identification of an influenza virus.

Mononucleosis or Glandular Fever. This is a febrile disease running an acute or chronic course, beginning with sore throat and cervical lymphadenopathy, and is thought to be caused by a type of herpesvirus (the Ebert-Barr virus). The reticuloendothelial system and often the liver are primarily affected. Varying degrees of bronchitis and pneumonitis may be present. Diagnosis is confirmed by a monocytic leukocytosis of 30,000 to 40,000, with atypical Downey cells (monocytes with vacuolated cytoplasm) and a positive heterophil antigen test in which the patient's serum agglutinates sheep erythrocytes. This disease is usually not included among the various forms of pneumonitis; however, it may produce roentgenographic changes and a clinical picture resembling primary atypical pneumonia but without elevation of the cold agglutinin titer.

Psittacosis. This is a pulmonary infection caused by an obligate intracellular parasite that passes through a coarse bacterial filter (Chamberland L-1). Because of its inability to propagate on nonliving media and because of its filterability, the coccal bodies, when stained with Giemsa, have been classed as large viruses although they resemble rickettsiae in size and staining reactions and are now considered to be a mutational form of bacteria (under the term Bedsoniae). The organisms are grown on embryonated eggs or tissue cultures and are susceptible to the broad spectrum antibiotics of which chlortetracycline is favored.

Psittacosis is an endemic disease of South American parrotts and parakeets, and in the United States turkeys are a reservoir of infection. The disease is usually transmitted to man from an avian host, the symptoms begin with fever, backache, prostration and cough after a variable incubation period of one to several weeks. The leukocyte count remains normal or subnormal and rales are audible in the lungs without evidence of consolidation. However, roentgenograms show a patchy bronchopneumonia with scattered zones of consolidation that tend to resolve slowly after the temperature subsides (by lysis), about the seventh or eighth day. Children have a better prognosis than adults. In adults, the mortality may reach as high as 20 percent, although prompt treatment with chlortetracycline aborts the illness.

In undiagnosed and untreated cases, the pneumonitis is accompanied by nausea, vomiting, diarrhea or constipation. Hepatosplenomegaly has been reported and at times, both jaundice and oliguria. In severe cases, there is disorientation or delirium. Death may result from respiratory failure or generalized toxemia. In the absence of serologic studies, the diagnosis is presumptive and based upon contact with birds (wild or domestc, living or dead) and the presence of bronchopneumonia without leukocytosis.

The presence of psitticosis is confirmed if the patient's serum (during convalescence) fixes complement and agglutinates the organism. Where several infective patients have been in contact with diseased or dead birds, the organism may be identified by cultivating on embryonated eggs.

Interstitial Pneumonitis With Upper Respiratory Viral Infections. Interstitial pneumonitis may accompany upper respiratory infections caused by the adenoviruses and echoviruses. The presence of pneumonitis is inferred in seasonal epidemics in patients with sore throat, fever, cough and at times cervical lymphadenitis. The extent of the bronchitis and pneumonitis with these "cold viruses" is difficult to ascertain but is assumed if the nasopharyngitis is relatively mild and the presence of postnasal drip is insufficient to account for the prolonged cough and fine rales which may continue for one to several weeks after subsidence of the nasopharyngitis. The roentgenogram is usually negative (positive in less than 10% of the cases). In most of these infections, absence of fever after the first few days of symptoms suggests that the viral infection is limited to a tracheobronchitis. (See chap. 3)

Interstitial Hemorrhagic Pneumonitis with Rickettsial Disease. Severe and at times fatal hemorrhagic interstitial pneumonitis occurs with scrub typhus and Rocky Mountain spotted fever. A less severe and less common form of pneumonitis is associated with rickettsial infection with the organism of Old World typhus. A diagnostic feature of rickettsial disease is the presence in the patient's serum of antibodies which agglutinate strains of proteus organisms such as OX19.

Pneumonitis, which is rarely fatal, is present in the Australian disease known as Q fever, caused by *Rickettsia burneti*. Ocular disease and thrombophlebitis may be complications. In America, it is a rare disease found among those who handle livestock.

Fibrosing Interstitial Pneumonitis. The concept of interstitial pneumonitis has been still further widened in recent years by including in this category fatal forms of interstitial pulmonary fibrosis, which produces progressive respiratory deficiency with increasing degrees of dyspnea and cyanosis. These cases have also been characterized as the Hamman-Rich

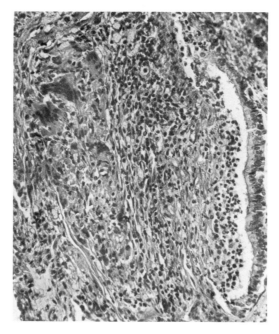

Fig. 7-11. Giant cell pneumonia. Photomicrograph ×200.

syndrome. Bilateral changes are found in the roentgenogram and characteristic features are present pathologically at biopsy or autopsy. These cases are of unknown etiology and are discussed subsequently under hypersensitivity diseases (Chap. 10).

Measles, Pneumonia and Giant Cell Pneumonitis. Infants and children dying of measles may have a characteristic bronchopneumonia in which the bronchial and bronchiolar epithelium show either proliferative or degenerative changes and in which granulation tissue with giant cells surrounds the bronchioles or invades them to produce partial occlusion. Not all forms of giant cell pneumonia have been traced to the measles virus but intracytoplasmic inclusion bodies have been found in giant cells found within the alveoli or within the bronchiolar lumen (Fig. 7-11). One of the unusual features of this type of viral or giant cell pneumonitis is the tendency for vascular occlusion and for pericapillary organization. The bronchiolar involvement, the hyperplasia of the bronchial epithelium, the presence of giant cells and the tendency to organization are characteristic. These cases are best referred to as giant cell viral bronchopneumonia, since the presence of the measles virus is not demonstrable in most cases.

Neonatal Pneumonitis. Pneumonitis occurring within the first 48 hours after birth is usually the result of inhaled amniotic fluid in which the fatty

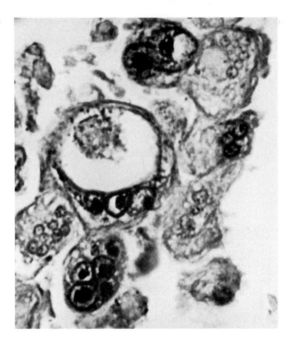

Fig. 7-12. Photomicrograph of pulmonary involvement in cytomegalic inclusion disease. (×300)

acids of the meconium are considered the irritant factor. Pneumonia starting within hours after birth may also result from pus inhaled from an infected birth canal. There is also a possibility of transplacental infection from the mother. The last-named cause has been confirmed by pneumonia occurring in an ectopic pregnancy in a small fetus. When pneumonia occurs after the first two days of life, it is apt to be an antibiotic-resistant staphylococcic infection acquired in the hospital, similar to that involving adults.

Cytomegalic Inclusion Disease. When this viral disease is acquired from the mother during the gestational period, the infant is severely damaged, suffering chorioretinitis, optic atrophy, mental retardation, microcephaly and cerebral calcifications. Postnatally, infants may suffer interstitial pneumonitis; a similar disease is found in debilitated patients dying of lymphoma or carcinoma. The infection produces inclusion bodies of large size within the nuclei or cytoplasm of infected cells which are desquamated into the alveoli. The appearance is distinctive (Fig. 7-12).

8

Pulmonary Tuberculosis

Tuberculosis is a disease with a worldwide distribution affecting all known populations regardless of race, sex or age. It may exist in latent, acute or chronic form and, although any organ of the body may be affected, its major portal of entry is in the lower respiratory tract and subsequent systemic spread is usually secondary to primary pulmonary involvement. The disease is caused by *Mycobacterium tuberculosis* or by a bovine strain, *M. bovis.* Other strains such as *M. avium, M. fortuitum* and *M. ulcerans,* rarely cause human infection other than ulcerating lesions of the skin. The spread of pulmonary tuberculosis is from man to man by droplet infection from coughed or expectorated secretions from a softened necrotic focus finding exit through an open bronchus from a patient with active disease.

Improved hygiene, periodic chest roentgenograms, vaccination with non-virulent strais of tubercle bacillus (BCG vaccine) and modern chemotherapy have greatly diminished the morbidity and mortality rates of pulmonary tuberculosis in Europe and North America in the past decade. In the United States, the death rate has fallen from 200/100,000 in 1900 to 4/100,000 in 1965. During 1967, 45,647 new cases were reported in the United States giving a total active number of 316,000.[61] Most of the new cases are in individuals 45 years of age and over, but nearly 20 percent are in children and young adults. In this country, the proportion of nonwhites with the disease has risen from 26 percent in 1953 to 37 percent in 1967 (Fig. 8-1).

Pulmonary tuberculosis is divided into two mayor types: (1) Primary infection of individuals in the nonimmune state; and, (2) reinfection or post-primary tuberculosis in individuals in the partially immune state.

Primary tuberculosis infection in children and young adults in most cases is followed by rapid healing either with complete resolution or with a residual "primary complex." This complex includes a small healed nodule

135

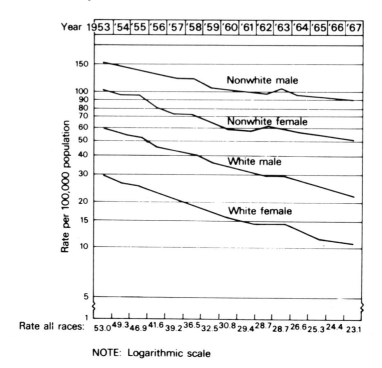

Year 1953 '54 '55 '56 '57 '58 '59 '60 '61 '62 '63 '64 '65 '66 '67

Rate all races: 53.0 49.3 46.9 41.6 39.2 36.5 32.5 30.8 29.4 28.7 28.7 26.6 25.3 24.4 23.1

NOTE: Logarithmic scale

Fig. 8-1. Declining rate of pulmonary tuberculosis in the United States from 1953 to 1967. (Lowell, A. M. *et al.:* Tuberculosis. Harvard Univ. Press, Cambridge)

(Ghon tubercle) within a lower lobe of the lung (at times calcified) and an enlarged healed hilar lymph node. Such individuals are usually tuberculin positive to 5 T.U. (0.1 mcg. P.P.D. tuberculin) injected intradermally. The positive reaction consists of a 5 mm. indurated zone at the injection site. A similar response occurs in individuals previously vaccinated with BCG vaccine (a strain of tubercle bacillus of low virulence). In a minority of individuals, primary pulmonary infection progresses with a rapidly spreading pneumonia or with diffuse miliary involvement of both lungs.

Reinfection tuberculosis, occurring in partially immune individuals with a *healed primary complex,* is the most common active form of the disease (Fig. 8-2). The lesion occurs in the apical or subapical position of one lung and, in most individuals, results from the breakdown and liquefaction of a previously healed focus in a lymph node, which discharges into a bronchus. More rarely, a similar reactivated focus gives rise to hematogenous spread and more rarely still, postprimary tuberculosis occurs from re-exposure to a patient with active disease. This is exogenous reinfection as opposed to the two endogenous forms.

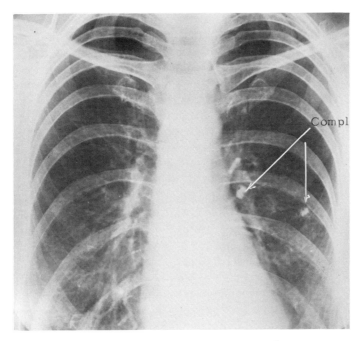

Fig. 8-2. Tuberculosis, primary complex.

The type of tubercle bacillus to which an individual is exposed is a major factor in the pathogenesis of the disease. Strains of tubercle bacilli have been classified into virulent forms, nonvirulent forms and forms with low virulence. *Virulent* strains of human and bovine tubercle bacilli (on culture media) form serpentine cords of varying thickness composed of strongly acid-fast bacilli wtih their long axis parallel to the cords. This characteristic of virulent strains is associated with a lipopolysaccharide antigen or toxic glycolipid, known as the "cord factor." *Avirulent* strains of mammalian tubercle bacilli in culture fail to form cords and grow in nonoriented fashion. Virulent tubercle bacilli, when repeatedly subcultured on artificial media, tend to become avirulent. During such subculture, some forms remain stable at an in-between stage and have *low virulence.* This is true of the bacillus of Calmette and Guerin, known as BCG strain, which is used for mass vaccination.

The other major factor determining the outcome of the infection is the individual's immune response. Cellular immunity on the part of the host's phagocytes is the chief defense. In the immunized host, macrophages ingest numbers of bacilli, which fail to multiply once ingested, although some remain viable for years. Such "sensitized" phagocytes oppose the "cord factor" of the virulent tubercle bacillus, which tends to immobilize and at times destroy the macrophage. The other immune factor is humoral. Certain protein factors of mycobacteria can be shown to stimulate precipitins, agglutinins and complement fixing antibodies which circulate in the serum. However, along with this antibody formation there is an anaphylactic type of sensitization (or allergy to the infection). It is believed that acquired sensitivity to the protein or polysaccharide components of the tubercle bacillus is responsible for the toxicity and the spread of the disease.

The intradermal injection of P.P.D. or the standardized tuberculin test is used to measure individual resistance. Individuals who respond negatively to 5 to 10 T.U. although they have a higher risk on re-exposure to the bacilli, are resistant to the breakdown of their healed lesions. In the United States, 30 percent of young adults among military and college personnel are in this category of *nonreactors*. In this same age group, approximately 60 percent will respond positively only when a high dose is used. These are termed *poor reactors* and it is believed they have acquired their natural immunity by previous exposure to some other form of mycobacteria, furnishing a cross-immunity. These poor reactors do not have a high degree of immunity to the human tubercle bacillus and should be followed by repeated chest films. In a third group of individuals, there is over-reaction to 5 T.U. of P.P.D. with an indurated dermal zone in excess of 10 mm. in diameter. These *hyperreactors* have an increased risk and are sensitized to the bacteria. The U.S. Public Health Service recommends these patients receive isoniazid therapy for the duration of one year. This is based upon an attack rate of 33/100,000 in military personnel showing hyperreaction.[34]

In America, endogenous reinfection tuberculosis in individuals over the age of 45 is the common form of active pulmonary disease. These individuals are considered either partially immune or sensitized to the products of the bacilli. The active focus usually appears in a single lobe in an apical or subapical position and a primary healed complex also can be visualized in the roentgenogram.

DIAGNOSTIC PROCEDURES

The time-honored symptoms and findings of pulmonary tuberculosis, which include cough, fever, hemoptysis, loss of weight and anorexia with lassitude and weakness, cannot be ignored but are not helpful for early diagnosis. A routine x-ray film of the chest with findings of infiltration or consolidation is indispensable as the initial screening procedure. Two confirmatory tests are needed: (1) a positive intradermal reaction to P.P.D. and (2) the demonstration of acid-fast bacilli in the sputum or on culture of the sputum. Cutaneous reactors whose chest films exhibit lesions but whose sputum fails to show bacilli on smear or culture, cannot be considered as having active disease. Patients with symptomatology resembling tuberculosis, but with a negative reaction to P.P.D. may have either sarcoidosis or bronchogenic carcinoma or a fungus infection such as histoplasmosis or coccidioidomycosis. Such patients may have roentgenographic findings that are difficult to distinguish from tuberculosis. Repeated search for the acid-fast bacilli must be performed as long as the diagnosis is in doubt and gastric washings are used when the sputum is scant or negative.

Roentgenographic Changes. In cases of active tuberculosis, the roentgenogram is employed to define the extent and the progress of the infection. The findings in the film correspond closely to the character of the lesions at autopsy in patients with the disease but dying of other causes or those dying with disseminated tuberculosis.

Active tuberculosis is a parenchymal infection with two outstanding characteristics. The active focus is a necrotizing pneumonitis. This tissue necrosis is at first a solid coagulative necrosis, but with progressive disease it becomes a liquefying or lytic process. The second characteristic is dependent upon the inflammatory monocytic defense in which macrophages (also termed epithelioid cells), many coalescing to form giant cells, defend against the infection with varying degrees of perilesional fibrosis.

Minimal or partially healed tuberculosis gives rise to a dense, partially fibrosed nodule with a central zone of solid caseation necrosis. This solidified lesion is known as a tuberculoma. It may be solitary, or it may give rise to satellite nodules. The solitary nodule is known as a "coin" lesion, varying in size from 2 cm. in diameter up to several centimeters or fifty-cent piece size. The total area involved is one fifth or less of one lung (Fig. 8-3).

Moderately advanced tuberculosis may include involvement of one or both lungs. In this form or stage of the disease, the margins of the lesions are ill defined or infiltrating. The dense or confluent lesions are confined to less than one third of the lung volume. Cavitation (or liquefied necrosis) if present is less than 4 cm. in diameter and may be absent. With modern chemotherapy, the prognosis is good with both minimal and moderately advanced forms of the disease (Fig. 8-4).

In *far advanced* tuberculosis, extensive cavitation and diffusely involved parenchyma in one or both lungs is present (Fig. 8-5). A *progressive fibroid* form may involve an entire lung (with or without a minimal rim of uninvolved tissue). With this fibroid variety, there is a shift of the mediastinum to the affected side, marked thickening of the pleura and elevation of the diaphragm. In another advancing and often fatal lesion, both lungs are stippled with small dense nodules, one to several millimeters in diameter. This is *miliary* tuberculosis with hematogenous spread, which in the past usually terminated with tuberculous meningitis (Fig. 8-6). Both the diffuse and fibroid miliary types (which are fulminant lesions) may

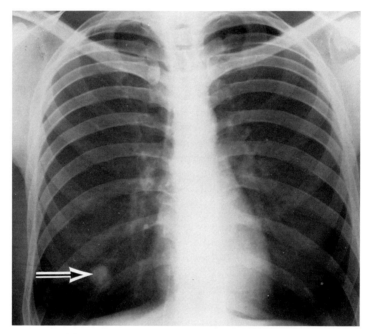

Fig. 8-3. Coin lesion in healed tuberculosis.

respond dramatically to antibiotic therapy, (isoniazid, streptomycin and PAS (para-aminosalicylic acid). A third and rare type of fulminant lesion is a rapidly *spreading caseous pneumonia,* which involves both lungs. This type of tuberculous pneumonia may be found in poorly nourished children suffering from a primary infection and is usually fatal.

In forms of advanced tuberculosis, pleural involvement may take the form of pleurisy with effusion or active tuberculous involvement with the seeding of nodules on the pleural surface, so-called tuberculous empyema (Fig. 8-5).

The miliary tuberculous infection may spread to both lungs via the lymphatics or the bloodstream. In the latter instance, multiple organs are involved, with only the muscular tissues escaping (Fig. 8-7).

Tuberculosis may coexist with other forms of pulmonary disease. In all forms of *pneumoconiosis,* in which silica is a component and in which heavy or chronic exposure to the effending dust has occurred, the incidence of pulmonary tuberculosis is much increased (Chap. 10). When asbestos or hematite are offending agents, pulmonary carcinoma also may occur. In such cases, bronchoscopic biopsy or transpleural biopsy may be required to distinguish the character of the advancing lesions.

Patients with active tuberculosis often suffer from pulmonary emphy-

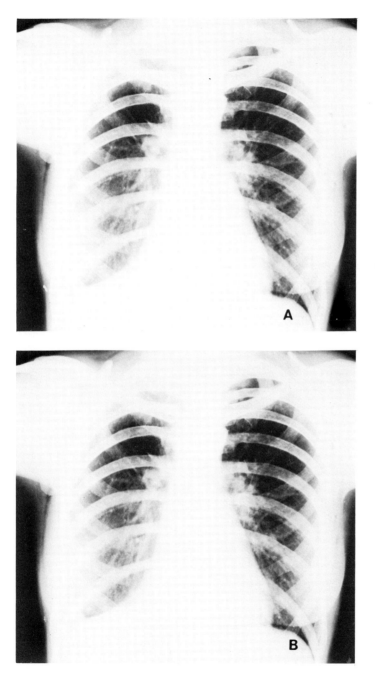

Fig. 8-4. Pulmonary tuberculosis. (*A*) Moderately advanced.
(*B*) Apical lesions.

Table 8-1. Major Features of Pulmonary Tuberculosis

Causative organism	*Mycobacterium tuberculosis* Human strain
Culture	Grows readily on standard media
Animal inoculations	All laboratory animals susceptible
Reservoir	Human cases with open lesions
Transmission	Droplet or airborne
Primary complex	Focal pneumonitis and hilar lymphadenopathy usually in childhood
Result of primary infection	Usually heals
Active primary tuberculosis	75% of cases in young adults 15 to 30 yrs. Usually exogenous
Active reinfection tuberculosis	71% of cases in individuals over 40 yrs. Usually endogenous affecting upper lobes
Dissemination of organisms	Early through lymphatics and later via liquefaction necrosis discharging along pre-existing anatomic channels — bronchi, serous surfaces, vessels, etc.
Early inflammatory response	Granuloma formation with epithelioid and giant cells
Healing response	Hyalinized tubercle formation, scarring and calcification
Progressive lesions	Caseation and liquefaction necrosis with endobronchial spread
Septicemia	Occurs in advanced cases; often fatal
Secondary involvement of other organs	Genitourinary tract, bones and brain
Prevalent type of active infection in USA	Endogenous reinfection in adults over 40
Predisposing factors	Diabetes, alcoholism, pregnancy, silicosis, malnutrition
Routine screening tests	Positive skin reaction to P.P.D. (purified protein derivative); Mantoux intracutaneous injection
Definitive diagnostic tests	Recovery of acid-fast staining tubercle bacilli from sputum or gastric washings

Definitive x-ray finding (early or moderately advanced)	Dense infiltrating zone in right or left upper lobe, zone of infiltration about spherical cavity formation
Additional pulmonic complications	Atelectasis, bronchiectasis, pleurisy and pleural effusion
Immunity after vaccination with BCG (Bacillus Calmette and Guerin)	Protection to 80% of cases for approx. 10 years
Statistics: Incidence rate (new, active)	37,187 cases in 1970 in USA 18.3/100,000
Mortality rate	5,560 deaths 2.7/100,000
Specific therapy	Isoniazid, streptomycin, and para-amino-salicylic acid

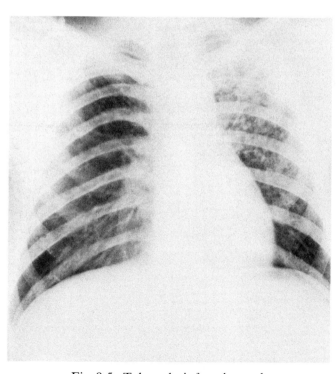

Fig. 8-5. Tuberculosis far advanced.

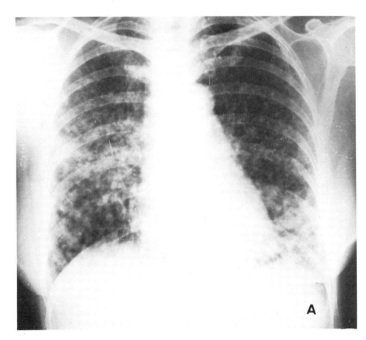

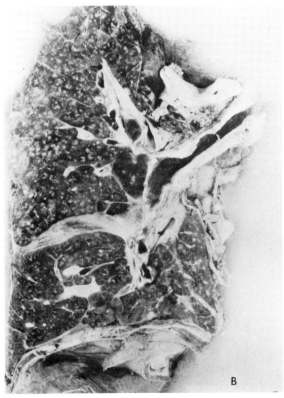

Fig. 8-6. Miliary tuberculosis. (A) Roentgenogram. (B) Gross specimen.

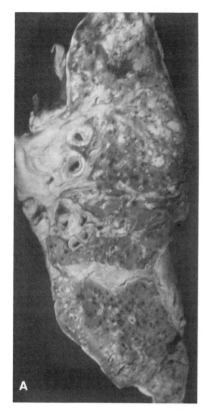

Fig. 8-7. (*A*) Advanced pulmonary tuberculosis with cavitation, calcified hilar nodes and pleurisy. (*B*) Advanced cavitary tuberculosis (gross specimens).

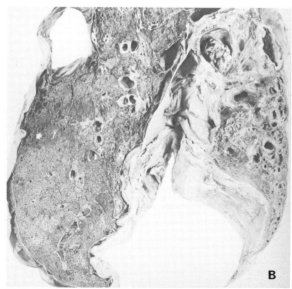

sema as determined by functional tests, and the accompanying cough, dyspnea and wheezing may be of emphysematous origin.[57] Bronchiectasis by second infection with pyogenic organisms may complicate tuberculosis arising in zones of atelectasis, either in the active disease or during healing.

Changes in ventilatory function in pulmonary tuberculosis depend upon the extent of parenchymal involvement, the presence or absence of pleural extension and the occurrence of bronchial stenosis complicating tuberculous bronchitis. Determination of reduced FEV_1 and arterial O_2 saturation may be helpful in evaluating the progress of the disease. In most cases of chronic pulmonary tuberculosis, there is little change in the blood gases unless there is diffuse fibrosis or secondary pulmonary emphysema. Bronchial stenosis with atelectasis is an exception. One of the features of active tuberculosis is the occurrence of pulmonary hypertension at a stage when ventilatory capacity is not reduced and when arterial oxygen saturation is within normal limits. But in other cases, ventilatory impairment occurs without hypertension.

FORM AND SEQUENCE OF PATHOLOGIC CHANGES *

The initial lesion in pulmonary tuberculosis, whether ultimately arrested or progressive, is a *microscopic focus of lobular pneumonia* caused by the inhalation of airborne particles contaminated by tubercle bacilli that have been coughed, sneezed, spat or otherwise extruded from a tuberculous patient (Fig. 8-8). The infective particles approximate 5 μ in diameter and contain three or more tubercle bacilli. This primary focus in many cases heals by complete resolution without scar formation. The initial inflammatory reaction (within one half hour to 24 hours) is composed of polymorphonuclear leukocytes, but by the second day (beginning at about 14 hours) these are replaced by macrophages and lymphocytes. The macrophages (termed epithelioid cells) are blood-borne monocytes or modified cells desquamated from the alveolar septa or endothelium of disrupted capillaries. In the initial pneumonic focus, both polymorphonuclears and macrophages are found and tubercle bacilli are sparse. Many macrophages contain anthracotic pigment if the patient is an adult urban dweller, indicating their origin from the septa or interstitium of the lung. If resolution occurs, the pneumonic focus lasts two to three weeks (Fig. 8-9).

If tubercle bacilli reproduce rapidly, tissue necrosis occurs. This necrotic focus, if small, may heal by lysis or by scarring and calcification.[65] If larger, it will progress, but if the patient's resistance is relatively high, tubercle formation results within three to four weeks. Most lesions in which

---

* This description is based on the studies of Medlar prior to the advent of antibiotic therapy.

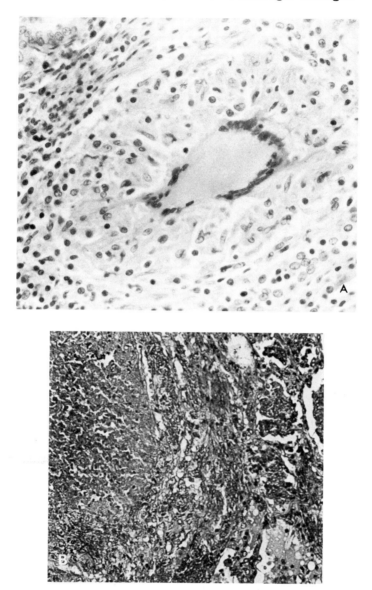

Fig. 8-8. Photomicrographs: (*A*) Hard tubercle with central Langhan's
giant cell. (×200) (*B*) Soft caseating tubercle. (×100)

tubercle formations predominate eventually heal by scarring and calcification after months or years.

The tubercle is a spherical granulomatous inflammatory response to the
tubercle bacillus. Its central portion contains modified histiocytes or

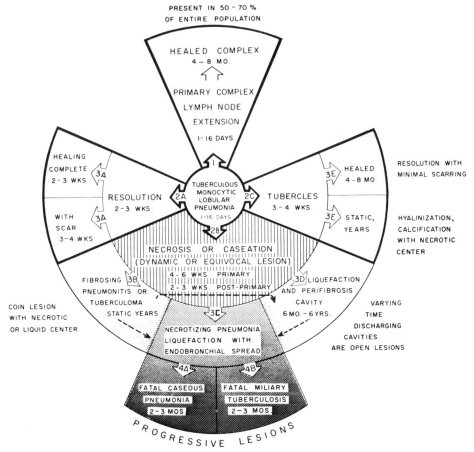

Fig. 8-9. Evolution of tuberculous pulmonary lesions.

epithelioid cells, radiating from the center as spokes in a wheel, with one or more giant cells near the center or at the periphery. Surrounding this mass of modified histiocytes, there is often a collar of lymphocytes and these, in turn, are surrounded by fibroblasts. If healing has begun, hyalinization often occurs at the center of the tubercle, associated with degenerated epithelioid cells. The peripheral fibroblasts send reticulum fibers into the tubercle, which is avascular.

Thus, the primary focus in primary tuberculosis in children and adults not previously exposed heals in the vast majority of cases by (1) resolution, (2) lysis or scarring, or (3) tubercle formation with calcification and scarring. The last named is the most frequent. Before complete healing, the disease has usually extended via the lymphatics to regional hilar lymph nodes that drain the infected area. The healed pneumonic lesions are usually in either the right or left lower lobes near the pleural surface and form either solitary or multiple Ghon tubercles. Such peripheral tubercles, together with the involved regional lymph nodes, form the *primary or Ghon complex.* In primary healed tuberculosis found at autopsy, over 90 percent is pulmonary in the form of a Ghon complex; less than 10 percent is healed intestinal tuberculosis caused by ingested bovine tubercle bacilli in contaminated milk or meat. Practically all of these patients develop a positive reaction to tuberculin.

In a minority of cases, the primary tuberculosis progresses from the localized pneumonic stage to the necrotic and caseous stage and then undergoes liquefaction and sloughing. The necrostic or caseous material forms a granular, slightly acidophilic homogenous mass that resembles cheese. When this caseating mass liquefies, it resembles porridge and may be purulent because of the degenerating granulocytes present. Necrotic lung tissue is often present. If the slough extends into an adjacent bronchus, endobronchial dissemination occurs with *acute progressive caseous tuberculous pneumonia.* If the slough extends into the parenchyma, vessels of appreciable size may be invaded and hematogenous spread gives rise to *disseminated miliary tuberculosis.* This may terminate with fatal cerebral involvement and tuberculous meningitis. Thus, unhealed primary pulmonary infection may eventuate in: (1) progressive necrotizing bronchopneumonia; (2) rapidly extending caseous pneumonitis (galloping consumption); (3) disseminated miliary tuberculosis. In miliary tuberculosis, the lung, liver, spleen, kidney are studded with small white tuberculous lesions about the size of a millet seed, hence the term "miliary" (Fig. 8-6).

Progressive primary tuberculosis is more common in childhood and more common in nonwhite than white races.

Reinfection Tuberculosis. The pathogenesis of primary pulmonary tuberculosis is well established, but this is not true of all cases of tuberculosis occurring in adults with a preceding healed primary complex. Usually, reinfection is endogenous—the result of the breaking down of an infected lymph node or ulceration of a formerly healed parenchymal focus. Spread most often extends to the right upper lobe by a lymphohematogenous route or rupture into a major bronchus. *A second exogenous infection is a rare cause of adult reinfection tuberculosis.*

Medlar [65] found that in patients dying between the ages of 16 and 30 of pulmonary tuberculosis, 75 percent had primary pulmonary tuberculosis. In patients dying of the disease after the age of 50 years, 70 percent had reinfection tuberculosis in addition to their primary complex. Such post-primary tuberculosis is chiefly a disease of white males over the age of 40 (often diabetics, alcoholics or poorly nourished individuals). In women, pregnancy may be a cause. The progressive lesion involves the apex of the upper lobe posteriorly (in about 85 percent of the cases) and may be bilateral. The regional lymph nodes may be actively involved, but this occurs far more rarely than in the healed primary complex. (In early lesions of reinfection tuberculosis, Medlar found the regional lymph nodes involved in only 2.5%.) Scattered progressive lesions in the lower lobes occur in advanced stages in 10 percent of all cases. Hematogenous spread is also rare and the main route of extension is endobronchial discharge of liquefied, infected, necrotic material usually associated with cavity formation. The histogenesis of the lesions in reinfection tuberculosis is similar to that described for primary tuberculosis except that the changes occur more rapidly. Thus, where breakdown and liquefaction of progressive caseous lesions occurs in seven to ten days in primary tuberculosis, this occurs in two to three days in reinfection tuberculosis. The susceptibility to and the acceleration of reinfection tuberculosis is thought to result from an acquired hypersensitivity.[77] In clinical management, it makes little difference whether the cases are primary or postprimary, except fatal hematogeneous spread is more common in primary cases.

Extrapulmonary Tuberculosis. This may be caused by the bovine tubercle bacillus, which localizes in the pharynx or intestine, or there may be a hematogenous spread from a pulmonary focus. Unpasteurized milk may infect the tonsils and cervical lymph nodes, producing scrofula, "the king's disease." Meat handlers and cooks contract tuberculous ulcers of the skin and infected axillary lymph nodes from handling infected beef. Tuberculosis of the bone is often of the bovine type, but it also occurs from the human tubercle bacillus via a hematogenous spread from the lungs. It localizes in the epiphysis or may spread from a joint. The bones of the spine, hip and knee are affected in that order of frequency. The vertebrae may collapse and produce a gibbus or "hunchback."

In the female genital tract, tuberculosis begins in the *fallopian tube* via hematogenous dissemination from the lungs. The wall of the tube is invaded, followed by invasion of the lumen and then the lining of the uterus. In the male genital tract, a corresponding hematogenous seeding usually begins in the seminal vesicles, whence it spreads to the prostate, the bladder or the epididymis. Renal tuberculosis is most common in young adults and is usually secondary either to a pulmonary focus or to tuberculosis of the genital tract.

Treatment of Tuberculosis. The combination therapy of three antituberculosis drugs—isoniazid, streptomycin, and aminosalicylic acid—has greatly reduced the mortality of tuberculosis in the past two decades. In addition, it has greatly reduced the number of surgical procedures required for renal and osseous tuberculosis and such procedures as pneumothorax and phrenicotomy. All patients except the far advanced cases of tuberculosis can have prolonged therapy (usually extending over a two-year period) administered on an out-patient basis.

Isoniazid is the most effective drug and is used alone over a one- to two-year period as a preventive measure in susceptible or exposed patients. It is not recommended alone as a therapeutic measure because of a small number of organisms resistant to this drug and the tendency of these resistant strains to dominate the infection when this is the only mode of therapy. Streptomycin must be given by injection. It may affect hearing and, at times, other cranial nerves, and hazardous retention of this drug may occur in patients with impaired renal function. Viomycin is sometimes substituted for streptomycin but is less effective and more toxic to the kidneys. Pyrazimamide is substituted for aminosalicylic acid and sometimes alternated with streptomycin (along with isoniazid). This drug is hepatotoxic in 15 percent of cases but has the advantage of being effective orally.

Isoniazid is the standard therapeutic agent. Overdosage produces peripheral neuritis and at times, cerebral damage. These effects may be neutralized or prevented by administering the antagonist, pyridoxine, in high doses.

Rifampicin and ethambutol are secondary agents in the treatment of tuberculosis. Ethambutol is not recommended alone but must be combined with one of the other three agents. Its most serious toxic effect is optic neuritis.

Rifampicin (Rifampin) has been used in combination with isoniazid, avoiding the use of streptomycin, particularly in those cases where drug-resistant tubercle bacillus have been found under standard therapy.

9

Pulmonary Mycotic Infections and Parasitic Diseases

Systemic mycotic infections frequently involve the lungs and may produce either chronic or fulminant pulmonary disease. These fungi imperfecti
grow in colonies with a complex of branching, threadlike structures termed
mycelia. The individual branches are known as hyphae. These hyphae
are capable of forming rounded or sporelike structures as a mode of replication but in some instances, replication is by spores alone or "budding"
without mycelia formation, referred to as yeast or yeastlike growth. As a
rule, only the sporulating forms survive and spread in human infections
and these forms may lead either to extracellular existence or multiply
within macrophages or giant cells. The infected tissue is destroyed although
no specific toxins have been described. At times, a hypersensitivity reaction is associated with the pulmonary involvement. The fungal pulmonary
infections most often found in the United States include histoplasmosis,
coccidioidomycosis, cryptococcosis, aspergillosis and blastomycosis.

Amphotericin B (Fungizone) is the treatment of choice for systemic
fungal infections which are resistant to the antibiotics used against bacterial
disease. It has a number of toxic side effects. Iodides, which were once
the only effective agents, are occasionally indicated.

HISTOPLASMOSIS

Pulmonary mycotic infection, caused by *Histoplasma capsulatum,* is
endemic in portions of the United States including western Pennsylvania,
Ohio, Indiana, Tennessee, Kentucky, Missouri and Arkansas. The portal of
entry may be via the respiratory mucous membrane or skin, and spread is to
the reticuloendothelial system. In the common benign form, scattered
miliary lesions in the lung simulate healed tuberculosis. In its rare and
progressive form, there may be ulcerated dermal and pharyngeal lesions

with invasions of the lungs and systemic spread to the brain and the meninges. Involvement of the lungs is patchy but widely scattered in lesions that fibrose and eventually calcify. Typical granulomas occur about the replicating organisms. In rare cases, these may undergo necrosis and cavitation, giving rise to hemoptysis. Such lesions may extend to the pleura, producing pneumothorax or empyema. The small calcified nodules in healed cases remain as tell-tale evidence of the pulmonary involvement (Fig. 9-1).

An antigenic substance obtained from tissue cultures of the organism, known as histoplasmin, is used for skin testing. It is obtained from either the hyphae or the yeast cell wall. Latex particles sensitized with histoplasmin have been used as an agglutinating test against the patient's serum.

In active cases, clinical symptoms resemble those of tuberculosis, with cough, fever, malaise and loss of weight. It has been estimated that four to five years is required for the healed calcified lesions to predominate. Hepatosplenomegaly may be present during the active phase of the disease, together with anemia and leukopenia. Smears obtained from sternal marrow or enlarged lymph nodes and stained with PAS show histoplasma organisms within macrophages. A fluorescent antibody technique has been used to test the sputum for the infectious agent.

The infectious spores can live in the soil of caves, storm cellars or silos, and pulmonary infection follows their inhalation. In spite of the agglutinins and complement fixing antibodies, passive transfer of immunity has not been accomplished.

COCCIDIOIDOMYCOSIS (VALLEY FEVER)

This mycotic infection of the lungs (at times associated with skin lesions) is endemic in the southwestern United States, northern Mexico and some regions of South America. Infection is usually through inhalation of the spore-laden dust, at times carried by cotton or wool dust exported from these regions.[2] Although the pulmonary infection (beginning after an incubation period of one to several weeks) is self limited in most cases, progressive systemic involvement occurs in from 5 to 10 percent of military personnel exposed in these regions. The fatal cases often are associated with meningitis (Fig. 9-2).

In the common benign course of the disease, there is fever, cough and an associated pleurisy. If pleural effusion is present, it usually resorbs within two weeks. The pulmonary lesions are typical granulomas which heal by fibrosis and calcification or resolve completely, but in progressive cases, may undergo necrosis and cavity formation similar to tuberculosis (Fig. 9-3). In these progressive cases, involvement of the lymph nodes, liver, kidneys, bones and meninges has been reported. Such cases, successfully

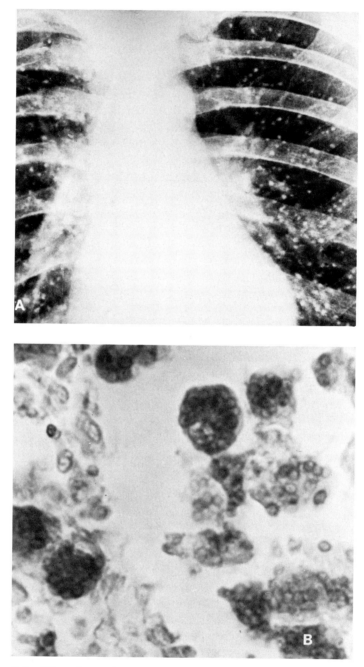

Fig. 9-1. Histoplasmosis. (*A*) Roentgenogram showing multinodular calcification. (*B*) Photomicrograph ×450.

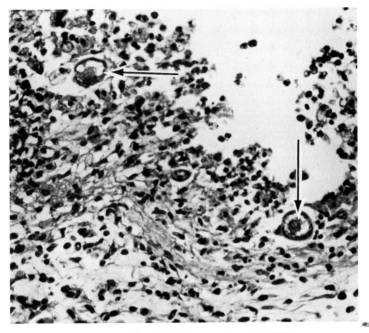

Fig. 9-2. Coccidioidomycosis. (×250)

treated with Amphotericin B, may relapse as long as ten years after treatment.[43]

The organism, which shows multiple spores encased in a double contoured spherical wall, is readily identified in the sputum or pleural fluid. Complement fixing antibodies and precipitants are present in the patient's serum in progressive cases. In such cases, the prognosis must be guarded.

CRYPTOCOCCOSIS (TORULOSIS)

This is a subacute or chronic systemic infection involving the lungs, usually the skin and also the central nervous system and visceral organs. The causative agent, *Cryptococcus neoformans,* is a yeastlike nonmycelial budding fungus with a thick spherical capsule which, in the tissues, is often embedded in giant cells and macrophages (Fig. 9-4). It is found in the soil in Europe and America and may be associated with pigeons. Inhalation of infected dust with primary pulmonary involvement is the mode of infection. The granulomatous lesions of the lungs are pseudotubercles and may resemble neoplasm or tuberculosis in the roentgenogram. In advanced cases, the infection spreads from the lung via the lymphatics and reticuloendothelial system to the meninges, producing brain lesions and a fatal

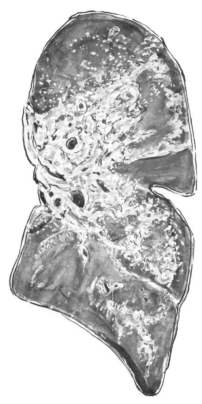

Fig. 9-3. Primary pulmonary coccidioidomycosis. Necrotizing and confluent granulomatous pneumonia with cavity formation. (After Forbus, W. D. and Bestebreurtje, A. M.: Military Surg. 99:653, 1946)

meningitis. Sputum, pus or centrifuged spinal fluid will reveal the organisms and establish the diagnosis, which can be confirmed by culture of the organism on Sabouraud's media. Successful treatment with amphotericin B has been documented, but relapses may occur after years. It is now possible (by using a rabbit anticryptococcus serum adherent to latex particles) to identify the organism and its antigenic polysaccharide by immunofluorescent staining technique.

Cryptococcosis was formerly considered a rare disease. However, Kuykendall et al.[56] found the number of recorded cases had risen from 43 in 1931 to more than 300 by 1955. The pulmonary infections in these cases were associated with bloody sputum, pleurisy with friction rub and effusion, elevated erythrocyte sedimentation rate and patchy bilateral zones of consolidation in the lower lobes by roentgenogram examination. In rare instances, the pulmonary involvement is fatal and occasionally patients have

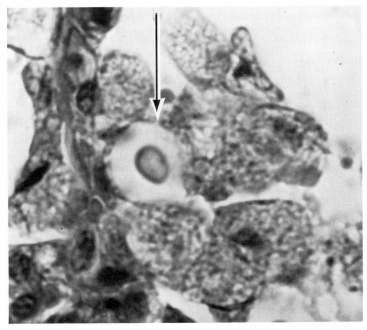

Fig. 9-4. Cryptococcosis. (×400)

been cured by lobectomy. Most frequently, however, death results from systemic spread and terminal meningoencephalitis.[56]

ASPERGILLOSIS

The spores of this fungus are usually present in grain, particularly spoiled grain and other forms of rotting vegetation. Inhalation produces pulmonary infection only in debilitated individuals or in previously diseased pulmonary structures such as tuberculous or bronchiectatic cavities. The infection has complicated vigorous cancer therapy with mustargens. In addition to the secondary invasion of other pneumonic lesions, aspergillosis may provoke an allergic response, producing attacks of asthma and eosinophilia. Diagnosis is made by the recovery of the characteristic hyphae in the sputum.

In a survey of sanitoriums in the south central United States, approximately 2 percent of patients had a positive titer for aspergillus organisms by the complement fixation test and approximately 1 percent also had positive sputum. In 54 patients harboring these organisms, 12 had active aspergillosis, producing pulmonary consolidation, aspergilloma, or cavity formation with positive culture. Patients with a positive titer for aspergillosis also had positive reactions for histoplasmosis and blastomycosis in some instances.[71]

BLASTOMYCOSIS

Blastomycosis in the form of chronic skin ulceration or primary involvement of the lungs is caused by *Blastomyces dermatitides,* which has branching forms of spores as well as yeastlike forms. The organisms, characterized by double contour yeastlike cells, often are enclosed within macrophages or giant cells and, in infected cases, can be demonstrated in the sputum or in pus. The patient's serum will fix complement in only about 50 percent of these cases in the presence of an extract of *B. dermatitides.*

In its primary pulmonary form, blastomycosis has been reported as a self-limited disease with healing similar to cases of histoplasmosis and coccidioidomycosis. However, progressive systemic involvement usually occurs unless treatment is promptly instituted. Metastasis to the internal viscera, bones and brain has been recorded. Lobectomy has been successful in some cases and in others, cures have been established by amphotericin B or Hydroxystilbamidine.

Although *Blastomyces dermatitides* presumably resides in the soil of North America, it has been isolated from this source only once. Transmission from animal to man or from man to man has not been demonstrated. Dogs are affected more than humans.

FARMER'S LUNG

Farmer's lung is an occupational disease produced by sensitivity to the spores of *thermophilic actinomyces,* usually those of the group known as micropolyspora. The patients suffer dyspnea, wheezing, cough, fever, chills and malaise. Rales are distributed over the lower two thirds of both lungs and the roentgenograms show an interstitial pneumonitis wtih varying degrees of fibrosis in chronic cases with persistent dyspnea. Pulmonary functional studies show decreased compliance and reduced diffusion. The pathologic changes of the disease show an inflammatory monocytic infiltrate of the alveolar walls with occasional foreign body giant cells. In some cases, the causative organism may be cultured.

In patients suffering from this syndrome, acute exacerbations follow exposure to moldy forage. There may be fever, chills and hemoptysis. Removal of the patient from contact with the offending material and administration of corticosteroids for the acute symptoms are the only effective treatment.

PARASITIC DISEASES

Parasitic diseases of the lungs are rare in America and are usually secondary to infestations elsewhere in the body. *Amebic abscess of the lung* (caused by *E. histolytica*) may complicate amebic dysentery with dissemination via the blood stream to the liver and lungs and more rarely to the bones. If the liver abscess is large, a sterile pleural effusion may occur on that side and organisms may reach the pleura via the diaphragmatic lymphatics and subsequently invade the lungs. More frequently, the organisms are carried by the venous circulation to form pulmonary abscesses. Amebic liver abscesses occur in approximately 5 percent of patients with amebic dysentery, and about one sixth of these cases with liver abscess develop pulmonary abscesses. Males are affected ten times more frequently than females by lung involvement. A secondary empyema is the rule in those cases which terminate fatally. Lung abscesses draining through a bronchial fistula are rarely fatal (less than 10%). Amebic infection is controlled by chloroquine therapy and the abscess is drained surgically.

Pulmonary Schistosomiasis (Schistosoma mansoni). It is believed that pulmonary involvement in schistosomiasis occurs only when hepatic fibrosis has diverted blood from the portal to the systemic circulation via the posterior mediastinal veins. The adult worms lodge in the pulmonary arteries and, upon their death and subsequent necrosis, incite a granulomatous reaction with giant cell formation, eosinophilic and histiocytic infiltrate surrounded by a zone of fibrosis. The lesions may eventually calcify. Severe vascular involvement may produce cor pulmonale. Ova from the parasites lodge in the smaller arteries (50 to 100 μ in diameter). Those that erode the vessel are ejected into the alveoli, where they incite a foreign body reaction. Some may be discharged into the sputum. Ova deposited in fresh water hatch free swimming larvae (miracidia) which must infect snails and be discharged in the water as cercariae. These penetrate the skin of man to renew the cycle. Infestation in the Western Hemisphere is found in Puerto Rico, the Caribbean and South America.

Stibophen (Winthrop) an organic trivalent antimonilial solution in 5 ml. ampules, is used to control schistosomiasis infections. An attempt has been made to decrease the pulmonary granuloma formation by the use of anti-lymphocytic serum. Neither form of treatment is effective if extensive liver involvement is present.[30]

Paragonimiasis. This is a trematode infection of the Far East which has been termed a "lung fluke" because of its tendency to involve the respiratory organs. The eggs and their larvae (a miracidium of *Paragonimus westermani*) are part of a complicated cycle in which fresh water snails are infected by the miracidium, which are liberated by the snail as cercariae to infect crayfish and crabs. Upon ingestion of these shellfish by the human host, these cercariae are liberated into the bowel which they penetrate, then travel from the peritoneal cavity through the diaphragm into the pleura and into the lungs. The pulmonic involvement produces fever, moderate dyspnea, cough, hemoptysis and severe anorexia with weight loss. Roentgenograms of the chest show varying degrees of patchy consolidation or cloudy infiltration with occasional calcified spots. Pleural thickening is relatively common and pleural effusion may occur more rarely. The disease may persist in chronic form for years after the patient has left an endemic area and usually is accompanied by eosinophilia. The diagnosis is confirmed by finding ova in the sputum. Emetine hydrochloride is used to control the infestation.

Hydatid Pulmonary Disease. This follows infestation with *Echinococcus granulosus,* the dog tape worm. The infected animal excretes innumerable ova which, upon ingestion, mature as embryos which penetrate the intestinal wall. On reaching the liver or lungs, a multilocular cyst with a characteristic blue capsule forms, which may grow to the size of an entire lobe. The cyst is lined by a syncytium of cells forming the germinal layer and has an outer laminated wall. This is supported by a fibrous layer of human reactive tissue, known as the pericyst. From the germinal layer of the parent cyst, the scolices (which give rise to separate worms) are derived (Fig. 9-5). The disease is particularly prevalent in sheep raising countries. The ruptured cyst may drain into a bronchus and produce death by anaphylactic shock. In most cases, the cyst tends to grow outward toward the pleural cavity. The erosion of the bronchi in this region may give rise to pneumothorax. The development of a large cyst is slow and usually takes a period of years.

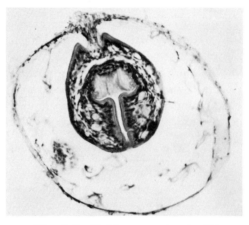

Fig. 9-5. Echinococcosis. (×50)

In most cases, the hydatid cyst develops in the liver, but in approximately 20 percent of infections the lung is involved. Bronchograms will show the smaller bronchi and bronchioles "grasping" the tumor. In the roentgenogram, the cyst is usually readily visualized with occasional calcification of its wall. Definitive diagnosis requires explorative cyst puncture, but the method is dangerous because of anaphylactic shock which may result from the escape of hydatid fluid. The surgeon should be prepared to perform radical removal. An eosinophilia of 20 to 25 percent in the presence of a positive roentgenogram is highly suggestive. An antigen has been prepared from sterile hydatid fluid in cases of animal echinococcosis. An intradermal test injecting 0.2 ml. of the antigen is used for diagnosis. A typical wheal will develop within 30 minutes if the test is positive.

Medical treatment is ineffective. A new surgical technique has been described to prevent the spillage of cyst fluid at the time of excision. The cyst wall is toughened by freezing and after removal of the cyst, the emptied exocyst space is sterilized by injecting 0.5 percent silver nitrate solution.[80]

10

Pneumoconiosis and Interstitial Fibrosis

The hazards of occupational dusts have been extensively documented in regard to pulmonary emphysema, pulmonary fibrosis, tuberculosis and cancer of the lung. Cor pulmonale, tuberculosis or carcinoma may complicate the lung changes produced by dust in ceramic industries, tool grinding or the mining of various minerals. The larger inhaled particles are arrested in the nose and nasopharynx while smaller particles of less than 100 μ enter the air passages and the minute particles (1 to 10 $\mu\mu$) are more readily inhaled than exhaled. With dimensions of 0.5 μ or less, exhalation tends to offset inhalation.

Silicosis. The chemical nature of the dust particle is equally important. Silica dust is one of the most harmful. In its natural state, it exists as the dioxide or tetraoxide. Among the occupations where this dust is a hazard, Spencer [87] lists:

1. Mining of gold, tin, copper, mica and graphite
2. Quarrying or stone masonry with granite, slate or sandstone
3. Use of carborundum wheel abrasives in metal grinding
4. Sandblasting
5. Pottery, ceramics and enameling industries
6. Work with blast furnaces or boiler scaling
7. Manufacture of rubber fillers and paint extenders.

It has been estimated for medicolegal purposes that each cubic foot of inhaled air must contain at least 5 to 10 million particles of silica dust smaller than 10 $\mu\mu$ of which 25 to 50 percent is free silica, in order to be hazardous to the exposed workers; and exposure during working hours must have continued for several years.

162

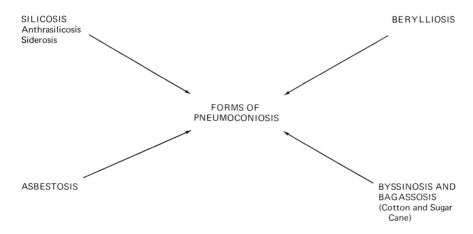

SILICOSIS
Anthrasilicosis
Siderosis

BERYLLIOSIS

FORMS OF
PNEUMOCONIOSIS

ASBESTOSIS

BYSSINOSIS AND
BAGASSOSIS
(Cotton and Sugar
Cane)

Silica is a fibrogenic agent that produces tough fibroid nodules which measure from a few millimeters to 5 to 10 cm. in diameter in the lung. They are found more often in the upper than in the lower lobes, but mainly are confined to the central or hilar region. In addition to the fibroid nodules, the fibrous septa of the lungs increase in thickness and toughness and dense pleural adhesions are formed. The larger fibroid masses extend across the interlobar fissures. Within their centers, small secondary cavities of a purulent nature or lined by tuberculous, granulomatous tissue may form. The microscopic changes include a mantle of phagocytes which ingest the silica, and the presence of increased amounts of bronchial mucus. The macrophages are soon surrounded by fibrous tissue which is adherent to the bronchioles and vessels and septa of the lungs. The silica particles often cause black pigmentation of the lung because they block the lymphatics and prevent anthracite pigments from reaching the lymph nodes. In advanced silicosis, the smaller branches of the pulmonary arteries are occluded and destroyed by the fibrous nodules. In the arteries thus obliterated, remnants of their elastic lamellae may be clearly demonstrated.

Clinical evidence of the disease in hazardous industries usually develops after 3 or more years of exposure, varying between 2 and 10 years, depending upon the industry. In the early stages, there is dyspnea and attacks of asthmatic bronchoconstriction. At other times, more severe symptoms are precipitated by superimposed infection. There is little correlation between the radiographic changes and the degree of incapacitation. The nodules in the roentgenogram (Fig. 10-1) are designated as "small" opacities when their diameter is under 1 cm. and "large" opacities when the nodules vary from 1 to 5 cm. These discrete nodules (Fig. 10-2) extend outward from the hilar region bilaterally, usually sparing the

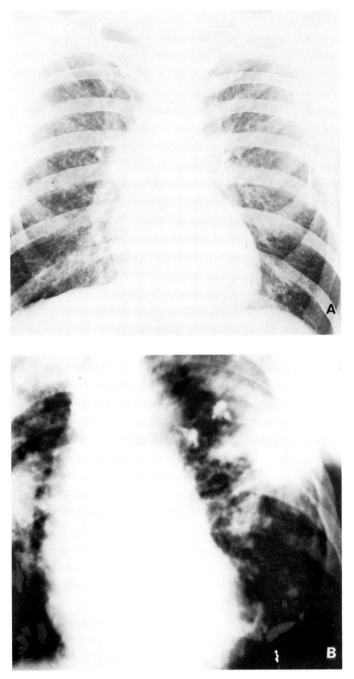

Fig. 10-1. Silicosis. (*A*) Moderately advanced. (*B*) Advanced.

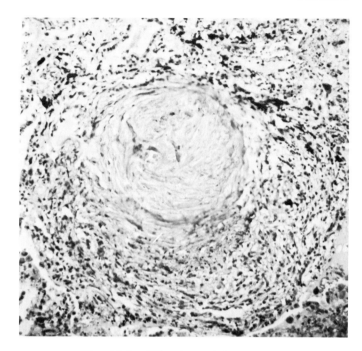

Fig. 10-2. Silicotic nodule. (×100)

apices and the lowermost regions of the lung bases. The spherical shadows may be hazy in outline or surrounded by a sharply demarcated calcified "egg shell." The hilar lymph nodes are enlarged and the mediastinal shadow widened. The linear lung markings are accentuated, and thickening of the pleura with or without calcification occurs. Cavitation may be visible within the dense nodules; enlarging cavities may be tuberculous, but this cannot be ascertained from the films.

Fluoroscopic examination shows limited diaphragmatic excursion in keeping with the emphysematous changes which are usually maximal at the lung bases. Increased sputum with fever and weight loss suggest the presence of complicating tuberculosis.

Death from right sided heart failure, from tuberculosis or from complicating bronchopneumonia occurs in advanced cases. The right ventricular strain is usually the result of pulmonary hypertension and is associated with varying degrees of polycythemia.

There is no specific therapy except by avoidance of further exposure. In some cases, symptoms thus are arrested but in others the pulmonary changes progress without further exposure.

The incidence of tuberculosis in silicosis is increased, and activated disease has been reported in as high as 65 to 75 percent of the fatal cases of silicosis (Spencer).[86] However, the incidence of bronchogenic carcinoma is not increased. The mechanism by which silica causes fibrosis is unknown. Some believe that the mineral itself forms protein complexes destroying collagen by linkage between amino acids and mucopolysaccharides, thus stimulating fiber formation. However, the deposition of fibers in the silicotic nodule bears no relation to the enclosed quartz crystals.

Another theory is that the macrophages ingesting silicates die and liberate phospholipids, which act as fibroblastic stimulants, or that the dying macrophages release previously ingested antigens which, together with silica, stimulate antibody formation and that these antibodies attack normal macrophages and the fibroblasts from which they are derived. In this way, an autoimmune reaction may become a component of the disease and stimulate massive fibrosis. This is suggested because immunoglobulins (IgG and IgM) are abundant in early progressive silicotic lesions and bind complement. Moreover, about one third of silicotic patients have a positive serologic test for rheumatoid factor.

In some cases, silicosis is accompanied by scleroderma (progressive systemic sclerosis), and antilung antibodies have been isolated.[64A] Such antibodies are rarely the initiating factor in disease and are usually secondary to prior tissue destruction.

Hematite Miner's Lung. The damaging ore in iron mining is FE_2O_3. This is hazardous when pulverized in drilling hard rock where the hematite and silica both act as irritating agents. The damage is similar to that produced by silicosis and increases the hazard of tuberculosis. In addition, lung cancers may arise in zones of scar tissue. Thus, the hematite is an added noxious agent when present in the fibrotic nodules. This condition is not synonomous with siderosis, since the mine dust contains minerals in addition to iron. As in silicosis, varying degrees of emphysema are present and damage to the smaller arteries occurs. This pattern of mixed inhalations may be found in steel workers as well as miners.

Asbestosis. Asbestos is a fibrous silicate of iron, magnesium and aluminum. The crystals formed by this mineral are large and needlelike and entirely different from the ordinary silica crystals. They provoke a more granulomatous response in the lung with less fibrosis and a different distribution, with a tendency to involve the lower lobes and the pleura (Fig. 10-3). The so-called asbestos bodies or particles have an elongated irregular dumb-bell shape and a distinct brown color. They can be found in the sputum. A foreign body giant cell reaction following a monocytic exudate precedes scarring about the particles, and the scar tissue does not hyalinize as it does in silicosis.

Radiologically, the lungs show a diffuse haziness which is bilaterally

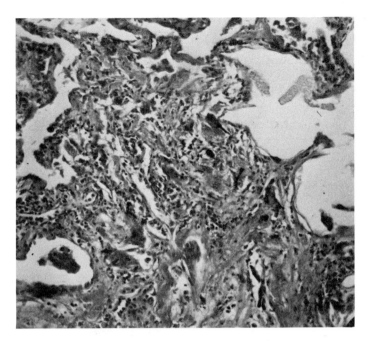

Fig. 10-3. Asbestosis. (×150)

symmetrical and accompanied by fine mottling or reticulation. There is pleural thickening, and the hilar lymph nodes may be slightly or moderately enlarged. In the thickened pleura, calcific plaque formation may occur, suggesting asbestosis, which is confirmed by finding the particles in the sputum. Dyspnea, cough and clubbing of the fingers are associated clinical findings and hyperkeratotic asbestos warts may be found on the hands and soles of the feet.

After termination of exposure, the condition may remain relatively stationary, the prognosis depending upon the degree of right ventricular strain. However, the remote complications include tuberculosis (occurring in approximately 30%), pulmonary carcinoma (approximating 10%), and pleural mesothelioma (10%).

It has been estimated that the pulmonary changes may be demonstrated in 50 percent of miners exposed for 5 years and in 100 percent of the personnel after exposure for 10 years whether in the mines or in related industries.

Coal Worker's Pneumoconiosis (Dust Reticulation). Workers in the soft coal mines develop pulmonary changes without a complicating exposure to silica dust. A fibrous reticulation extends outward from the hilum, enclosing parenchyma with overaerated emphysematous patches.

Although the majority of coal particles are removed in the sputum by ciliary action, some particles eventually become fixed to the walls of bronchioles and of alveoli, and to blood vessels, fibrous septa and the pleura. The dust-laden phagocytes adhere to these structures. At these sites, minute areas of destruction occur and adjacent areas show compensatory overaeration. The end result to such exposure is central lobular emphysema (Fig. 10-4).

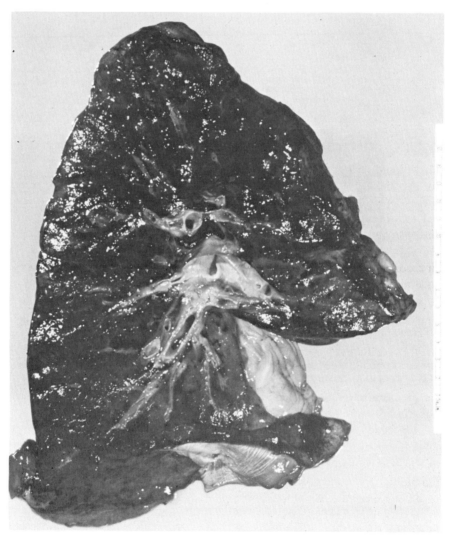

Fig. 10-4. Coal miner's lung (anthracosilicosis).

In the forms of pneumoconiosis discussed above, changes in the ventilatory capacity of the lungs depend upon the degree of emphysema present. In silicosis, because of the central location of the nodules, pulmonary function studies may remain normal (20% of the patients) in spite of marked roentgenographic changes. In all types of pneumoconiosis, there is a tendency for reduced lung compliance and diminished total lung volume and residual functional volume, but these changes may not be marked until emphysema occurs. However, in asbestosis, the changes in lung compliance and reduced diffusion and reduction in ventilation/perfusion ratios are more marked than would be expected from the roentgenographic changes.

Berylliosis. Berylliosis is a systemic poisoning caused by the inhalation of finely divided beryllium compounds. The inhalation of a sufficient number of particles produces an acute pneumonitis, with changes in the roentgenogram visible toward the end of the first week. The parenchymal injury causes an outpouring of granulocytes accompanied by congestion and edema and the formation of a hyaline-alveolar membrane. The acute pulmonary manifestations are more apt to be provoked by the soluble compounds such as beryllium fluoride or sulfate. The acute pneumonitis occasionally may prove fatal, or it may resolve, or be followed after several years by chronic berylliosis. The acute exudate in such cases is supplanted by an attempt at resolution by macrophages, and, if sufficient lung tissue is destroyed, this is followed by fibrous scarring.

Chronic exposure to beryllium compounds in the atmosphere produces a chronic interstitial pneumonitis, with the formation of miliary granulomas containing macrophages and giant cells resembling the lesion seen in pulmonary sarcoidosis. The interstitial tissues are thickened. In the x-ray films of the chest, there is diffuse bilateral infiltration studded with fine nodularity, with a tendency for the apices of the lung and the bases adjacent to the diaphragm to escape. Compensatory emphysema forms about the granulomatous nodules. This chronic pulmonary condition has an insidious onset, with dyspnea, loss of weight and weakness, and cyanosis and clubbing of the fingers; chronic cor pulmonale develops in the later stages.

The metal remains in the tissues for years, but is slowly excreted. Patients with the disease have elevated gammaglobulinemia (IgG) and a positive skin patch test for beryllium, but the relation of these antibodies to the disease is unknown.[76]

Symptoms are benefited by adrenocorticoid therapy. Only a small proportion of these patients develop emphysema with reduced ventilatory capacity and increased residual volume. These features result from advanced interstitial fibrosis late in the disease.

Table 10-1. Diseases with Immunologic Reaction in the Lungs

DISEASE	SOURCE	ANTIGEN
Farmer's lung	Moldy hay	*Micropolyspora faeni*
Mushroom worker's lung	Mushroom compost	*Thermoactinomyces vulgaris*
Bagassosis	Moldy sugar cane	*Thermoactinomyces vulgaris*
Malt worker's lung	Germinating barley	*Aspergillus clavatus*
Maple-bark disease	Dry, moldy bark	*Cryptosporium corticale*
Suberosis	Moldy cork dust	?
Sequoiosis	Moldy sawdust	Graphium, pullularia
Mill worker's lung	Mill dust	*Sitophilus granarius*
Coffee worker's lung	Coffee-bean dust	?
	Vegetable dusts	Fungal & other flora
Byssinosis	Cotton	Cotton antigens
Bird breeder's lung	Feathers, droppings, egg white	Derived from species (parakeets, pigeons, chickens, etc.)
Pituitary snuff taker's lung	Powdered pituitary extracts	Bovine and porcine serum and pituitary tissue
Hypersensitivity pneumonitis	Contamination of air conditioning and heating systems	Thermophilic actinomycetes

From: McCombs, R. P.: Disease due to immunologic reactions in the lungs. New England J. M. *286:*1245, 1972.

Inhaled Organic Dusts. Cough, dyspnea and bronchitis with varying degrees of airway resistance are produced by exposure to organic dusts. This occurs in workers in cotton mills, in sugar cane workers and in farmers who harvest grain. The pulmonary injury has been variously attributed to hypersensitivity to the organic material and to fungal spores contaminating the dust. In addition to the bronchitis, varying degrees of a low-grade pneumonitis occur. These patients are benefited by the use of masks and cortisone therapy.

Byssinosis is a respiratory disorder caused by the inhalation of cotton dust over prolonged periods. Chronic exposure produces a low-grade fever and reduced ventilatory capacity when contact with the dust is renewed. Workers in the cotton mills improve over the weekend, but have recurrent disability on Mondays, the symptoms being referred to as "Monday fever." Most of the pathologic studies show, in addition to the chronic bronchitis, varying degrees of emphysema and the formation of dust bodies which stimulate an increase of reticulum and collagen fibers. These dust bodies with a diameter of about 10 mμ are the central core of yellowish black material surrounded by macrophages. The adjacent bronchial epithelium may show squamous metaplasia. Schrag and Gullet [82] found that the intensity of symptoms correlated with the protein content of the cotton dust and demonstrated an antibody against the cotton protein in the patient's serum.

Bagassosis. A low-grade fever, dyspnea and cough associated with a presumed broncheolitis occurs from exposure to bagasse, a residuum of cane after the sugar has been extracted. It has been reported that chronic exposure may produce interstitial fibrosis and emphysema.[86]

Farmer's lung is caused by a mycotic infection from spores inhaled from moldy hay (See Chapter 9).

Sarcoidosis is a disease of unknown etiology with its primary manifestations in the mediastinal lymph nodes and lungs, accompanied by skin lesions that often resemble erythema nodosum. Fever, dyspnea and articular swellings are frequent complications. A number of authors have found bilateral hilar lymphadenopathy to be the earliest manifestation of the disease. This hilar "lymphoma" with erythema caused by hypersensitivity is known as Lofgren's syndrome. When parotitis and uveitis are present, the condition is known as Heerfordt's syndrome. Other manifestations may include nodular granulomatous lesions in the soft tissues, the bones and the meninges of the spine and liver involvement. Mather *el al.*[63] found histologic evidence of hepatic sarcoidosis in 59 of 93 patients with pulmonary manifestations by means of liver biopsy and recommended this as a means of diagnosis (Fig. 10-5). When hilar nodal involvement is prominent, there is moderate cough, a feeling of substernal compression and usually, a low-grade fever. Perihilar fibrosis and skin nodules may show progression, but in over 80 percent of the cases, spontaneous healing occurs in the following 18 months and the lesions may disappear under steroid therapy or following irradiation.[74]

Histologically, the presence of tubercle formation without zones of necrosis is characteristic. Initially, monocytes and foreign body giant cells predominate and, later, epithclioid cells and fibrous tissue are prominent. The fibrous tissue undergoes hyalinization and para-amyloid infiltration in advanced lesions. The giant cells contain stellate inclusions, the so-called Schaumann-Boeck bodies, which, however, are not pathognomonic for the disease. In a majority of patients, serum globulins are elevated and hypercalcemia may occur. A number of investigators have suggested that the disease is an allergic response to pine pollen because of its frequency in regions of pine forests. The digestion of pine pollen in the tissue liberates material that produces granulomatous response

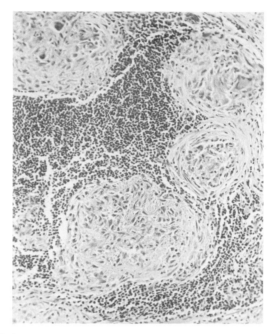

Fig. 10-5. Sarcoidosis in supraclavicular lymph node. ($\times$100)

resembling sarcoidosis in rats injected intratracheally with pine pollen suspensions in buffer. However, the relation of these experiments to the human disease remains unestablished.[1]

Roentgenograms of the chest are variable in appearance and may present (1) hilar masses produced by lymphadenopathy with negative findings in the pulmonary parenchyma; (2) reticular infiltration of both lung fields with moderate or absent linear markings or fibrosis; (3) a combination of (1) and (2); (4) fibrosis of the pulmonary parenchyma only.

Studies of ventilatory capacity in patients with sarcoidosis usually indicate reduced FEV_1 or lowered maximal breathing capacity. The diffusing capacity, measured by carbon monoxide, is usually reduced, whereas perfusion studies are normal.[91]

PULMONARY AMYLOIDOSIS

Patients with productive cough, dyspnea and recurrent attacks of hemoptysis and persistent wheezing who show deformity of the tracheal bronchial tree in the bronchograms may suffer from diffuse nodular infiltration, caused by the deposition of amyloid. Diffuse tracheobronchial amyloidosis may occur as a primary pulmonary disease unrelated to the familial hereditary form of amyloidosis. Antunes and DaLuz reported 18 cases from Portugal.[5] The recurrent attacks of respiratory symptoms with wheezing show mild ventilatory obstruction, as determined by FEV_1. The bronchographic studies show deformity of the walls of both the trachea and main bronchi, with evidence of thickening of their walls extending to the smaller ramifications. Diagnosis is confirmed by biopsy of the bronchial mucosa by means of bronchoscopy. In a case reported by Mainwaring *et al.,*[62] the roentgenograms showed increased translucency of the left lung, produced by nearly complete obstruction of the left main bronchus, which shifted the mediastinum to the opposite side. At necropsy, the trachea was inflamed and partially ulcerated. All of the larger branches of the bronchial tree showed localized thickening with varying degrees of obstruction, producing over-distention or complete collapse of the various lobes, with terminal bronchopneumonia in the left lower lobe.

FORMS OF INTERSTITIAL PULMONARY FIBROSIS (ALVEOLAR-CAPILLARY BLOCK SYNDROMES)

A variety of pulmonary diseases produce progressive interstitial fibrosis that destroys both alveoli and capillary blood supply. Most of these are of unknown cause or attributed to hypersensitivity. Some are a part of generalized systemic involvement such as pulmonary scleroderma, lupus erythematosus, periarteritis, Goodpasture's syndrome, Wegener's granulomatosus or rheumatoid lung (Caplan's syndrome). Other disturbances such as sarcoidosis or Hamman-Rich syndrome may remain confined to the lung and their relation to hypersensitivity is unknown.

Two types of pulmonary allergy are related to extrinsic causes. These are extrinsic bronchial asthma, which stimulates the anaphylactic antibody (IgE) known as Type I allergy, in response to inhaled pollens, danders or

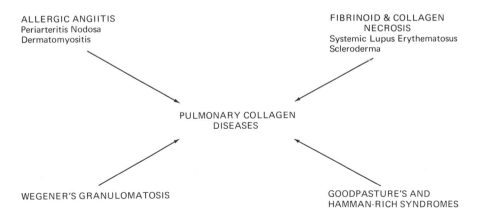

ALLERGIC ANGIITIS
Periarteritis Nodosa
Dermatomyositis

FIBRINOID & COLLAGEN
NECROSIS
Systemic Lupus Erythematosus
Scleroderma

PULMONARY COLLAGEN
DISEASES

WEGENER'S GRANULOMATOSIS

GOODPASTURE'S AND
HAMMAN-RICH SYNDROMES

dusts; the second is extrinsic allergic alveolitis produced by the spores of fungi (Table 10-1). These create circulating antibodies (IgG, IgA and IgM immunoglobulins) combining with complement to produce immune complexes. This is Type III allergy. Another cytotoxic or auto-immune antibody (Type II) which requires complement destroys cells and has been proved only for Goodpasture's syndrome in pulmonary disease. Such cytotoxic tissue-specific antibodies are characteristic of hemolytic anemia and thrombocytopenic purpura but are difficult to establish for systemic diseases. No prior exposure to a specific antigen is demonstrable and prior tissue damage is postulated. A fourth type of antibody which is cell mediated via lymphocytes is classified as delayed hypersensitivity and was first demonstrated in the study of tuberculosis and is the basis for the tuberculin test. It is also present in systemic mycotic diseases involving the lungs, such as histoplasmosis, coccidioidomycosis and cryptococcosis. In these cases of infectious origin, delayed hypersensitivity is mediated by sensitized lymphocytes whose sensitivity is acquired by a transfer factor derived from previously exposed leukocytes. The sensitized lymphocytes arriving at the infection release a "migratory inhibitory factor" immobilizing thousands of macrophages, which, together with the lymphocytes, form the granulomas or tubercles characteristic of these infections. This type of delayed immunity is also involved in host-graft rejection of transplanted tissues or organs.

Complement is involved in Type II and Type III tissue allergies but only in Type III do the immune complexes precipitate and as such, result in vasculitis or tissue damage (Table 10-2).

Hamman-Rich Syndrome. (Diffuse Interstitial Fibrosis) This is an in-gravescent disease, usually of adults and of unknown etiology, which is accompanied by cough, dyspnea and fever and progressively diminishes respiratory capacity. The patients develop cyanosis, clubbing of the fingers and polycythemia. Within several months to several years, death results from respiratory failure. As additional cases have been reported in the literature, the age distribution has widened, spanning from 12 to 77 years, and numerous descriptive terms have been proposed such as fibrosing alveolitis and interstitial fibrosis pneumonitis.

Pathologically, the lung is stiffened and nonaerated in appearance be-cause of an interstitial fibrosis which produces knoblike projections in the alveolar walls and obliterates their lumens. The small pulmonary arteries show medial hypertrophy and zones of parenchyma are permeated by an inflammatory exudate, although the alveolar pattern persists with an epithelial lining resting upon widened bands of connective tissue in which capillaries are sparse or absent. In places, the epithelium of the alveoli rests upon a hyaline membrane, although an obliterating sclerosis pre-dominates in the late stages (Fig. 10-6).

Table 10-2. Forms of Immune Response Involved in Tissue Allergy

CLASS OF ANTIBODY	SOURCE	ACTION	DISEASES
Type I Anaphylactic or skin sensitizing	IgE globulin serum	Releases histamine and kinins acting on smooth muscle	Asthma Eczema Hayfever Hives
Type II Cytotoxic antibodies	IgG and IgM serum	Destroys basement membranes or cells in presence of complement	Goodpasture's syndrome Hemolytic anemia Erythroblastosis Fetalis Thrombocytopenia
Type III Complex precipitating antibodies	IgG, IgA, serum	Combines with antigen and complement to form precipitated complexes at endothelial surface	Hypersensitivity vasculitis, Serum sickness Periarteritis, Wegener's granulomatosus Glomerulonephritis Lupus disseminata
Type IV Delayed hypersensitivity	Cell mediated sensitized lymphocytes	Immobilizes macrophages to form granulomas	Granulomatous infections in response to tuberculosis or fungi Sarcoidosis(?) Contact dermatitis Thyroiditis

Modified from Bellanti, J.A.: Immunology, Philadelphia, 1971, W.B. Saunders

In the roentgenogram, coarse webs of trabecular markings extend from the base toward the upper lobes while the hilar and mediastinal shadows are relatively unchanged. As the process advances, less aerated tissue is visible between these dense trabeculations. Eventually, this alteration of normal pattern reduces the ventilatory and perfusion capacity of the lungs to the point of asphyxia.

Although the oxygen saturation of the blood is lowered, the degree of dyspnea usually exceeds the degree of hypoxia because of loss of lung

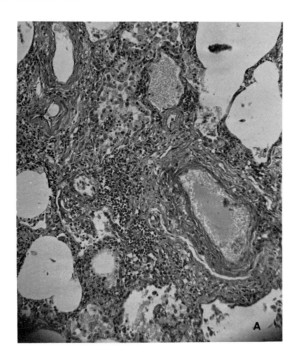

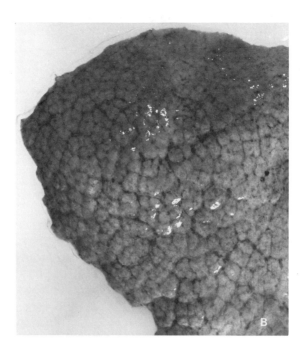

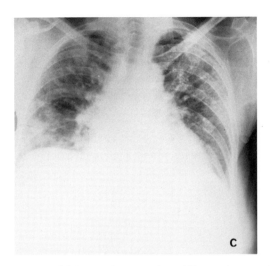

Fig. 10-6. Hamman-Rich syndrome. (*A*) Photomicrograph. ($\times 100$)
(*B*) Gross specimen. (*C*) Roentgenogram.

compliance. The established disease reduces both vital capacity and total lung volume, although the reserve volume remains within normal limits. In spite of lowered FEV_1, P_{O_2} and P_{CO_2} remain within normal limits until late in the disease. The outstanding feature of the progressive pulmonary fibrosis, which may resemble scleroderma or sarcoidosis roentgenologically, is the absence of systemic manifestations other than the polycythemia and right ventricular hypertrophy. The disease is attributed to a hypersensitivity response but only six patients have been reported with elevated gamma globulin. Neither autoimmunity nor viral infection has been demonstrated. Several cases have been complicated by bronchogenic carcinoma and some have had rheumatoid arthritis, but in the approximately 50 cases recorded, these may be coincidental. Nearly one half of the recent cases have responded symptomatically to cortisone therapy, but the prognosis remains grave.

Cases pathologically similar to the Hamman-Rich syndrome have been reported in children on an hereditary basis complicated by fibrocystic changes in the lungs. This entity, termed *familial fibrocystic pulmonary dysplasia,* is an independent disease and is not related to pancreatic fibrocystic disease (mucoviscidosis).

Wegener's Granulomatosis. This is a disease of the upper respiratory tract which produces granulomatous destructive lesions in young adults in which sinusitis and involvement of the orbit are often initial findings. Blindness may result. Secondary to this upper respiratory involvement, there is widening of the mediastinal shadow in the roentgenogram (Fig.

10-7) followed by progressive pulmonary granulomatous lesions which may terminate fatally. However, accompanying the sinopulmonary lesions there is a widespread arteritis and glomerulitis so that necrotizing renal lesions may terminate in death from uremia. The progress of the disease is accompanied by fever, elevated erythrocyte sedimentation rate and anemia. There is only transient benefit from steroid therapy. The lesions involving the sinuses and orbit may extend upward, invade the brain and occlude the carotid vessels. Cerebral softening secondary to intracranial vasculitis has been described along with necrotizing granuolomas of the liver. There is no established cause. Some type of bacterial toxin with a systemic Schwartzman reaction has been suggested.[59]

The interpretation of the granulomatous response as a form of hypersensitivity has led to the use of immunosuppressant agents for the treatment of this disease. Successful clinical results with cyclophosphamide (Cytoxan) have been reported by Novack and Pearson.[70]

LUNG INVOLVEMENT IN SYSTEMIC HYPERSENSITIVITY DISEASES

The pulmonary vasculature is rarely involved in hypersensitive states or so-called collagen diseases other than scleroderma. The most common

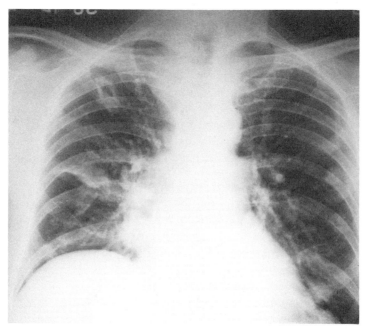

Fig. 10-7. Pulmonary lesions in Wegener's granulomatosis.

major involvement occurs in polyarteritis nodosa and the incidence has been variously given as from 4 to 20 percent. The lesions in the pulmonary vessels are similar to those in the systemic circulation with the characteristic fibrinoid necrosis of the vessel wall and an abundant exudate of polymorphonuclear and eosinophilic leukocytes, which extends through the entire wall and pervades the adventitia and surrounding spaces. Intravascular thrombosis and infarction may result. The incidence of pulmonary polyarteritis overlaps with the cases of Wegener's granulomatosis described above in which vasculitis is often a prominent manifestation.

Disseminated lupus erythematosus rarely involves the lung. Interstitial pneumonitis has occasionally been described in fatal cases, with a basophilic mucinous edema in the alveolar walls. Rarely fibrinoid necrosis of the smaller pulmonary arteries and arterioles has been described. In cases of rheumatic fever, the vascular changes are secondary to rheumatic valvular disease. In rheumatoid arthritis, fibrinoid degeneration of small vessels has also been described as a rare complication, but is in no way characteristic or specific.

In cases of *dermatomyositis,* sclerosis of the pulmonary vessels, beginning with intimal fibrosis and muscular hypertrophy, have been described. However, these findings are identical with those found in scleroderma and apparently are a separate stage of this disease.

Pulmonary Scleroderma—Honeycombed Lung. Pulmonary involvement is unusual in scleroderma, but when it occurs it produces a characteristic gross appearance the so-called honeycomb lung (Fig. 10-8). There is a fibrous thickening which involves the pleura and the major septa and extends into the interstitial tissue, replacing the alveolar walls and their capillaries with dense hyalinized partitions. Tears occur in the parenchyma so that clusters of alveoli form cysts one to several centimeters in diameter. Later, the cystic dilatation includes the bronchioles. The arterioles and the muscular arteries of the pulmonary circulation show intimal sclerosis which tends to obliterate their lumina. The veins show adventitial rather than intimal fibrosis. Thrombi form and may be recanalized. This type of change in the lungs accompanies dermal involvement and has been described also in patients with Raynaud's disease. The generalized vascular sclerosis that occurs in scleroderma and the tendency for the fibrosing process to replace smooth muscle in the gastrointestinal tract are the reasons for the term *progressive systemic sclerosis.* Vascular changes are widespread and produce characteristic lesions in the kidneys. Roentgenograms of the soft tissues in longstanding cases reveal calcinosis of the ligaments and tendon sheaths (calcinosis universalis). When such calcinosis is combined with telangiectasia (caused by venular obliteration),

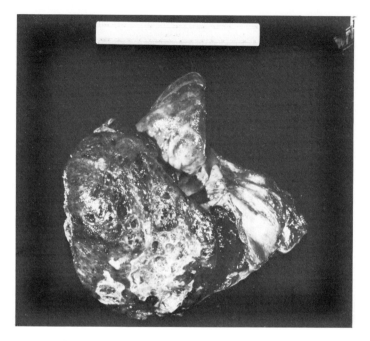

Fig. 10-8. Honeycombed lung in scleroderma.

the condition is known as *Thibierge-Weissenbach* syndrome. Arthritis is common and may resemble the rheumatoid variety. Lung involvement produces pulmonic hypertension and right sided failure. The disease usually lasts for years, but pursues an unremittingly fatal course.

GOODPASTURE'S SYNDROME

The septa of pulmonary alveoli and the basement membrane of glomerular capillaries may undergo progressive thickening in patients who develop hemoptysis from small multiple pulmonary hemorrhages, apparently following an unrecognized minor upper respiratory infection (Fig. 10-9). As the disease progresses, the respiratory symptoms may be overshadowed by renal insufficiency and fatal uremia. The application of fluorescent-labeled antibodies to the histologic studies at autopsy demonstrate that deposits along the alveoli septa and in the glomerular capillaries are similar and, apparently, are precipitated antigen-antibody complexes.[55] A number of these patients have died of pulmonary hemorrhage. Bilateral nephrectomy has been performed and, if the patients have been maintained by dialysis for 5 to 6 months, renal transplantation has been successful.

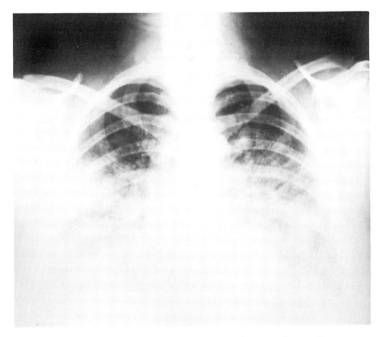

Fig. 10-9. Pulmonary lesions in Goodpasture's syndrome.

PULMONARY ALVEOLAR PROTEINOSIS

This is a rare, chronic and usually fatal condition of the lungs, which progressively fills the alveolar spaces with a proteinacious material which stains positive with PAS (Fig. 10-10). The septal cells of the alveolar wall show proliferations, sloughing and degeneration, occasionally forming laminated bodies in the proteinacious material. There is remarkably little inflammatory response, but occasional fibrosis may develop late in the disease. Respiratory distress results from alveolar-capillary block. Roentgenograms show bilateral butterfly infiltration of the lung extending out from the lower mediastinal region. In the early phase of the disease, the roentgenographic findings appear before symptoms. The occasional cures reported have followed the administration of fairly large doses of potassium iodide.[64]

PULMONARY HEMOSIDEROSIS (CEELEN'S DISEASE)

Two types of pulmonary hemosiderosis are described. The adult form is secondary to mitral stenosis or pulmonary venous hypertension from chronic forms of left sided heart failure. The initial cause is diapedesis

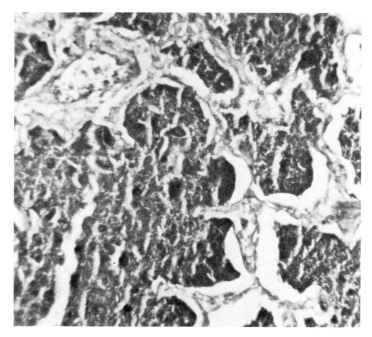

Fig. 10-10. Alveolar proteinosis. (×150)

of erythrocytes from the walls of the congested capillaries. The disintegration of these cells and the release of blood pigment result in the characteristic induration of the lungs. However, in longstanding cases, the hemosiderosis results in iron impregnation of the walls of the pulmonary arteries and arterioles and veins, the pigment being deposited in the elastic and reticulum fibrils. The alveolar septa are similarly affected. The combination of both calcium and ferric encrustation of elastic lamellae of the pulmonary vessels is characteristic of hemosiderosis secondary to pulmonary venous hypertension.

Idiopathic pulmonary hemosiderosis was first described by Ceelen in children, but has since been found in adults. These patients suffer from hemoptysis, tachycardia, anemia and petechial hemorrhages of the skin. Later, cyanosis and jaundice occur. Histologically, the lining of the pulmonary alveoli by hemosiderin-laden macrophages is similar to brown induration of the lung in heart failure and a similar deposition of iron and calcium salts in the elastic and reticulum fibrils of the pulmonary vessels results. Some authors believe the primary disturbance is in the capillary wall which has excessive fragility resulting in repeated small hemorrhages. There is a fibrotic reaction around the focal deposits of hemosiderin. The primary disorder of capillary structure has been suggested because of the coexistence of glomerulonephritis as part of the syndrome of idiopathic pulmonary hemosiderosis. Granulomatous response in the lung to iron pigment associated with calcium phosphates is thought to be similar to the response to iron oxide in the lungs of iron ore miners.

ENDOGENOUS PNEUMOCONIOSIS

In patients with chronic left ventricular failure, progressive fragmentation of the elastic tissue of the lungs may develop and provoke a granulomatous foreign body reaction causing death from respiratory failure. Foreign body giant cells surrounded by epithelioid cells and dense fibrous tissue are sufficiently extensive to destroy the parenchyma and its blood supply. The resultant pathologic changes of the lung have been compared to the anthracosilicosis in coal miners and the disease termed endogenous pneumoconiosis.[99]

11

Congenital and Hereditary Pulmonary Diseases

Both gestational disturbances and hereditary defects combine to make respiratory disturbances of the newborn relatively common. The frequency is increased if there have been maternal difficulties such as toxemia, diabetes or hormonal insufficiency or if the baby is premature, with a gestation of 34 weeks or less, a weight between 1 and 2 kilos or if there is a history of premature rupture of the membranes.

The human lung during gestation and before the period of "viability" is a glandular organ in which the ramifying tubules, which form numerous outpouchings about the 20th week, are lined by cuboidal epithelium. At about the 28th week, capillary loops develop in the mesenchyme between the alveolar ducts and groups of alveolar structures are lined by attenuated epithelium in apposition to the capillary walls. In most cases, the fetus (weighing above 1,000 Gm.) has sufficient capillary exposure within air spaces to support extrauterine life.

In fetal life, the patent foramen ovale between the right and left atria and the patent ductus arteriosus furnish mixed arterial-venous blood to the lungs. Thus, the pulmonary circulation of the fetus has a relatively high Po_2* and also a relatively high systolic pressure. This elevated systolic pressure produces a capillary transudate † which fills the alveoli and bronchi and aids in distention of the alveolar structures.

In the fetus at term, occlusion of the cord raises left atrial pressure above the right, closing the foramen ovale and forcing the entire fetal

---

* The blood coming from the placenta to the fetus via the umbilical vein is about 65 percent oxygen saturated.

† Whether the pulmonary fluid in the fetus is contributed by the amniotic fluid or whether the secretions of the lung contribute to the amniotic fluid has been debated but recent evidence is in favor of the origin of fetal pulmonary fluid as an active secretion or transudate supplied by an exchange of lung liquid and plasma.

circulation through the lungs. At the same time, a transient period of hypoxia constricts the ductus arteriosus, leading eventually to its fibrous occlusion. During the first hour of birth, pressure in the pulmonary artery is equal to or higher than systemic pressure and, thereafter, gradually falls over the next few days. If the umbilical cord is clamped relatively late after birth, pulmonic artery pressures are higher than aortic pressures. The mechanism for constriction of the ductus arteriosus and the umbilical vessels at birth in preference to other vessels is unexplained.

The reabsorption of pulmonary fluid at term is via both the lymphatics and the capillaries and presupposes a low alpha-1 antitrypsin, so that trypsin or fibrolysin can aid in the absorption of the fluid by preventing its precipitation and the formation of a hyaline membrane. This chemical secretion, along with surfactant secretion by the pneumonic epithelium, is essential to adequate neonatal pulmonic function.

RESPIRATORY DISTRESS SYNDROMES

Massive Inhalation of Amniotic Fluid. Premature respiratory movements of the fetus in the birth canal or in utero may lead to inhalation of the contents of the amniotic sack, flooding the bronchi and alveoli in the lungs of the newborn. In these cases, respiratory distress is apparent at or within 24 hours after birth. Quantities of meconium debris can be aspirated from the trachea and radiologic evidence of foci of consolidation are present. Metabolic acidosis is common. This condition is found in approximately 12 percent of newborn infants with severe respiratory distress. Approximately two thirds have a normal period of gestation with a normal birth weight. About one fourth are delivered by cesarean section, and abnormalities of the cord are present in about 15 percent. The breathing rate is between 50 and 80 per minute and is of the superficial "flutter respiration" type. Cyanosis, an abnormal cry and varying degrees of neurologic inertness are present. The radiologic signs are nodular opacities of variable density and relatively large size. They may be unilateral or bilateral, accompanied at times by signs of atelectasis or pneumothorax. Laboratory signs include lowered pH, hypercapnia and severe hypoxia.

The mortality in these cases is over 10 percent. Treatment is with aspiration, artificial ventilation, oxygenation, correction of acidosis and antibiotics.

Acute Respiratory Distress Syndrome in Premature Infants. Fetal atelectasis and hyaline membrane disease have long been recognized as major causes of mortality in prematurely born infants. In recent years, respiratory distress in these neonates has been traced to a lack of alveolar stability caused by a deficiency of surfactant. Surfactant is a phospholipid pulmonary secretion which lowers surface tension at the air and fluid interface of the alveolar walls, preventing their collapse at the end of expiration. Both fetal atelectasis and hyaline membrane disease are now considered fatal complications of this syndrome.

In the healthy child born at full term, the first inspiration expands the chest and supplies 40 percent of the lung volume as residual air at the end of the first expiration. In "prematures" born before the 38th week and weighing 2 Kg. or less, the alveolar walls tend to approximate and collapse at the end of expiration and thus, fail to retain residual air. The infant must repeat the gasping inspiration of his first breath, since he is unable to maintain sustained pulmonary inflation within normal limits. This syndrome appears in 33 to 50 percent of premature neonates while the infant is still in the delivery room. It is characterized by rapid respiration, expiratory grunting varying degrees of chest wall retraction, nasal flaring and cyanosis. Analysis of the blood gases may show a P_{O_2} of 40 mm. Hg or below and a P_{CO_2} of 50 to 60 mm. Hg or above. Roentgenograms show a fine reticulation and dense foci of atelectasis (Fig. 11-1).

While there are other causes of respiratory distress syndrome (RDS) in the premature infant, this is the common form and is regarded as the specific consequence of *surfactant deficiency*. Premature infants with this form of RDS are unable to synthesize adequate amounts of surfactant which, during normal late fetal life is present in two forms—a surface active lecithin derivative in which myristic acid predominates before term and palmitic acid predominates at term. These derivatives are phosphatidyl methyl ethanolamine and the dimethyl ethanolamine (PME and PDME). Unless PDME is available in sufficient quantities as a surfactant component, alveolar stability is not maintained. According to this concept, the alveoli are viewed as spherical gas bubbles within a fluid envelope in which the surface tension follows the LaPlace equation:

$$P = 2T/R$$

Surface tension (T) is inversely related to the radius (R) of the sphere and proportional to the pressure (P) of the gas therein. Thus, the alveolar surface tension increases when the radius of the alveoli decreases on expiration and the presence of surfactant is required to reduce the tension, which otherwise causes collapse.

If premature labor is imminent, the probability of the respiratory distress syndrome can be evaluated by a test of the amniotic fluid (sampled by amniocentesis) for surfactant.[22a] Treatment of the acute respiratory distress syndrome consists of assisted ventilation, oxygen therapy and control of respiratory acidosis to tide the infant over until increased secretion of surfactant occurs with maturation.

Babies dying within 72 hours with hyaline membrane disease complicating this syndrome have adrenals that weigh approximately 20 percent less than normal. The administration of corticosteroids or ACTH to rabbits and lamb fetuses accelerates lung maturation and the use of such therapy in neonates with acute RDS to aid in maturation may be indicated.

Unilateral Hyperlucent Lung Syndrome in Infants. This unusual disease has been described in infants who develop severe and unresolved pneumonitis before the age of 15 months.[27a] Infection with adenovirus may be indicated by rise in serum antibody titers. The original pneumonia is bilateral but worse on the side developing the hyperlucency. The unilateral hyperlucid lung is not recognized until six months to five years following the original infection. The affected lung has decreased vascular markings, a mediastinal shift away from the affected side on expiration and bronchograms show a "pruned tree" appearance. Lung scans show practically no perfusion on the affected side and reduced P_{O_2} in blood coming from the abnormal lung. However, the patients tend to improve with age despite deficient perfusion on the affected side. In some patients, this is not the case and cylindrical bronchiectasis develops. It is probable that this postpneumonic unilateral lung syndrome is the forerunner of cases previously considered as congenital atelectasis.

Congenital Lobar Emphysema. Overinflation of one or more lobes of the lung (usually on the right) with acute respiratory distress may be present in the newborn. The cause may be expiratory collapse due to deficiency of bronchial cartilage, aspirated mucus acting as a ball-valve obstruction, or compression of a bronchus by abnormal cardiovascular structures. The symptoms are wheezing, dyspnea, cyanosis and retractions. The chest film shows a radiolucent lobe with a mediastinal shift compressing the opposite side. Bronchoscopy is indicated to rule out a mucus plug. Lobectomy may be required.

CHRONIC RESPIRATORY DISTRESS IN PREMATURE INFANTS

Pulmonary Dysmaturity (Wilson-Mikity Syndrome). This is an infantile form of pneumonitis which most often appears in premature infants (average weight 1,500 grams) with gestational ages ranging from 24 to 36 weeks and with onset of respiratory symptoms usually between the first and third weeks of life. The symptoms are milder than those with the acute respiratory distress syndrome and are more chronic. They are not present at birth. The hypoxia may develop in severe form and, although recovery usually occurs within 3 to 24 months, the child may suffer mental retardation on recovery. The outstanding features are the late onset, the chronicity and the prematurity of the infant. Radiographs of the chest during the first week show multiple punctate densities, which may enlarge during the next several weeks. Because of the hypoxia and respiratory distress, the lower lobes of the lungs become overexpanded and hyperlucid and the diaphragm flattened. Biopsies and postmortem examinations have shown bronchiolitis or interstitial pneumonitis with zones of alveolar hyperinflation. In fatal cases, a hyaline membrane may be present at autopsy. There are no criteria at the present time to distinguish this form of respiratory distress from surfactant deficiency in prematures.

Hyaline Membrane Disease. This is a pathologic diagnosis rather than a clinical disease entity and is a fatal end-stage in the respiratory distress syndromes of premature infants. Whether the membrane, which consists of fibrin and precipitated cellular debris, is accentuated by the type of treatment (assisted ventilation and oxygen therapy) has not been determined. This diagnostic term often is used interchangeably with acute respiratory distress syndrome.

While surfactant deficiency with hypoxia leading to the formation of the membrane is used to explain the association of hyaline membrane disease with prematurity, decreased alveolar fibrinolysins associated with high alpha-1 antitrypsin, has also been considered to play a role. Thus, term infants do not develop the disease because of high levels of surfactant and low levels of antitrypsin.

Regardless of the etiology of the disease, the following features are considered part of the syndrome: (1) Absence of the disease in the stillborn; (2) frequent occurrence in immaturity in neonates weighing from 1 to 2 Kg.; (3) increased incidence in offspring of diabetic mothers; (4) prevalence in the first 72 hours of life with death prior to the fourth day; (5) presence of fluid leakage from pulmonary capillaries with membrane derived from the fibrinogen of the blood plasma associated with desquamated alveolar epithelium and disintegrated red cells; (6) association with varying degrees of atelectasis (Fig. 11-1).

Residual Wet Lung of Prematurity. Studies of the fetal lung in rabbits and lambs indicate that the lung is initially expanded by fluid in the alveolar spaces and respiratory ducts. Whether such pulmonary edema persists in some cases of respiratory distress in the premature has been postulated but not proved.

Immature Lung in the Full Term Infant. Respiratory distress caused by surfactant deficiency can occur in full term infants if the development of the lungs is retarded. At present, these are termed "Small for Gestational Age" babies (SGA). The causes of retarded pulmonary development are similar to those for other forms of congenital anomalies and include malnutrition and specific vitamin deficiency of the mother during gestation and perhaps forms of transplacental viral infection.

Neonatal Pneumonitis—Placental Infection. Transplacental infection via the hematogenous route may occur in mothers infected with toxoplasmosis, cytomegalic inclusion disease, Coxsackie virus and *Listeria monocygenes*. Bacteria are also found in transplacental infections, including staphylococci, streptococci, pneumococci and, at times, congenital tuberculosis or syphilis. In the last two, the placenta itself is usually infected. Premature infants are more susceptible than term infants to such maternal spread. The infant may be stillborn or desperately ill at birth if pneumonitis is present. The onset of respirations may be delayed and, once initiated, breathing is labored and adequate aeration is impossible. The infants remain hypothermic for abnormally long periods and, if surviving after several hours, they may develop a fever. Leukocytosis is not often present, but leukocytic infiltration of the cord on frozen section, once respiratory difficulty is manifest, may be diagnostic. The chest film shows ill defined streak densities with occasional confluent opacities. If death occurs, diffuse heavy congested lungs are the rule with

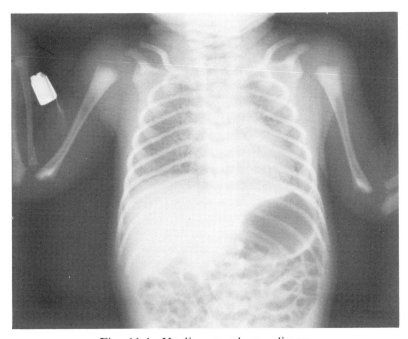

Fig. 11-1. Hyaline membrane disease.

or without pleuritis. Although not always effective, penicillin is the safest antibiotic in the newborn.

Syphilitic Pneumonia. Congenital syphilis of the lungs is usually a fatal disease in which the lungs are consolidated by increased interstitial fibrous tissue and widening of the pulmonary septa, reducing the size and number of the alveoli. Small gummas usually are present and numerous treponema can be demonstrated by silver stains. The gross appearance of the firm, white pulmonary tissue on sectioning has led to the term "pneumonia alba."

Congenital Cystic Disease of the Lung. In newborn infants, a lethal maldevelopment of the lungs characterized by the appearance of numerous cystic spaces lined by bronchial epithelium may occur. The microscopic and gross appearance is that of fetal lung in which diffuse widening of the alveolar ducts has occurred instead of the elaboration of alveolar spaces. The pattern of the cystic change is extremely variable and cases have been reported as bronchiolectasis, fetal bronchiectasis, honeycombed lung and congenital cystic malformation. When the disease is localized to a single lobe, it is compatible with life and is most often referred to by radiologists as congenital honeycombed lung.

HEREDITARY DISEASES

Hereditary Deficiency of Alpha-1 Antitrypsin. The pulmonary disease produced by this enzymatic deficiency is transmitted as an autosomal recessive trait. The affected individuals in adulthood have airway obstruction, chronic bronchitis and emphysema. Although the changes of destructive emphysema are found only in adults, respiratory symptoms appear earlier. The Alpha-1 AT values in the serum of homozygotes is less than 20 percent of normal, with averages of 40 to 80 percent in heterozygotes. In both, there is a high frequency of upper respiratory infections and severe bronchopulmonary infections. At autopsy, the emphysema is of the panlobular destructive type complicated by bronchopneumonia with foci of fibrosis and pulmonary abscesses. The predisposition to sinusitis and pneumonia is well documented. The organisms most frequently cultured are Pseudomonas, Proteus and *Staphylococcus aureus*. Chest roentgenograms showing destructive emphysema may be preceded by evidence of pulmonary perfusion deficiency, determined by scintigrams using radioisotopes. The panacinar emphysematous changes have been associated with progressive liver failure and portal hypertension in some of the siblings. The degenerative changes in the lungs are associated with destruction of elastic tissue in the alveolar septa. There is also obstructive lung disease resulting from expiratory collapse following the interruption and disappearance of bronchiolar elastic lamellae. Digestion of these lamellae by serum trypsin is postulated. Liver biopsies in the first year of life show perilobular cirrhosis and bile plugging. The hepatocytes are swollen and have PAS-positive cytoplasmic granules. Death may occur from massive intraperitoneal as well as intrapulmonic hemorrhage because of liver disease.

Avoidance of aerosols and tobacco and the prompt treatment of infections with antibiotics have been recommended, but nothing seems to prevent the ultimate changes of emphysema.

Pulmonary Changes With Cystic Fibrosis. Cystic fibrosis is the most common genetically transmitted fatal disease in childhood. It affects the exocrine secretion of the pancreas, the intestinal glands, the bile ducts, the bronchial glands and the sweat glands. The high salt content of the sweat is diagnostic as well as the fatty diarrhea or meconium ileus that may be observed in neonates. In such patients, the mucoviscidosis resulting in tenacious bronchial secretions leads to obstruction and infection of the airway passages with foci of parenchymal damage. Aerosol therapy and humidified air (sleep in mist tents) have slowed the progression of pulmonary changes, delaying some of the severe manifestations to adulthood. In such survivors, episodes of severe hemoptysis have been reported, associated with respiratory infections with *Staphylococcus aureus* or *Pseudomonas aeruginosa* producing bronchiectasis. Low prothrombin times may be a factor, since these patients suffer a form of hepatic cirrhosis. The hemorrhages may be severe enough to require transfusion. Aerosols, antibiotics and mist tent therapy are recommended to slow the progress of the pulmonary complications in cystic fibrosis; however, no form of therapy has proved highly effective.

The tenacious mucus secreted by the bronchial glands and other exocrine glands in cystic fibrosis has been attributed to abnormal glycoproteins together with a disturbed pattern of ionic constituents. L-Argenine has been used to combat the viscosity of the secretions.

Fibrocystic Pulmonary Dysplasia. This is a rare hereditary disease transmitted as an autosomal dominant. The affected patients suffer progressive dyspnea, cyanosis, clubbing of the fingers, pulmonic hypertension and polycythemia. Roentgenograms show progressive pulmonary fibrosis. A Canadian family with eight cases in four generations has been reported.

Pulmonary Alveolar Microlithiasis. Multiple bilaterally distributed minute foci of calcification may rarely appear in the roentgenograms of individuals affected with this disease. The occurrence in several members of the same family in which there is consanguinity of parents has been reported and a disproportionate number of cases occur in Spanish families. The disease is unrelated to parathyroid disturbance and is usually not associated with other symptomatology. It may be an incidental autopsy finding.

Hereditary Telangiectasia—Rendu-Osler Disease. This hereditary defect in the wall of capillaries with the formation of multiple small angiomas is transmitted as a Mendelian dominant. Bleeding from these lesions (epistaxis, melena, hemoptysis, or hematuria) and the development of anemia (with pallor, dyspnea, and weakness) are the leading symptoms. Repeated nosebleeds may be present in childhood, but more frequently, the lesions appear and become worse in adulthood. They form small red papules visible on the face or neck or in the oral cavity.

Telangiectases in the pulmonary circulation produce recurrent hemoptysis and are responsible for multiple arteriovenous shunts. The multiple small shunts are the equivalent of a single large communication and result in cyanosis. Polycythemia, clubbing of the fingers, emphysema and pulmonary fibrosis may develop. A history of bleeding and "red spots" in other members of the family aids in diagnosis.

Treatment is directed at controlling local bleeding, freezing, or electrocoagulation to destroy the angioma and transfusions, iron and vitamins to control the anemia.

Inherited Agammaglobulinemia with Sinopulmonary Infections. Two types of inherited agammaglobulinemia occur. The more common is an x-linked recessive disorder affecting males; the other is sporadic autosomal recessive. Infants suffering from pulmonary infections are well for the first 9 months (because of retained maternal gammaglobulin) and some have no serious difficulties until 5 or 6 years of age. A striking clinical feature, suggesting this disorder, is the tendency to develop repeated respiratory infections to encapsulated pyogenic organisms (*M. pyrogenes, D. pneumoniae, H. influenzae,* and *S. pyrogenes*), while no impairment to recovery or to immunization exists for the viral infections such as measles, mumps and varicella. Protection against the bacterial infections requires circulating gamma globulins, but if the organism is unencapsulated, leukocytic phagocytosis provides some resistance. On the other hand, protection against viral infections is via interferon and possibly to such substances as properdin. (Bellanti, J. A.: Immunology, Philadelphia, W. B. Saunders 1971.)

Repeated infections with pneumococci is the most common clinical finding. These include pneumonia, otitis, and sinusitis. Some children may suffer four to five such infections annually. The diagnosis of agammaglobulinemia and the antibody deficiency syndrome can be established by electrophoretic or immunologic methods.

Treatment is by intramuscular injections of commercial immune serum globulin. These must be repeated about once monthly.

Other forms of hereditary immune deficiency include dysgammaglobulinemias, in which a deficiency of one or two of the gamma globulins (G, A, or M) is present. These patients are also susceptible to recurrent skin and pulmonary infections. One of these is the Louis-Bar syndrome of hereditary ataxia telangiectasia in which a dwarfed cerebellum and oculo-cutaneous hemangiomas are associated with hypoplasia of the thymus and lymphoid tissue with deficient IgA globulin. Sinopulmonary infections and lymphosarcoma are complications.

12

Neoplasms of the Lung

BENIGN TUMORS OF THE LUNG

Benign neoplasms of the lung include mesenchymal tumors arising from the bronchial walls and epithelial tumors derived from the lining cells and their glandular appendages. The mesenchymal tumors are not peculiar to the lung and may be either intralumenal in their growth or intramural. The most common are chondromas derived from the bronchial cartilages, and leiomyomas. The location of the growth is readily depicted by roentgenograms, but its nature is determined only by biopsy. Airway obstruction with cough or bloody sputum are leading symptoms.

The common epithelial tumors of benign nature are exophytic squamous cell papillomas, which at times are transplants from papillomatosis of the larynx and benign argentaffine tumors (carcinoids). More rarely, salivary adenomas resembling the mixed tumors of the parotid gland occur. These may have low-grade basal cell foci of proliferation, but are nonmetastasizing. They are treated by excision.

Benign bronchial carcinoids may produce obstructive wheezing and cough complicated by purulent bronchitis and, if of long duration, by secondary bronchiectasis. Hemoptysis is common in the long-standing, infected cases. The roentgenographic findings are more often produced by obstruction and atelectasis than by the visibility of a tumor mass. Diagnosis is accomplished by means of bronchoscopy. Microscopic examination shows cords or islands of epithelial cells of moderate size with small nuclei embedded in thin strands of connective tissue. Carcinoids of the bronchus contain argyrophilic cells but rarely the brown granules of carcinoids found in the intestine. Malignant change occurs in a small percentage of these cases and these may be associated with Cushing's syndrome or pleuriglandular adenomatosis.[37, 100]

In past decades, since peripheral carcinomas have become as common as those of the main stem bronchus, benign peripheral adenomas have been recognized as small occult tumors in areas of atelectasis or in relation to bronchiectasis.[54] These are found accidentally at autopsy or following lobectomy.

Pulmonary Adenomatosis. Reduplication of the lining layers of respiratory bronchioles and alveoli to produce papillary growth of cuboidal or columnar cells that may have ciliated margins or contain mucus, is referred to as adenomatosis. The lesions are usually multiple and may be benign or malignant. The diffuse multiple lesions frequently undergo malignant change, although microscopic differentiation cannot be made with certainty. When these tumors are multiple and malignant, they are also classed as bronchiolar carcinoma or alveolar cell cancers. These multiple peripheral tumors of the lung are distinguished in regard to their tissues of origin by means of the electron microscope [69a] (Fig. 12-1).

Mesotheliomas of the Pleura. Mesotheliomas of the pleura are relatively rare tumors and protrude inwardly from the chest wall, compressing the underlying lung and casting a dense shadow in the roentgenogram. Their origin from the pleura can be verified by a diagnostic pneumothorax on the affected side preliminary to repeated roentgenographic examinations. Although the tumor grows by extension, focal distant metastases occur after a period of several years. More rarely, the tumor disseminates widely to the pleura and lungs, resulting in massive effusion.

Microscopically, the fusiform tumor cells surround small clear spaces giving an appearance closely resembling synovial sarcomas arising in the joints. The mesenchymal nature of the growth is revealed by the elaboration of collagenous processes by tumor cells. Dense fibrous bands divide the growth into lobules (Fig. 12-1).

These tumors usually appear in mid-adult life and are more frequent in miners exposed to asbestos (chapter 10). They are treated by wide excision or resection.

CARCINOMAS OF THE LUNG

Once considered a rare form of malignancy, the incidence of lung cancer among men in the large cities of industrialized countries has risen to epidemic proportions in the decades between 1930 and 1970. The attack rate for men exceeds 50 per 100,000 while that for women is about 10 per 100,000, in the United States.[86] Fatalities from lung cancer were estimated at 72,000 for 1972.

The average age incidence of carcinoma of the lung in a series of 500 to 1,000 cases varied between 48 and 56 years. However, there are exceptions. Adenocarcinoma of the lung in patients under the age of 20 years has been reported by Sawyer et al.[82] The disease has also been reported among four siblings in one family (Brisman et al.).[17] All four cases were exophytic squamous cell cancers and extended into the bronchus in papillary fashion. All were still living after resection (16 to 33 months).

MAJOR FORMS OF LUNG CANCER

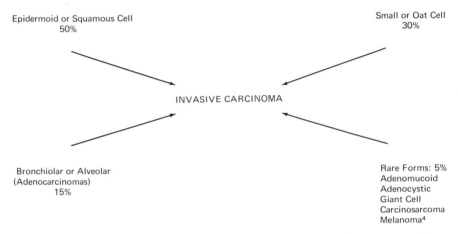

Epidermoid or Squamous Cell
50%

Small or Oat Cell
30%

INVASIVE CARCINOMA

Bronchiolar or Alveolar
(Adenocarcinomas)
15%

Rare Forms: 5%
Adenomucoid
Adenocystic
Giant Cell
Carcinosarcoma
Melanoma[4]

The relation of this form of cancer to air pollution, cigarette smoking and to laborers in heavy industry has been much emphasized. Both cigarette smoking and urban life increase the risk, but cigarette smoking is the greater danger and is more hazardous for men than for women.[16] The

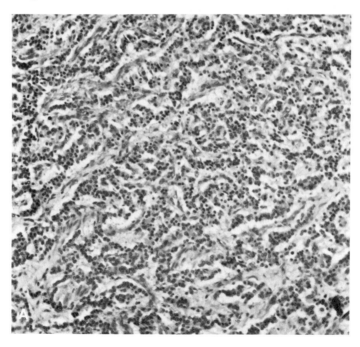

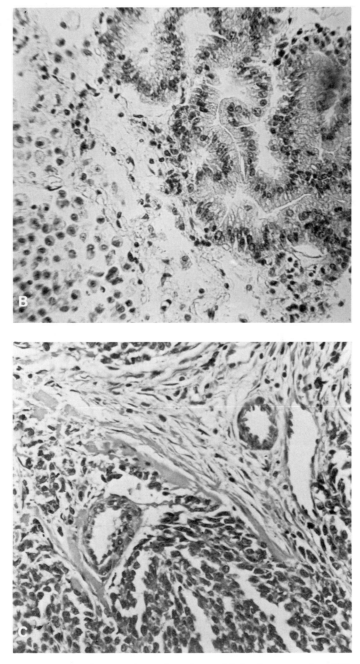

Fig. 12-1. Photomicrographs: (*A*) Bronchial adenoma. (×150) (*B*)
Pulmonary adenomatosis. (×200) (*C*) Pleural mesothelioma. (×150)

heavy cigarette smoker has five times the risk of the nonsmoker and, between the ages of 65 to 74, the risk is ten-fold for those starting the habit in their twenties. Among the other proved etiologic factors are exposure to industrial dusts or irritants including nickel, chromium, arsenic, cobalt, asbestos, hematite and radioactive ores. The intravenous administration of thorium dioxide for diagnosis, the use of antileukemic drugs such as busulfan and exposure to coal distillates containing 3,4 benzpyrene are similar hazards. The former use of arsenicals (Fowler's solution) for prolonged periods has been associated with lung cancers. (Robson, A. O. and Jelliffe, A. M.: Brit. Med. J., 5351:207, 1963.) The latent period between severe or chronic exposure and clinically detectable lung cancer varies from 7 to 19 years.

The carcinogenic action of most of the agents listed have been proved by the production of corresponding malignant tumors in animals. A particularly potent method is to absorb benzpyrene or other cancerogenic hydrocarbons on metallic dust and administer these intratracheally to the experimental animal.[52]

The incidence of lung cancer is both sex- and dose-dependent. It is five to six times more common in men and occurs a decade earlier. The peak of age incidence is between 50 and 60 years. Multiple tumors occurring in the same individual have become more frequent. This indicates increased severity of environmental exposure (regardless of the nature of the noxious inhalants), since it has been demonstrated experimentally that increasing the dose of the carcinogen increases the number of animals affected and the number of cancers per animal and shortens the time required for the appearance of malignancy within the limits of tolerance.

Precancerous Lesions. The more widespread use of roentgenograms of the chest in health surveys and of bronchoscopic examination for obtaining lung biopsies has added information regarding the histogenesis of these tumors. Loss of specialized function and structure in bronchial and alveolar epithelium is the earliest change. This is followed by squamous metaplasia and then atypical proliferating cellular foci in regions of scarring. These changes are multifocal in the respiratory tract in cigarette smokers and have been produced by cigarette smoke in dogs exposed for 410 days.[7] Hammond and Auerbach [47] trained beagles to inhale cigarette smoke (through tubes inserted in their throats) from nonfiltered cigarettes daily for 2.5 years (equivalent to about 18 years for humans) and produced typical precancerous changes.

No symptoms are present in the early stages of the disease and 25 to 35 percent of pulmonary cancers discovered in chest films are asymptomatic. In the roentgenogram, the lesion may be at the hilum where it resembles the structure of enlarged lymph nodes or it appears as a solitary peripheral lesion resembling the "coin" lesion of healed tuberculosis. Less than 15 percent of the tumors are under 2 cm. in diameter at the time of diagnosis suggesting a duration of over one year. The characteristic symptoms are nonspecific and include a combination of dyspnea, cough, chest pains, hemoptysis, wheezing and a low-grade fever. If the radiograph is inconclusive, additional methods of diagnosis are available. Radioisotopic scanning of the lung by the perfusion technique may be confirmatory (Chap. 3). If the lesion is small and peripheral, isotopic scanning is without value, since lesions under 2 to 3 cm. are not detected by this technique. However if the lesion is central and must be differentiated from mediastinal lymph nodes, the area of hypoperfusion by scanning is usually greater than the shadow depicted in the radiograph. The reason for hypoperfusion in the cancer stems largely from the fact that the cancer receives its blood supply from the bronchial rather than the pulmonary artery. The malignant lesion, therefore, tends to compress the vessels in the pulmonic circuit or, by bronchial obstruction, causes reflex vasoconstriction. In recent decades both central and peripheral forms of lung cancer are common (Fig. 12-2).

In a number of cases, diagnosis may be confirmed by finding malignant cells in the sputum or in bronchial washings obtained by means of the bronchoscope (Fig. 12-3). An additional refinement is to utilize bronchial catheterization in which brushing is employed to obtain exfoliated cellular

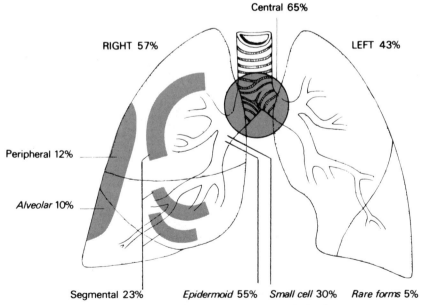

Fig. 12-2. Distribution of cancers of the lung.

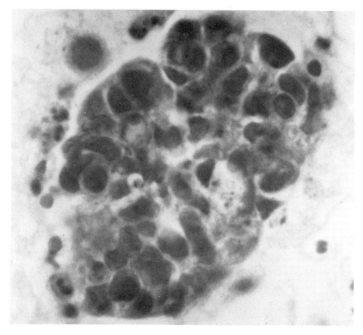

Fig. 12-3. Epidermoid bronchogenic carcinoma. Cells obtained from
bronchial washings. (×450)

material for microscopic examination.[92]   In the final analysis, biopsy by
the transthoracic technique is required if the tumor is considered resectable.

Pathologic Varieties of Lung Cancer. The major pathologic varieties of
lung cancer include *epidermoid carcinoma* of the large bronchi (45 to
55%) with a 5-year survival rate of 15 percent; *oat- or small cell carcinoma* from the reserve cells of the large bronchi (20% to 30%), with a
survival rate of 5 percent; and *adenocarcinoma* arising from the bronchioles
or alveolar lining (10% to 15%), with a survival rate of 12 to 14 percent.
Whereas epidermoid and oat-cell carcinomas are usually central or hilar in
location, the adenocarcinomas are usually peripheral. These peripheral
lesions are often associated with pulmonic scars, may appear as coin lesions
simulating healed tuberculosis or, in about 10 percent of the cases, arise as
bilateral multiple nodules.

The *epidermoid variety* (a hilar tumor) in its more differentiated forms
shows increasing degrees of keratinization or pearl formation and intracellular bridges of tonal fibrils and occurs in the right or left hilus (Fig.
12-4). Mitotic figures are atypical and conspicuous. The nucleus contains
a large nucleolus. A less differentiated variety resembles basal cell carcinoma of the epidermis. This type is more prevalent in men who are heavy

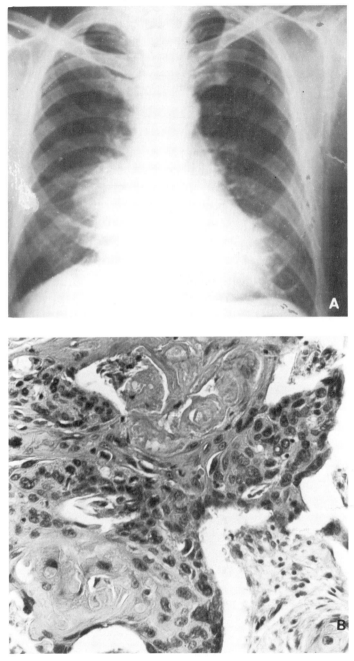

Fig. 12-4. Epidermoid bronchogenic carcinoma. (*A*) Roentgenogram;
(*B*) Photomicrograph. (×250)

smokers, usually produces bronchial obstruction with a zone of atelectasis and is often accompanied by bronchitis with fever, hemoptysis and severe loss of weight because of secondary infection.

The *small cell carcinoma* of the lung is also found at the hilum. It is highly malignant and often fatal within less than one year. The cells are only slightly larger than a lymphocyte and grow in sheets or trabeculae separated by fibrous strands. Small tubular structures or rosettes are formed in scattered areas (Fig. 12-5). Under the electronmicroscope, secretory granules resembling those found in argentaffine tumors of the gastrointestinal tract identify these as arising from argentaffine cells normally found in the bronchus and the bronchial mucous glands. Similar secretory droplets have now been identified in tumors of the adrenal medulla, in chemodectomas and in pancreatic islet tumors. Mast cells are often attracted to the tumor. The malignant carcinoid syndrome and Cushing's syndrome may occur in these patients and gonadotropins have at times been identified in the urine.[12]

In the three major types of cancer of the lung, epidermoid, oat-cell and adenocarcinoma, the plasma corticoids may be elevated, the result of the stimulating effect of the tumor on the pituitary-adrenal axis and increased binding of plasma corticoids to the plasma protein. Elevated plasma ACTH

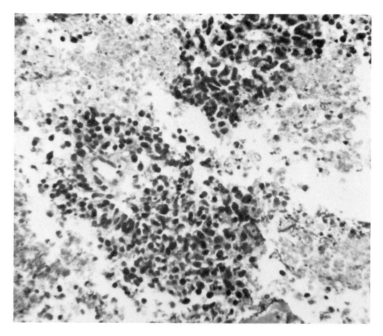

Fig. 12-5. Oat- or small-cell carcinoma. Photomicrograph. ($\times 150$)

may be an aid to diagnosis and also in following the result of treatment. The administration of prednisone or dexamethasone fails to suppress these plasma levels. In rare cases, ACTH-like material may be extracted from the tumor.

Adenocarcinoma and Bronchiolar Carcinoma. These tumors may give rise to papillary structures and irregular acinar formations. They invade the blood vessels and other portions of the lung early and, because of their usual peripheral location, show pleural invasion in approximately 80 percent of the cases. Metastasis to the mediastinal lymph nodes is demonstrable at the time of operation in over 40 percent of the cases. This tumor is less definitely related to smoking than other forms and the ratio of men to women is about 3:1. When arising in the smaller bronchi, the tumor extends downward into the alveoli, using the alveolar septa as its stroma for extension and growth. Examined with the electronmicroscope, these adenocarcinomas have elongated microvilli, numerous secretory vacuoles, abundant mitochondria and rough endoplastic reticulum.

Alveolar or adenomatous carcinoma is apparently a complication of benign alveolar adenomatosis in many instances. It is the one form of cancer in which malignant cells are apt to be found in the sputum. The nuclear membrane of the cell is irregular and the cytoplasm contains numerous vacuoles and blunt microvilli.[23]

Among the rare forms of cancer of the lung are adenomucoid, giant cell and carcinosarcoma. These are pathologic curiosities but do not differ from the standpoint of the patient from other forms of carcinoma of the lung (Fig. 12-6).

Cancers of the lung spread to other portions of the lung via the bronchi and tissue spaces, invade the pleura and result in hemorrhagic effusion, metastasize to the hilar lymph nodes and also disseminate via the blood stream to other organs such as the brain and bones (Fig. 12-7). In about 3 to 5 percent of the cases, a mediastinal shadow in the roentgenogram may not be clearly demonstrated and yet the tumor may metastasize widely to other organs, its origin from a bronchus being demonstrated only at autopsy.

The preferred treatment for carcinomas of the lung is resection of a lobe or lung. In the peripheral bronchiolar carcinomas, the number of operable cases is particularly high and has been reported as 80 percent. The peripheral coin lesions give the best results, with 5-year survivals ranging from 20 to 45 percent. The higher figure is for asymptomatic lesions discovered on routine x-ray films. Truly resectable epidermoid or squamous cell cancers of the large bronchi occur in less than 50 percent of the cases. In those resectable, about 25 percent will survive 5 years, which is about 12 percent for the entire group. Palliative lobectomies may be performed

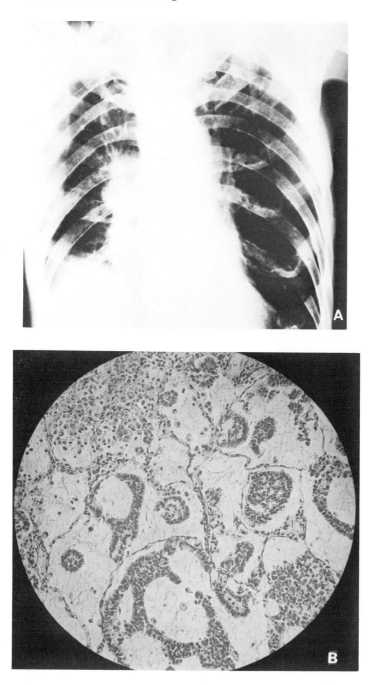

Fig. 12-6. (*A*) Adenomucoid carcinoma with rib involvement. (*B*) Bronchogenic adenomucoid carcinoma. Photomicrograph. (×100)

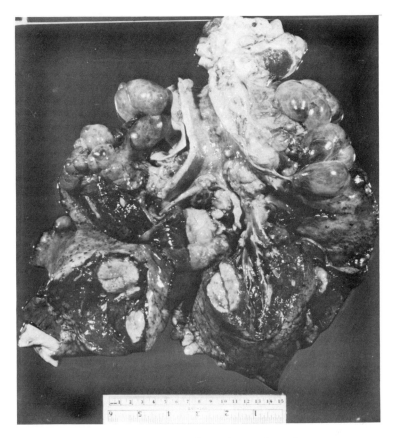

Fig. 12-7. Multiple nodules from intrapulmonic metastases.

in a number of these cases where mediastinal lymph nodes with involvement cannot be totally removed. With postoperative irradiation and chemotherapy, the survival time for these averages about two years.

The small or oat-cell carcinomas have the worst prognosis. Resectable forms are found in only one third of the cases and of these, only 5 percent, or approximately 1.5 percent of the series, survive 5 years. Postoperative irradiation and chemotherapy are used extensively in those cases where there is recurrence or where complete resection cannot be performed. The overall 5 year survival of all types is 9%.

Preoperative irradiation of cancer of the lung has been evaluated in a large series of cases. In over 500 patients with this disease, approximately one half received immediate surgery and the other half were given preoperative radiotherapy followed by surgery. The 3-year survival rates were the same in both groups and hence, no advantage was found for the preoperative treatment. In a like manner, 425 patients were considered inoperable and received extensive radiotherapy. In this group, 152 were considered resectable after treatment. These were again divided into two equal groups; one group was subjected to radical surgery, the other was not. Again, no difference was seen. It has been established that clinically inoperable cases cannot be rendered operable by radiotherapy. These are the results reported by the Committee for Radiation Therapy Studies,* established by the National Cancer Institute, of the U.S. Public Health Service covering the clinical years from May 1963 to December, 1966 at 17 medical centers.

Rare Forms of Juvenile Bronchogenic Carcinoma. Although intrathoracic sarcomas occur in the young, bronchogenic carcinoma of the lung in children is exceedingly rare and occurs before the age of 14 in less than 1 percent of the cases of all forms of bronchogenic carcinoma. Cayley and his coworkers state that in a review of 4,307 cases of bronchogenic carcinoma by Ochsner et al., 0.16 percent occurred in the first decade and 0.7 percent in the second. In the single case reported by Cayley et al., the patient (aged 13 years) had a small cell undifferentiated carcinoma of the left lung and was considered the 16th verified case in the literature.

In the case reported by Hauser,† the cancer appeared in a boy, 5½ months old. The tumor was of the undifferentiated type and was verified at autopsy. This case was not listed in the series reviewed by Cayley. It had been treated for 5 months under a diagnosis of whooping cough and was not suspected until the roentgenogram showed a homogenous shadow occupying the entire left hemithorax.

Among the cases in the literature, three have been associated with congenital malformations such as cystic disease of the lungs. This relation of infantile or juvenile cancer to anomalies of development is similar to the associated forms of malformation found in Wilm's tumor of the kidney in infants and in cancers in the first few years of life involving the liver. The association of these juvenile cancers with phases of retarded development is probably higher than recorded, since the associated malformation (such as absence of the iris with tumors of the kidney in infants) need not affect the organ in which the cancer appears. Instead, a functional immaturity of the affected organ may be of a biochemical nature (such as fetal hemoglobin in anemia) and not be apparent on microscopic examinations. None of the infantile forms of lung cancer has been diagnosed early enough to warrant an attempt at surgical resection.

Pulmonary Metastases. The lungs are a common site for metastatic growths. About 50 percent of all carcinomas at autopsy have pulmonary metastases, a percentage of involvement exceeded only by the lymph nodes

---

* Cancer, 23:419, 1969.
† Hauser, H.: Cancer of the Lung in Infancy. Radiology 89:33, 1942.

and liver. Sarcomas disseminating via the blood stream produce secondary deposits in the lung and in nearly 100 percent of the cases. With such metastatic involvement, the pleura and the ribs are frequently invaded accompanied by a bloody pleural effusion. If thoracentesis is performed and the fluid centrifuged, embedded, and sectioned, malignant cells are usually demonstrable. As metastatic involvement progresses, a persistent nonproductive cough and pleural pain are distressing symptoms. When the pulmonary lymphatics are involved by multiple miliary metastases, paroxysms of coughing terminating in vomiting may be uncontrollable. If the diaphragmatic surface is involved by extension from the pleura, (or from hepatic extension), pain on respiration may complicate the picture.

No therapeutic regime is helpful in these advanced stages of disseminated cancer. At times, irradiation or removal of the primary site of the cancer has resulted in the regression of metastases. This is excessively rare but has been reported for carcinoma of the kidney. With pulmonary metastasis from mammary carcinoma, testosterone therapy in women under age 55 or estrogen therapy in women past age 60, may produce temporary regression of these secondary deposits. Oophrectomy and/or adrenalectomy occasionally produce similar results. Chemotherapy rarely produces more than short-term, symptomatic results (2 to 4 months).

13

Therapy in Pulmonary Disease

In the past several decades, major therapeutic advances have changed the incidence and mortality of pulmonary diseases. The four major advances include: (1) antibiotics (penicillin, tetracycline and amphotericin B) for the control of pneumonitis; (2) combined isoniazid and streptomycin therapy with aminosalicylic acid for the control of tuberculosis; and, (3) cortisone and its synthetic derivatives for allergic bronchitis and alveolitis and forms of hypersensitivity. (4) The availability of oxygen therapy.

In spite of symptomatic relief by bronchial dilators in asthma and in emphysema, three major therapeutic voids persist. These are lack of specific treatment for viral infections and for emphysema, and the absence of chemotherapy to control bronchogenic carcinoma. The accompanying tables list the major drugs or therapeutic modalities available for the treatment of lung diseases.

MANAGEMENT OF RESPIRATORY FAILURE IN ADULTS

Respiratory failure is accompanied by changes in the blood P_{O_2}, P_{CO_2} and pH. It is important to determine whether or not there is a functional airway and, if the patient is conscious he should be encouraged to cough. The possibility of laryngeal edema or the presence of a foreign body must be ruled out. In severe cases of emphysema complicated by pneumonitis, tracheostomy (which is lifesaving if there is airway obstruction) may also be indicated. It allows better control for assisted ventilation, permits suction or cleaning out of the airway and reduces the volume of the anatomic dead space. Drowsiness or impending coma usually signifies CO_2 narcosis with a P_{CO_2} of 80 to 100 mm. Hg. Many of the manifestations of

Table 13-1. Antibiotic Therapy in Forms of Pneumonitis

Condition	Drug
Bacterial Pneumonitis	
Pneumococcal, streptococcal	Penicillin
Pneumococcal with complications	Penicillin or tetracycline
Staphylococcal	Synthetic penicillin salts Methicillin, Nafcillin, Oxacillin
Tularemia	Streptomycin, tetracycline, Chloramphenicol
Plague	Streptomycin, Chloramphenicol
Brucellosis	Streptomycin, tetracycline
Friedlander's bacillus	Sulfadiazine, streptomycin
Mycoplasma pneumoniae	Tetracycline
Hemophilus influenzae	Chloramphenicol, sulfonamides
Fungal or Mycotic Pneumonitis	
Histoplasmosis	
Coccidioidomycosis	Amphotericin B
Cryptococcosis	Iodides
Blastomycosis	
Pulmonary Tuberculosis	Isoniazid, streptomycin, aminosalicylic acid, Reserve Drugs Rifampicin, ethambutol
Schistosomiasis	Antimony potassium tartrate
Viral Pneumonitis Associated with the Common Cold (Palliative only)	Antipyretics Antihistamines Decongestants, expectorants Combinations of antihistamines adrenergic agents and codeine

respiratory failure are the result of acidosis, particularly if cardiac action is retarded and renal shutdown may be caused by the high P_{CO_2}. When the P_{CO_2} is higher than 100 mm. Hg, it is safe to reduce the level to about 60 mm. Hg, while maintaining oxygen saturation with 30 percent oxygen inhalation. This is to allow for the excretion of bicarbonate, which, if unusually high, will cause retention of serum potassium with cardiac damage. THAM-E is administered to control the pH level. In hospital practice, assisted ventilation by means of either a time-cycled or volume-cycled respirator may be used in severe cases.

The five major conditions for which such therapy is lifesaving are extensive pulmonary consolidation with pneumonitis, advanced emphysema

Table 13-2. Corticosteroid Therapy, Bronchial Dilators and Expectorants in Forms of Pulmonary Allergy and Hypersensitivity

CONDITION	DRUG
Bronchial Asthma Acute episodes	Cortisone or prednisone Isoproterenol inhalation Epinephrine injectable Aminophyllin intravenously
Bronchiectasis	Potassium iodide Pancreatic dormase (inhalant)
Extrinsic Allergic Alveolitis Organic dusts and spores	Cortisone or prednisone
Sarcoidosis	Cortisone or prednisone

Fibrosing Alveolitis
    Subacute—Hamman-Rich syndrome
    Desquamative interstitial pneumonia
    Scleroderma
	Cortisone or prednisone

Systemic Hypersensitivity with
    Lung Involvement
        Systemic lupus
        Periarteritis
        Wegener's granulomatosus
        Rheumatoid nodules
        Caplan's syndrome
	Cortisone or prednisone

Equivalent doses:
    Cortisone or hydrocortisone, 25 mg.
    Prednisolone or prednisone, 5 mg.
    Fluprednisolone, 2 mg.
    Dexamethasone, 0.75 mg.

usually complicated by pneumonitis, status asthmaticus, barbiturate poisoning and hypovolemic shock.

In nearly all cases of respiratory failure, there is a tendency to retain fluid in the lungs with resultant pulmonary edema. No adequate explanation is available, but the effect on the nervous system is associated with increased secretion of antidiuretic hormone (so-called "inappropriate secretion"). More specifically, anoxemia from any cause tends to produce increased permeability of the capillary bed. For this reason, the intake of fluids per os or intravenously should be limited in respiratory failure and the patient should be weighed repeatedly to guard against fluid retention. Diuretics should be administered. Increasing the intravascular volume with salt-poor albumin is not recommended because this fluid may leak

Table 13-3. Antibiotic Therapy in Bronchial Infections

CONDITION	DRUG OR OTHER THERAPY
Broncheolitis (Pertussis)	Chloramphenicol Oxytetracycline Gamma globulin
Chronic Bronchitis	Oxytetracycline Methacillin Bronchial dilators
Bronchiectasis	Oxytetracycline Methacillin Postural drainage Lobectomy (prolonged cases)

Table 13-4. Treatment of Pulmonary Edema and Thromboembolism

CONDITION	DRUG OR OTHER THERAPY
Pulmonary thromboembolism	Heparin (intravenous or intramuscular) Emergency embolectomy

Edema	Intravenous aminophylline
	Intravenous diuretics
	   (Ethacrynic acid-furosemide)
	Digitalis
	Intermittent tourniquets to
	   extremities with cardiac failure

into the alveolar spaces. In artificial respiration (with respirators or with a mask), it has been found helpful to maintain positive expiratory pressure at end of expiration in patients with severe hypoxemia. (Attachments to ventilators for producing adjustable expiratory plateau pressure are available commercially.) This has the effect of decreasing venous return to the right heart and to the lungs and preventing pulmonary venous engorgement and the pressure on the pulmonary capillaries inhibits pulmonary edema. During artificial ventilation, there is an increased tendency to pulmonary edema. In patients in shock or in cardiac failure, the administration of diuretics may be without the desired effects if renal blood flow is markedly decreased. The intravenous administration of vasopressor substances (such as Levophed, Aramine, or adrenalin) is indicated when renal function is depressed in this manner (Pontappidan).[71A]

TREATMENT IN THE RESPIRATORY DISTRESS SYNDROME OF THE NEWBORN

Prematurity, maternal diabetes, prolonged or abnormal labor or prolapsed cord are common causes of respiratory distress and threatened asphyxia in the newborn. Whereas a chest roentgenogram is the single most useful diagnostic aid in distinguishing cause, the establishment and maintenance of an airway by intubation and the artificial inflation of the lungs with air or oxygen can be undertaken immediately. Laboratory biochemical determinations of P_{CO_2}, pH and P_{O_2} from the capillary blood of the infant are important follow-up procedures. Oxygen tension in the arterial blood and hematocrit are helpful in determining the rational use of oxygen in the treatment of cyanosis and the significance of the cyanosis.

External cardiac massage, intubation, intermittent positive pressure by mask, correction of acidosis and hyperbaric oxygen are accepted emergency procedures for the treatment of respiratory distress in the infant.

In maternal drug addiction or with overdosage during labor, a morphine antagonist (N-allynormorphine or levallorphan, 0.2 mg./Kg. intravenously) is recommended.[7a]

Bibliography

1. Adams, D. O.: Experimental pine pollen granulomatous pneumonia in the rat. Am. J. Path., *49*:153, 1966.
2. Albert, B. L., and Sellers, T. F.: Coccidiomycosis from fomites. Arch. Int. Med., *112*:253, 1963.
3. Alexander, J. K., *et al.:* Studies on pulmonary blood flow in pneumococcal pneumonia. Cardiovasc. Res. Cent. Bull., *1*:86, 1963.
4. Allen, M. S., Jr., and Drash, E. C.: Primary melanoma of the lung. Cancer, *21*:154, 1968.
5. Antunes, M. L., and DaLuz, J. M. V.: Primary diffuse tracheo-bronchial amyloidosis. Thorax, *24*:307, 1969.
6. Attwood, H. D., and Park, W. W.: Embolism to the lungs by trophoblast. J. Obstet. Gynaec., *68*:611, 1961.
7. Auerbach, O., *et al.:* Histologic changes in bronchial tubes of cigarette smoking dogs. Cancer, *20*:2055, 1967.
7a. Avery, M. E.: The Lung and Its Disorders In The Newborn Infant, ed. 2. Philadelphia, Saunders, 1968.
8. Barnhard, H. J., *et al.:* Roentgenographic determination of total lung capacity. Am. J. Med., *28*:51, 1960.
9. Bates, D. V., and Christie, R. V.: Respiratory Function in Disease. Philadelphia, Saunders, 1964.
10. Baum, G. L., *et al.:* Left ventricular function in chronic obstructive lung disease. New Eng. J. Med., *285*:361, 1971.
11. Beerel, F. R., and Vance, J. W.: Daily PCO_2 and pH fluctuations in pulmonary emphysema with carbon dioxide retention. Am. Rev. Resp. Dis., *92*:894, 1965.
12. Bensch, K. G., *et al.:* Oat-cell carcinoma of the lung. Its origin and relation to bronchial carcinoma. Cancer, *22*:1163, 1968.
13. Blackford, S. D., and Casey, C. J.: Pleuro-pulmonary tularemia. Arch. Int. Med., *67*:43, 1941.
14. Bower, G.: Bronchial adenoma. Am. Rev. Resp. Dis., *92*:558, 1965.
15. Buckberg, G. D., *et al.:* Pulmonary changes following hemorrhagic shock and resuscitation in baboons. J. Thorac. Cardiov. Surg., *59*:450, 1970.

16. Buell, J., *et al.:* Carcinoma of the lung and Los Angeles type of air pollution. Cancer, *20:*1259, 1967.

17. Brisman, R., *et al.:* Carcinoma of the lung in four siblings. Cancer, *20:*2048, 1967.

18. Burrows, B., and Kettel, L. J.: Important considerations in emphysema —chronic bronchitis syndrome. Geriatrics, *24:*72, 1969.

19. Canetti, G.: Pathogenesis of tuberculosis in man. Ann. N.Y. Acad. Sci., *154:*13, 1968.

20. Canter, H. G., *et al.:* Dynamics of major airways in patients with lung disease. Am. Rev. Resp. Dis., *92:*932, 1965.

21. Cayley, C. K., *et al.:* Primary bronchogenic carcinoma of lung in children—Review of literature; report of case. Am. J. Dis. Child., *82:*49, 1951.

22. Chernick, V., *et al.:* Estimation of differential pulmonary blood flow by bronchoscopy and radioisotope scanning during rest and exercise. Am. Rev. Resp. Dis., *92:*958, 1965.

22a. Clements, J. A., *et al.:* Respiratory-distress syndrome: rapid test for surfactant in amniotic fluid. New Eng. J. Med., *286:*1077, 1972.

23. Coalson, J. J., *et al.:* Electron microscopy of neoplasms of the lung with special emphasis on alveolar cell carcinoma. Am. Rev. Resp. Dis., *101:*181, 1970.

24. Committee of Diagnostic Standards in Respiratory Diseases. Am. Rev. Resp. Dis., *101:*116, 1970.

25. Comroe, J. H. *et al.:* The Lung. Clinical Physiology and Pulmonary Function Tests. New York, Year Book, 1960.

26. Connell, J. T.: Asthmatic deaths. Role of the mast cell. JAMA, *215:*769, 1971.

27. Cullen, J. H., and Formel, P. F.: The respiratory defects in extreme obesity. Am. J. Med., *32:*525, 1962.

27a. Cumming, G. R. *et al.:* Unilateral hyperlucent lung syndrome in children. J. Pediat., *78:*250, 1971

28. Dayman, H. G., and Manning, L. E.: Pulmonary atelectasis—physical factors. Ann. Int. Med., *47:*460, 1957.

29. Dennis, J. M., and Bondreau, P. P.: Pleuropulmonary tularemia. Radiology, *68:*25, 1957.

30. Domingo, E. O., and Warren, K. S.: The inhibition of granuloma formation around Schistosoma mansoni eggs. Am. J. Path., *52:*613, 1968.

31. Drinker, C. K.: Pulmonary edema and inflammation. Cambridge, Mass., Harvard University Press, 1945.

32. Eaton, M. D., *et al.:* A virus from cases of atypical pneumonia; relation to the viruses of meningopneumonitis and psitticosis. J. Exp. Med., *73:*641, 1941.

33. Ebert, R. V., and Pierce, J. A.: Pathogenesis of pulmonary emphysema. Arch. Int. Med., *111:*34, 1963.

34. Edwards, L. B., and Palmer, C. F.: Identification of the tuberculous-infected by skin tests. Ann. N.Y. Acad. Sci., *154*:140, 1968.

35. Einthoven, W.: Ueber die Wirkung der Bronchialmuskeln nach einer neuen Methode untersucht, und ueber Asthma nervosum. Arch. ges Physiol., *51*:367, 1892.

36. Eriksson, S.: Studies in alpha$_1$-antitrypsin deficiency. Acta Med. Scand. [Supp.], *432*:6, 1965.

37. Escovitz, W. E., and Reingold, I. M.: Functioning malignant bronchial carcinoid with Cushing's syndrome and resultant sinus arrest. Ann. Int. Med., *54*:1248, 1961.

38. Evans, J. A.: Sliding hiatus hernia. Am. J. Roentgen., *68*:754, 1952.

39. Finegold, M. J.: Pneumonic plague in monkeys. Am. J. Path., *54*:167, 1969.

40. Finley, T. N., *et al.:* The cause of arterial hypoxemia at rest in patients with "alveolar-capillary block syndrome," J. Clin. Invest., *41*:618, 1962.

41. Fishman, A. P.: Respiratory gases in the regulation of pulmonary circulation. Physiol. Rev., *41*:214, 1961.

42. Fowler, W. S.: The respiratory dead space. Am. J. Physiol., *154*:405, 1948.

43. Gardner, P., and Fuller, E. W.: Fatal relapse of coccidioidomycosis ten years after treatment with amphotericin B. New Eng. J. Med., *281*:950, 1969.

44. Geschickter, C. F., and Popavichi, A.: Phrenic or postemphysematous hypertension. AMA Arch. Int. Med., *92*:767, 1953.

45. Geschickter, C. F.: Quinoline therapy in asthma. Southern Med. J., *48*:497, 1955.

45a. Gluck, L. *et al.:* Diagnosis of the respiratory distress syndrome by amniocentesis. Am. J. Obstet. Gynec., *109*:440, 1971.

45b. Gordon, H. W. *et al.:* alpha-antitrypsin (A, At) accumulation in livers of emphysematous patients with A_1-At^1 deficiency. Human Path., *3*:361, 1972.

46. Guyton, A. C., *et al.:* Basic oscillating mechanism of Cheyne-Stokes breathing. Am. J. Physiol., *187*:395, 1956.

47. Hammond, E., and Auerbach, O.: Brief communication. Today's Health News, May, 1970.

48. Hicken, P., *et al.:* The relation between the weight of the right ventricle and the percentage of abnormal air space in the lung in emphysema. J. Path. Bact., *92*:519, 1956.

49. Hill, J. D., *et al.:* Extracorporeal oxygenation for post-traumatic respiratory failure. New Eng. J. Med., *286*:629, 1972.

50. Holland, R. A. B.: Physiologic dead space in the Hamman-Rich syndrome. Physiologic and clinical implications. Am. J. Med., *28*:61, 1960.

51. Howell, D. S.: Hypertrophic osteoarthropathy and developmental connective tissue disorders. *In* Hollander, J. L.: Arthritis and Allied Conditions, ed. 7. Philadelphia, Lea & Febiger, 1966.
52. Humberger, F.: Chemical carcinogenesis in the Syrian golden hamster. Cancer, *23*:313, 1969.
53. Kapanci, Y.: Hypertensive pulmonary vascular disease. Am. J. Path., *47*:665, 1965.
54. Kay, S.: Histologic and histogenic observations on the peripheral adenoma of the lung. AMA Arch. Path., *65*:395, 1958.
55. Koffler, D., *et al.:* Immunologic studies concerning the pulmonary lesions in Goodpasture's syndrome. Am. J. Path., *54*:293, 1969.
56. Kuykendall, S. J., *et al.:* Pulmonary cryptococcosis. New Eng. J. Med., *257*:1009, 1957.
57. Lancaster, J. F., and Tomashefski, J. F.: Tuberculosis as a cause of emphysema. Amer. Rev. Resp. Dis., *87*:435, 1963.
58. Latham, E. F., *et al.:* Pulmonary hyalus-like membrane. Bull. Johns Hopkins Hosp., *96*:173, 1955.
59. Liliequist, B., and Link, H.: Wegener's granulomatosis. Report of a case. Angiology, *19*:215, 1968.
60. Lillie, R. D.: Histopathologic Technique and Practical Histochemistry, ed. 3. New York, McGraw-Hill, 1965.
60a. Lindsay, M. I., Jr., *et al.:* Hong Kong influenza. JAMA, *214*:1825, 1970.
61. Lowell, A. M., *et al.:* Tuberculosis. Sections I & II. Cambridge, Harvard University Press, 1969.
62. Mainwaring, A. R., *et al.:* Localized amyloidosis in the lower respiratory tract. Thorax, *24*:441, 1969.
63. Mather, G., *et al.:* Liver biopsy in sarcoidosis. Quart. Med. J., *24*:331, 1955.
64. Mather, C. L., and Hamlin, G. B.: Pulmonary alveolar proteinosis. New Eng. J. Med., *272*:1156, 1965.
64a. McCombs, R. P.: Diseases due to immunologic reactions in the lungs. New Eng. J. Med. *286*:1186, 1972.
65. Medlar, E. M.: The behavior of pulmonary tuberculosis lesions. A pathologic study. Amer. Rev. Tuberc. *2*:1, 1955.
65a. Morgan, T. E.: Pulmonary surfactant. New Eng. J. Med., *284*:1185, 1971.
66. Morgan, W. K., and Lapp, N. L.: Cardiopulmonary function in uranium miners. Amer. Rev. Resp. Dis., *102*:124, 1970.
67. Morse, S. I.: Staphylococci and other micrococci. *In* Dubos, R. and Hirsch, J.: Bacterial and Mycotic Infections of Man, ed. 4. Philadelphia, Lippincott, 1965.
68. Naeye, R. L.: Advanced pulmonary vascular changes in schistosomal cor pulmonale. Am. J. Trop. Med., *10*:191, 1961.
69. ————: Hypoxemia and pulmonary hypertension. Arch. Path., *71*:447, 1961.

69a. Nash, G., *et al.:* Alveolar cell carcinoma: does it exist? Cancer, *29*:322, 1972.

70. Novack, S. N., and Pearson, C. M.: Cyclophosphamide therapy in Wegener's granulomatosis. New Eng. J. Med., *284*:938, 1971.

71. Parker, J. D., *et al.:* Pulmonary aspergillosis in sanitoriums in South Central United States. Am. Rev. Resp. Dis., *101*:551, 1970.

71a. Pontappidan, H., *et al.:* Acute respiratory failure in the adult. New Eng. J. Med., *287*:690, 743, 799, 1972.

72. Potter, E. L.: Pathology of the Fetus and Newborn. Chicago, Year Book, 1953.

73. Pushpakom, R., *et al.:* Experimental papain-induced emphysema in dogs. Am. Rev. Resp. Dis., *102*:778, 1970.

74. Rakower, J.: Sarcoidal bilateral hilar lymphoma. Lofgren's syndrome. Am. Rev. Resp. Dis., *87*:518, 1963.

75. Read, J., and Williams, R. S.: Pulmonary ventilation. Blood flow relationships in interstitial disease of the lungs. Am. J. Med. *27*:545, 1959.

76. Resnick, K., *et al.:* Immunoglobulin concentrations in berylliosis. Am. Rev. Resp. Dis., *101*:504, 1970.

77. Rich, A. R.: The Pathogenesis of Tuberculosis. Springfield, Thomas, 1951.

77a. Robson, A. D. and Jelliffe, A. M.: Medicinal arsenic poisoning and lung cancer. Brit. Med. J., *5351*:207, 1963.

78. Rotsztain, A., *et al.:* Blood gas changes during voluntary hyperventilation in normal and disease states. Am. Rev. Resp. Dis., *102*:205, 1970.

79. Roughton, F. J. W.: Average time spent by blood in human lungs. Am. J. Physiol., *143*:621, 1945.

80. Saidi, F., and Nazarian, I.: Surgical treatment of hydatid cysts by freezing of cyst wall and installation of 0.5% silver nitrate solution. New Eng. J. Med., *284*:1346, 1971.

81. Sasahara, A. A., *et al.:* Problems in the diagnosis and management of pulmonary embolism. Sem. Nuclear Med., *1*:122, 1971.

82. Sawyer, K. C., *et al.:* Fatal primary cancer of lung in teen age smoker. Cancer, *20*:451, 1967.

83. Schrag, P. E., and Gullet, A. D.: Byssinosis in cotton textile worker. Am. Rev. Resp. Dis., *101*:497, 1970.

84. Searcy, R. I.: Diagnostic Biochemistry. New York, McGraw-Hill, 1969.

85. Siebert, F., and Fisher, E. R.: Bronchiolar emphysema. Am. J. Path., *33*:1137, 1957.

85a. Siegel, H.: Human pulmonary pathology associated with narcotics and other addictive drugs. Human Path., *3*:55, 1972.

86. Silverberg, E., and Grant R. N.: Cancer statistics, 1970. CA, *20*:11, 1970.

87. Spencer, H.: Pathology of the Lung. New York, Macmillan, 1962.

88. Stein, I., *et al.:* Living Bone in Health and Disease. Philadelphia, Lippincott, 1955.

89. Stevens, P. M., *et al.:* Regional ventilation and perfusion after lung transplantation in patients with emphysema. New Eng. J. Med., *282*:245, 1970.

90. Storstein, O.: Circulatory failure in metastatic carcinoma of the lung. A physiologic and pathologic study of its pathogenesis. Circulation, *4*:913, 1951.

91. Svanborg, N.: Studies on the cardiopulmonary function in sarcoidosis. Acta. Med. Scand. [Suppl.] *366,* 1961.

91a. Swanson, E. W. *et al.:* Unilateral hypoventilation in man during temporary occlusion of one pulmonary artery. J. Clin. Invest., *40*:828, 1961.

91b. Szentivanyi, A.: Beta adrenergic therapy of the atopic abnormality in bronchial asthma. J. Allergy *42*:203, 1968.

91c. Taplin, G. V., and MacDonald, N. S.: Radiochemistry of macroaggregated albumin and newer lung scanning agents. *In* Freeman, L. M. and Blaufox, M. D.: Seminars in Nuclear Medicine, *1*:132, 1971.

92. Thiede, W. H., and Banaszak, E. F.: Selective bronchial catheterization. New Eng. J. Med., *286*:526, 1972.

93. Thurlbeck, W. M.: Incidence of pulmonary emphysema: With observations on relative incidence and spatial distribution of various types of emphysema. Am. Rev. Resp. Dis., *87*:206, 1963.

94. Tigertt, W. D.: Soviet viable Pasteurella tularensis vaccines. A review of selected articles. Bact. Rev., *26*:354, 1962.

95. Walsh, J. J.: Spontaneous pneumothorax. Dis. Chest, *29*:329, 1956.

96. West, J. B.: Oxygen transfer by the lung. *In* International Anesthesiology Clinics: Oxygen Measurements in Blood and Tissues and Their Significance. Boston, Little Brown, *4*:13, 1966.

97. ———: Causes of carbon dioxide retention in lung disease. New Eng. J. Med., *284*:1232, 1971.

98. White, B., and Geschickter, C. F.: Diagnosis in Daily Practice. Philadelphia, Lippincott, 1947.

99. Wilford, R. L., and Kaplan, L. A.: Pulmonary fibrosis and giant cell reaction with altered elastic tissues—endogenous pneumoconiosis. Arch. Path., *63*:75, 1957.

100. Williams, E. D., and Celestin, I. R.: Association of bronchial carcinoid and periglandular adenomatosis. Thorax, *17*:120, 1962.

101. Williams, M. H., Jr., and Zohman, L. R.: Cardiopulmonary function in bronchial asthma. Am. Rev. Resp. Dis., *81*:173, 1960.

102. Wilson, J. W., *et al.:* The lung in hemorrhagic shock. Am. J. Path. *58*: 337, 1970.

103. Winternitz, M. C., *et al.:* The Pathology of Influenza. New Haven, Yale Univ. Press, 1920.

Index

Numerals in italics indicate a figure, "t" following a page number indicates a table concerning the subject mentioned.

219

Wrestle Radio USA

Grapplers Speak

Ed Symkus and Vinnie Carolan

Published by ECW PRESS
2120 Queen Street East, Suite 200, Toronto, Ontario, Canada M4E 1E2

NATIONAL LIBRARY OF CANADA CATALOGUING IN PUBLICATION

Carolan, Vinnie
Wrestle Radio U.S.A.: grapplers speak / Vinnie Carolan and Ed Symkus.

ISBN 1-55022-646-0

1. Wrestlers — Interviews. 2. Wrestling. I. Symkus, Ed II. Title

GV1196.A1C37 2004   796.812'092'2   C2004-900614-2

Editor: Michael Holmes
Cover and Text Design: Darren Holmes
Cover illustration: Getty Images
Production & Typesetting: Mary Bowness
Printing: Transcontinental

This book is set in Goudy and Legacy.

The publication of *Wrestle Radio* has been generously supported by the Canada Council,
the Ontario Arts Council, the Ontario Media Development Corporation, and the
Government of Canada through the Book Publishing Industry
Development Program. **Canadä**

DISTRIBUTION
CANADA: Jaguar Book Group, 100 Armstrong Avenue, Georgetown, ON, L7G 5S4
UNITED STATES: Independent Publishers Group, 814 North Franklin Street,
Chicago, Illinois 60610

PRINTED AND BOUND IN CANADA

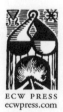

ECW PRESS
ecwpress.com

Wrestle Radio USA
Grapplers Speak

Ed Symkus and Vinnie Carolan

ECW PRESS

Acknowledgments

This whole experience, from doing the show to transcribing the interviews and watching the whole process of a book taking shape, has been a trip. My whole-hearted thanks go out to so many people who helped make it all happen: to my wife Lisa, for giving me all those precious Saturday afternoons to do the show and for still letting me have the TV on Monday and Thursday nights (when "Survivor" isn't on), I love you baby; to my mother and father, Jean and Ray, looking down from above, who probably never knew exactly what fascinated me about wrestling, but did watch with me from time to time; to my brother Alan, who went with me to plenty of matches, but can't remember the night George Steele lunged at us in the stands; to my grandfather, Hyman Oldsman, who watched religiously, yelled at the heels on TV, and always thought it was real; to Don Sandler, for giving us all that WMSX airtime and the freedom to do whatever we wanted with it; to Sheldon Goldberg, the best substitute host on the East Coast and quite the wrestling historian; to Bruno Sammartino and Killer Kowalski, because they were in the first match I remember seeing; and to every single person who took part in making the show a success, from engineer extraordinaire Dan Collier to Bruce "Mr. Breaking News" Mitchell to the greatest fan we could ever have hoped for, the Democratic Cowboy. And to Vinnie — Hey, pardner, I still can't figure out who was the comic and who was the straight man, but we made a hell of an entertaining team, didn't we?

— *Ed Symkus*

I can't express how proud I am of this book. Reading the final manuscript was one of the most joyous things I've ever done. And in reflecting on how I've gotten to this point, I need to thank many people.

I first want to thank my oldest brother, Kenny. Had he not turned me on to the radio show "Talking Trivia" in 1981, I would not have become friends with the host and producer of the show and would never have had the opportunity to co-host a wrestling radio program. Thank you, Ken.

I want to thank Neil Flicker and Morgan White Jr. for breaking me into commercial radio at an early age. I cannot express how grateful I am, as much was learned by watching you two work. And if it wasn't for Neil introducing me to WMSX General Manager Don Sandler, the program most likely would never have happened in the first place.

I want to thank Don Sandler for taking a chance on a young guy who simply had an idea. You didn't have to, but you did. Also to Dan Collier, Pat McDonough, Rich, Jeff, Neil, Mike and all of the other engineers that helped produced the show.

I want to thank Bruce Mitchell for being a loyal contributor to the program during its final years. Hey Bruce, the Pats may have won the Super Bowl, but you'll always be a champ in Boston.

A big thanks to Lou "PPV" Fortuna for allowing me to watch the big shows at his home (hey, I'm cheap).

I want to thank Mick Foley for setting the trend for good commercial wrestling books.

I want to thank the *Observer* for keeping me interested and informed for all these years.

And I absolutely want give a big bear hug to Jack David and Michael Holmes for the opportunity to write this book. It's been a dream come true and it wouldn't have happened without you two. Thank you.

I want to thank my mom, dad, Sean, Billy, Ken, Greg, Chrissy, Weezy Wallace, Lisa Becker (for keeping Ed in check), Grandma Doris and Nana Kathleen for their inspiration over the years. I love you guys.

And the two incredibly important people in my life who are the reason I could give 110% effort to help make this book so good.

To my love, Tracy. Your idea for the microphone was superb. Thank you for being there. I owe you lots of dinners. I love you!

And to my buddy and pal, Ed. What can I say? We make a fantastic team. I am the luckiest guy in the world to have met you and to be able to call you my friend. I've learned a lot. You really are the best and I'm going to finish it off with two simple words for you: "RE-UNION?"

— *Vinnie Carolan*

Photo Credits

2 Cold Scorpio, Chris Benoit, Mick Foley, Terry Funk, Eddie Gilbert, Jim Ross, Sandman, Pez Whatley: photos by Pete Lederberg (plmathfoto@hotmail.com). More rare and important photos from the Pete Lederberg collection can be found at http://home.bellsouth.net/p/PWP-flwrestlingpix.

Ric Flair, Terry Funk and Dusty Rhodes, Killer Kowalski, Fabulous Moolah, Fabulous Moolah and Vicky Williams, Bruno Sammartino, Kevin Sullivan, Terry Taylor, Lou Thesz: photo by Ruth Oman, courtesy of Pete Lederberg collection.

Lou Albano, Gordon Solie and Dusty Rhodes, Gordon Solie and Superstar Billy Graham, George Steele (page 123): photo by Brian Berkowitz, courtesy of Pete Lederberg collection.

Ricky Steamboat: photo by Don Freedman, courtesy of Pete Lederberg collection.

Hacksaw Jim Duggan: photo by Emanuel Melo.

George Steele (page 131): photo by Ed Symkus.

Chris Benoit (page 230), Jim Ross (page 219), Jim Ross and Paul Heyman, Triple H: photos by Mark Fissette.

Johnny B. Badd, Missy Hyatt, Sherri Martel: photos by Marko Shark.

Marcus Bagwell, Booker T, Eddie Guerrero, Shawn Michaels, Madusa Miceli, Kevin Nash, Steven Regal, Tony Shiavone, Vader: photos by Dr. Mike Lano, courtesy of the Dr. Mike Lano collection.

Contents

The Announcers

The Wrestlers Part 3: December 1995–January 1997

Introduction

When "Wrestle Radio USA" was first broadcast from the Brockton, Mass., ranch-house studios of WMSX-AM in August, 1992, the show ran for one hour, and consisted of news culled from Dave Meltzer's "Wrestling Observer Newsletter" and Wade Keller's "Pro Wrestling Torch"; notes and opinions on recent wrestling TV shows; a handful of phone calls from curious listeners; and two very green hosts who had only met each other about an hour before their first show.

By the time the show ended its run in January, 1997, it ran for two hours, and consisted of: news phoned in each week by wrestling journalists; notes and opinions of recent wrestling TV shows; live interviews with wrestlers, announcers, referees, and bookers; wrestling-related trivia games; a great deal of studio production work; an endless line of callers waiting to come on; and two seasoned producer-writer-host-interviewers who made an incredible tag team.

It was an odd and exciting period to be fans of pro wrestling. Around the time the show went on the air, Vince McMahon Jr.'s World Wrestling Federation was just beginning to fall into a tailspin that would bring it from the full houses and high Nielsen figures of its Hulk Hogan-led renaissance in the 1980s to half-empty arenas and lower television ratings. The WWF wouldn't fully recover until around 1996. And a year or two into the show, Ted Turner's upstart World Championship Wrestling — an offshoot of the National Wrestling Alliance — started building up a fan base. Perhaps it was McMahon's arrogance that led to a turning of the tide. But for whatever reason, by late 1995, WCW was starting to outscore the WWF in the weekly TV ratings. Coincidentally, WCW readily provided guests to be interviewed on the show, while the WWF rarely bothered to return phone calls, only jumping on the bandwagon a couple of years into the show's tenure, and even then only occasionally.

But there wasn't any hesitation from the marketing department of WCW. They knew a good opportunity when they heard it. Initial contact with them revealed relatively few concerns: what kinds of questions would be asked, how many people would be listening and where, and how powerful the signal was. Told that questions would be "inside" but respectful of the business, that listeners were all over Eastern Massachusetts, and that the station had a small 1,000-watt signal, they immediately started offering up guests.

Those guests were usually contacted the day before a broadcast, and they were asked to do the interviews out of character, to discuss behind-the-scenes situations, and be as honest and open as possible. Amazingly, almost every one of them agreed. If memory serves, the only ones who didn't cooperate, and either stayed in character or pretended wrestling was "real," were Chief Jay Strongbow and Colonel Rob Parker, whose interviews do not appear in this book. Highlights, for reasons that will be clear after reading them, were interviews with Mick Foley, Madusa Miceli, and Eddie Gilbert.

It's still surprising that so many people did agree to our requests, as these were the days when the wrestling business was still pretty much protected by everyone involved. Maybe it was a breath of fresh air for these men and women to talk as real people instead of playing a character—especially when management clearly did not object.

Wrestle Radio USA interviews worked for multiple reasons. We were not only longtime fans; we were also students of the game. We did a great deal of research and preparation. And often, just for kicks, one of us would book an interview but not tell the other who it was until they were on the phone, live. The idea sounds reckless, but it kept us on our toes, led to some wonderfully spontaneous questions, and made for great listening.

A decision was made early on not to let our callers talk with wrestlers. We would take calls before the guests came on and write down any questions they had, but the wrestlers would only speak with us. We had two reasons for this policy — we wanted to avoid the possibility of embarrassing our guests and, selfishly, we wanted them all to ourselves.

The following interviews are presented, almost verbatim, in the question-and-answer format we used on the show. They're of a specific time, when change was in the air, and pro wrestling was about to become more popular than any promoter could have dreamed possible. Looking back, we're still happily stunned at the way almost all of them played out.

— Ed Symkus and Vinnie Carolan

The Wrestlers Part 1: June 1993–April 1994

Professional wrestling is not the sport it used to be. Showbiz long ago superseded simple displays of athletic skill — creating careers for talented writers and bringing in much larger audiences. But there's no doubt that today's performers are also in better shape and able to do wilder and more dangerous moves than their predecessors ever were. There's more high flying; there are crazier, "hard core" matches; and the profession's smaller, more agile stars can do things the big men of yesteryear never even considered.

Of course, some things never change. Yesterday and today, three things remain constant: the winner of the match is predetermined, the contestants know what the finishing move will be, and they know how long the match is supposed to take. One major difference these days is that some wrestlers don't just tease the audience about doing a suplex from the ring to the floor. There are times when they actually fly over the top rope and hit that floor.

But the biggest change in the business is that the performers talk openly about themselves, obviously in scripted form, but with a wink of the eye, letting the truth play into the storyline. This was rarely done, even up to the days when "Wrestle Radio USA" was first on the air. Aside from a few other insider radio shows, the unspoken rule was to play the character and protect the business.

Perhaps it was just the right time to ask the wrestlers interviewed here to open up and share some inside, backstage information. Maybe they were itching to get the stories out there; maybe it was because there were no bosses around to tell them not to do it.

In presenting themselves out of character, most of these folks came across as sharp and funny and well aware that they were involved in a very odd profession. They also seemed to have a ball talking about it.

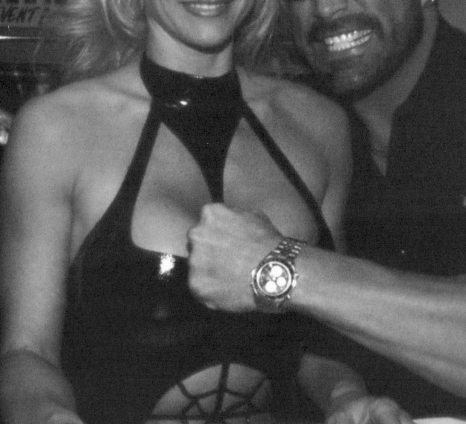

Johnny B. Badd
June 1993

Marc Mero will always be remembered by insiders for his marriage to Rena Mero aka Sable. But during his career in wcw, Johnny B. Badd was regarded as an entertaining mid-carder. When he later joined the wwf, his gimmick flopped. In this interview, he talks about winning the Golden Gloves boxing title in New York, and how he broke into wrestling. He also shared some revealing thoughts on morale in wrestling as well as on drug usage in the business — others' and his own. He was one of the few guests who remained partly in character, probably for entertainment value, but he answered all of the questions in a straightforward manner.

Johnny B. Badd, where are you right now?

I'm calling from Columbia, South Carolina. I'm going to be wrestling in Bishopville, 45 miles outside of Columbia. I was out working out at the gym and just got back to my hotel room.

Who are you going up against tonight?

I'm going against Michael P.S. Hayes and I'll tell ya, it's going to be a blessin' to teach him a lesson.

Who's been an influence?

I was born in Macon [Georgia], but I grew up in Buffalo and Syracuse, New York. When I was a young boy, my dad used to take us to matches and there was a guy named Chief White Owl and there was Johnny Powers, Ernie Ladd, and Fritz Von Erich. I grew up on these guys. Seeing old tapes of Gorgeous George and of course, Dusty Rhodes.

How has WCW changed in the two years you've been there?

Well, it's tough. There have been some ups and downs in not just World Championship Wrestling, but in all of professional wrestling. It's hard, because you get some new bosses in and they come and they go and they look like they're on track and things kind of fall apart. Right now, we're in a rebuilding process and I've got faith in our leaders now and I'm really hoping that Bob Dhue and Bill Shaw can really make this work now.

How is morale with the company as opposed to six months ago?

Much better. It's more relaxed, there's a lot more laughter. Guys are kind of back to themselves. Wrestlers have kind of been known for having fun and pulling ribs on each other, and all that's kind of back right now. So morale is up again.

Not a lot of laughter going on toward the end of the Bill Watts regime?

No, there wasn't. It got a little too serious, with all the fines and different things. It was more like boot camp, you know? We're grown men, and I don't think you talk to grown men like that. We know what we've gotta do out there. We know that wrestling is a tough business because you're wrestling probably 200–275 times a year.

Is that your schedule?

Yes, I'm under contact where I have to wrestle 200 times a year. I hope to get about 250 in this year. God willing, and I don't get hurt.

Now, you've officially renewed your contract?

Yes, I am renewed with World Championship Wrestling. I'm glad because I want to be a part of a rebuilding process and I want to see this become something. And I'm hoping that I'm going to be a big part of that.

It's no secret that at one point there was talk of you going to the World Wrestling Federation. In fact, Hulk Hogan personally had a discussion with you and tried to persuade you to go to the opposing organization. How far did those negotiations go and how serious were they?

It was very close. I had talked with Vince and I was just about there. It was that close. I had one more meeting with Bill Shaw and Bob Dhue and we all sat down and I told them what I wanted. I wanted to be a part of this organization. I didn't want to be the guy that was always looking in. I wanted to be a big part. And that's the only reason I wanted to stay, because I wanted to be a part of it. I put a lot of effort into learning — I've only been doing it for two years and, just like anything else, it's not something you can grasp overnight. It takes time to learn a lot about wrestling. I was a former boxer and going from boxing to wrestling is a very hard transition.

Well, can you tell us about that? Apparently you were involved with the Golden Gloves?

I won the New York State Golden Gloves. I won the state title five times, including the State Golden Gloves, the Empire State Games and also the EAU. I was 48-2 with 37 KOs, 16 in the first round, and I was a member of the U.S. Boxing team. Boxing was always my true love. I retired from boxing in 1986 and I decided to — well, after a long layoff, I was building round swimming pools in Florida — and then I gave wrestling a try in 1991. I feel so blessed to be in wrestling, especially meeting the fans. I have such a good time with the fans.

What got you in there? Why wrestling?

Well, you know, boxing is a sport. It's a one-on-one competition. You're out there in the limelight. It's kind of a do-or-die situation. Wrestling gave me that same competitive spirit. I went to a wrestling camp in Florida, Boris Malenko's training school in Tampa. And shortly after that, I was only there for a couple of weeks, I got a shot with World Championship Wrestling.

Just a couple of weeks?

Yeah. I think it was a total of six weeks working with WCW before I got a contract. I was really blessed, very lucky. But it's also very hard because you're basically learning and it's kind of on-the-job training. It was a little difficult at first and still is. Not that it's difficult completely, but I put a lot of effort into it. On my days off, I try to get down to the school and work with Jody Hamilton to keep upgrading my skills. I realize that I've got a long ways to go in every aspect of wrestling and I really want to put forth the effort to be a great wrestler.

Was it Dusty Rhodes who brought you in originally?

Yes. Dusty Rhodes first took a look at me and said, "Geez, you look just like Little Richard." And I said, "Oh hush, you big ol' ugly bear."

Now when you came in 1991, Jim Herd was running things. How would you compare working for Jim Herd, Kip Frey, and Bill Watts?

Well, I never really got to know Jim Herd, and Kip Frey wasn't there long enough to get to know, and Bill Watts I really didn't want to know.

It's a shame that Kip Frey didn't get more time because people were pointing fingers at him, claiming he was only a lawyer, when it appears that he really didn't get a fair shake.

The thing I liked about Kip Frey was that he had a vision and he realized that wrestling had to have entertainment involved with it. And he started to get us involved with people in Hollywood; he was going in that direction, which I thought was the right move.

And he would give incentives to the wrestlers who were working harder.

That's right. That's great for morale. I'll tell ya, Kip Frey I think had the right vision, but I don't think he had the experience to really put it all together. But I believe right now that Bob Dhue and Bill Shaw have a vision also. I sat and talked with these guys many times in meetings and I really believe that it's going to take some time now. It's going to take some time to really pull this together. There are some people that are going to have to put forth the effort, not just the wrestlers, but also the people in the office. I really believe that it's going to be a whole team effort right now. And if the guys aren't working hard, I think they should get rid of them. There's got to be a real standard in wcw if you want to make this work.

How was the transition for you of going from heel to babyface and whose idea was it?

Well, even in the other sports that I played — I was All-State in football and All-State in hockey, I liked to do different things. I used to get in trouble for wearing different pieces of equipment that I wasn't supposed to be wearing. I used to have long hair and I'd wear these bandanas coming out of the back of my football helmet and the coach would go crazy when I wore this stuff, but I would continue to do it. Now I can wear whatever I want and it's just crazy.

But let's stick with the transition for a second. Did you have trouble winning over the crowd as a babyface?

Well, the thing about wrestling is that people pay to have a good time. If they see someone having a good time, they're going to have a good time. So when they first saw me, they saw I was having a good time. People see me having fun and then they start to have fun.

Any chance of having a boxing match with Paul Roma, who's recently done some bouts?

Not sure who he is.

He just joined the Horsemen after Slamboree.

Oh, he's a Horseman. I'd love to be the first one to knock him off that horse.

OK. What would have been your role with Vince? Would you have gone up against Hogan early on?

No, they'd slowly build me. That's fine, because I'm still learning. Sometimes in this business people get thrown in where they don't belong. And then there's no future interest. I think if you build something slowly, it stays around a little bit longer.

What part do you have in the growth of your character at this point?

I control all of it right now. From costumes, to everything, they let me do pretty much what I want to do right now.

That's got to be a nice feeling.

It is because I have a lot of fun outside of this. I visit schools and tell kids the importance of an education and staying in schools and staying away from drugs.

Do you travel with Teddy Long doing this?

Teddy and I do a lot together but I do a lot on my own. It's a similar message that Teddy sends, but I also visit a lot of nursing homes. These are our forgotten generation, you know? They are wonderful and they're such big wrestling fans. I've gone to so many nursing homes. I went to one nursing home and they were all elderly black folks. I walk in and they were going crazy. I looked at the director because I couldn't believe it. This little lady came out of the wheelchair and hugged me and wouldn't let go. I looked at the director, because I couldn't understand it. "This is unbelievable and they must love wcw," I thought. Then the lady looks at me and says, "I've been watching you grow up in Macon, Georgia and I have all your albums." Then it hit me that she and all the friends thought that I was Little Richard. So, I sang "Tutti Frutti" to 45 elderly folks.

What kind of message did you give them?

I let them know that I love them and give them hope and we just have fun. They're so great, and it's sad to see them alone and looking out the window, so I put my arm around them and give them the kiss that don't miss and that makes their day.

Now, you just mentioned that you talk to kids about drugs and so forth. It seems that Vince's testing system is working in the WWF because wrestlers are getting smaller. Will this ever be successfully introduced in WCW?

I've got to commend Vince in the wwf, and I talked to Bill Shaw about this because we've got to have mandatory testing in wcw.

It's going to come to the point where someone's going to get sick.

Yeah, and these kids are the ones that look up to them, and if wrestlers in wcw start doing steroids, those kids are going to do steroids. One thing is that I don't do steroids, I don't want to do any drugs.

Have you ever done steroids?

Yes, I have done steroids. It was a mistake that I made and I regret doing it, and I tell these kids that. I'm honest with these kids, because I don't want to lie, 'cause it comes back, and then I let these kids down. But I have made mistakes, I have used steroids in the past and I will never do another steroid again. I'm blessed — I'm not as big as I used to be — I'm only 225 pounds.

No one should be against that. In Japan, they push you on ability and that should be reflected over here.

Right, and I really hope they start testing in wcw.

Any ideas if WCW will implement a plan soon?

There's lots of rumors that we'll be getting one soon and we'll have to weed the bad apples out.

Do you think there are wrestlers in the WCW office using steroids now, not mentioning any names?

There's a lot of speculating, but the main thing is to start testing and get these guys help or get them out of professional wrestling because they won't be able to go to New York (the wwf).

It's not needed.

We really don't need it. Guys might complain that we're in the ring and get hurt a lot, but wrestlers 20 to 30 years ago and before that, they never used steroids and they were as rough as we are.

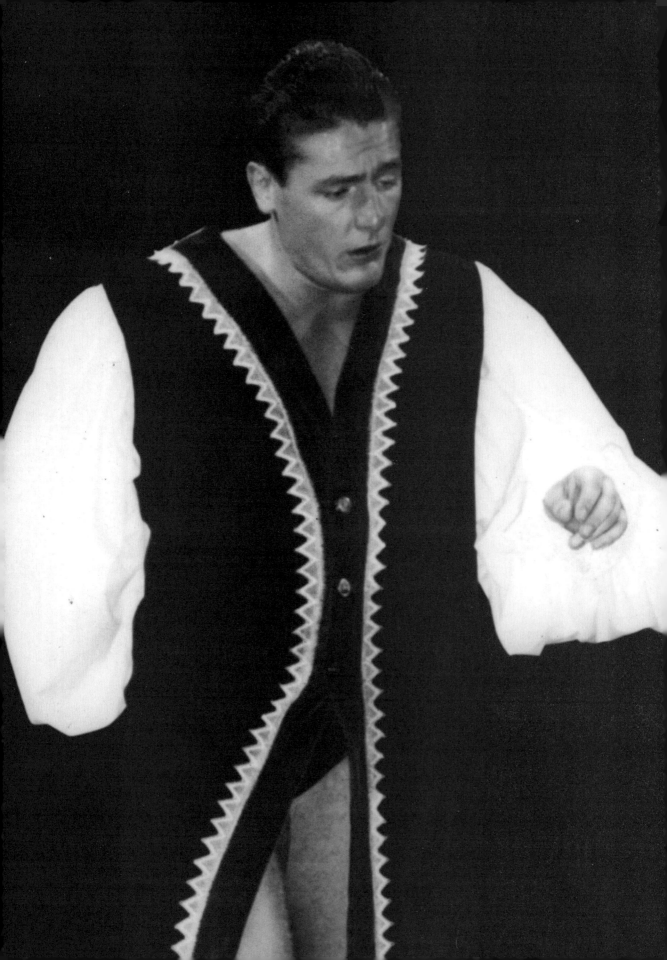

Steven Regal

September 18, 1993

These days he's called William Regal, but back when he was still Lord Steven Regal, he came on the show, keeping the haughty part of his character about him, and spoke about his early days in England and how he got started wrestling in the carnivals. He also talked about his British contemporaries, from "Fit" Finlay to Marc "Rollerball" Rocco, as well as the various promoters he worked for, including a horror story about how one promoter had a few wrestlers jailed while working in South Africa, just to skip payment. A very good technical wrestler, he hooked up with Bobby Eaton at one point during his stay in wcw and they were the Blue Bloods. At the time of this entertaining interview, he had just become wcw tv champion, winning the title from Rick Steamboat. He later lost it to Larry Zbyszko.

Mr. Regal, what is the proper way to address you?

His lordship will be fine, or Lord Regal.

Let's talk about England a little. There are a lot of accomplished wrestlers there. Could you comment on Mark "Rollerball" Rocco and David "Fit" Finlay?

Do you know what *happened* to Mark "Rollerball" Rocco?

He retired, but he'll be back in a while?

No, he's not coming back. He's having a heart operation. I was with him one night when he collapsed in a dressing room. And they found his heart was only working at 30 percent efficiency. Not good at all. But what an incredibly talented athlete he was. Most people know him as Black Tiger in Japan. He had some tremendous battles with Tiger Mask. I don't think the fans here in the United States know him. The same with Mr. Finlay, an incredibly talented wrestler. I'm sure the fans would appreciate his style. I'll go on record as saying that Fit Finlay is probably the best wrestler in the world today. He's the best wrestler I've ever seen.

You've worked independently throughout England and Europe . . .

I've worked in 20 different countries.

Did you once go by the name of the Hellraiser?

Yes, I had rather a bad back for a while, and I couldn't straighten up. I was walking around like a hunchback. So I took that guise to save any embarrassment on my own name. That was just for a while when we were doing television shows in France for Eurosport.

How long have you been in this business?

Ten years. I had my first match when I was 15, in 1983. Most of the English wrestlers start very young. I've been wrestling pretty much full time since I was 16.

How did you get into World Championship Wrestling?

Well, Mr. Bill Watts wanted a European-style wrestler because the World Championship Wrestling television show is so immensely popular in Europe. In fact, in England alone, it gets higher ratings than it does in America. But European style is just not accepted here, in this light. So I had to alter it a little. But I still keep it. Everybody has to be different, and I like my style. It took me a long time to learn, so I refuse to completely change.

It's a craft you don't just learn overnight.

You're right. Everybody talks all about the Japanese style, and so forth, in America. But it doesn't seem to be drawing a lot here. The different style doesn't seem to be putting people in the houses.

It's all about promoting.

But if certain individuals are as talented as they're supposed to be, then that alone is a draw.

One big difference for you is that in England you work in rounds.

Yes, but as I said, I've worked in 20 countries, and I'm used to working different styles. I've wrestled in sand pits in Pakistan. I can adapt pretty much to any kind of system.

Tell us about working with Giant Haystacks.

I must have wrestled that disgraceful person about 300 or 400 times, maybe more.

Were you usually the victor?

Certainly not. I ended up flat on my back most of the time.

What about Big Daddy?

Oh, he's a disgrace to the wrestling profession. He's like an outbreak of rabies in a guide dog's home.

Who have been some of the better promoters you've worked with?

Otto Wanz and Peter Williams, who run the CWA, have been very, very good to me. A man called Dara Singh was also very nice. I've had not many problems, apart from one dubious fellow in South Africa called Shane Gipollo. He's horrible. He got my friend Dave Taylor and an American wrestler named George Weingeroff thrown in prison for two weeks. It was just because he didn't want to pay them and he made some horrendous story up. As soon as it went to court, they threw it straight out and they were on the plane. And I had a lot of problems with him, too. In fact, I had him around the throat once. I don't think anyone realizes what a great company the CWA is. Right now they're running in Hanover. And they do nine weeks in the same building every single night. Most of the guys that work there are very talented athletes.

We recently saw a match on TV with you and Eric Watts. There were no flashy moves, there was solid mat wrestling all the way through, and the announcers were sitting there wondering why people weren't applauding.

Obviously people didn't want to applaud, otherwise they would have. That was basically a match for my entertainment, and anybody that was interested in the European style. But that was really for me.

Why don't we see more of those types of matches here?

People are just not used to seeing it. I didn't get many nice comments from people, but I read where somebody said it was just a way that big shows like that can have different variations and be entertaining in different ways. It's very good for certain guys to do these horrendous bumps and things. But if everybody did them, then they wouldn't mean anything. I have a role. Everybody has their own role. I just wanted to show that, at 6'4" and 250 pounds, I can wrestle better than most of the lightweights around. Every match is just clothesline after clothesline. From what I can gather, 10 or 15 years ago here, there were 30 different regional promotions, everybody seemed to make a good living, and there was plenty of money when people actually wrestled more. Now there are clotheslines and that other stuff. Certain guys are very good at it. Let them do that. Everybody else should try to adopt their own style and just wrestle. Nobody seems to want to do that. There are certain guys, such as Big Van Vader, who work tremendously hard, the same way Cactus Jack works tremendously hard. But everybody tries to copy these kind of things, and they can't — they're one and onlys. I do my style, Ricky Steamboat has his style, Ric Flair has his style. They're all tremendous, but almost everybody else seems to be becoming the same.

You mentioned the name Ricky Steamboat, who you will be fighting soon. He has a very different style than you. You work with submission moves, he uses martial arts moves. How do the two come together?

Once you learn how to be a good professional wrestler, you can pretty much adapt to anything, in a style that will please anybody. I've wrestled a lot of Japanese wrestlers and a lot of kick boxers in other countries — in an unprofessional manner, if you catch my drift. And I've never been beaten yet by any of them.

Have you ever worked shoot matches?

Lots of them.

Who would you rate the toughest?

I suppose I've been lucky up to now. There are lots of men that are far better than me. Gary Albright is very, very good at that. I'm not an amateur wrestler. I'm a submission wrestler, and there's a big difference. I've never done amateur wrestling at all. I started by jumping into the ring with a professional wrestler at a carnival when I was 15, and got the life beaten out of me. But by the time I was 18, I had his job. I was put on top, taking on any challengers for money. Drunks, rugby players, anybody that wanted to. That was how I made a career.

What do you think about the UWFI? Will it make a profit on a pay-per-view?

It's an acquired style. And I don't think so. I would like to see it because it's tremendous, but not enough people know about it. It took a long time in Japan to build up, maybe 10 years. It might take five or six here, but it also might never get off the ground. I hope it does.

Was it an idea of Bill Watts' to bring Bill Dundee in to play your second, Sir William?

No, Mr. Watts had left long before that. Actually it was my idea. Most people think Mr. Dundee is Australian, but he's Scottish. So I just wanted somebody who was authentic.

You had an injury lately?

Yes, I sprained my ankle, and I'm still suffering with it now.

So will you be working lightly now?

I never work lightly. Once it's taped solid, it's fine.

Do you know the other Steve Regal?

No I don't. I've heard about him for many years, but I never met the fellow.

What do you think about the fact that World Championship Wrestling is disbanding the National Wrestling Alliance?

I don't really know a lot about it. I've only been here a few months, and I don't really understand how it works.

What do you think of Eric Bischoff's abilities as an announcer?

As an announcer? I've never seen him announce. To be around this business as much as I have, and in as many different places, all I really worry about is myself now. I don't take a lot of notice of what else is going on.

How do you compare yourself to other British wrestlers that have come to the States and made it big — such as Davey Boy Smith and Chris Adams?

They left England at rather an early stage of their careers. Their styles are completely different than mine. I think Smith left for Calgary when he was 17 and never came back to England. I'm not sure how long Chris Adams has been here. There are people who actually like the European style. People who like it, that's all well and good — people that don't, fine. Just watch what you like. What it's all about is people coming to watch wrestling. If they like Big Van Vader, then come to watch him. If they like Steve Regal's style or Ricky Steamboat's — it's all about entertainment. People need to be entertained in various ways.

Do the crowds in Europe react as loudly as they do here?

They do, and my style is the kind that gets over there. We wrestle in tournaments. And people like to watch the competition in them. The American style doesn't suit well there at all.

How do you intend to defend your newly won belt against Ricky Steamboat?

Basically with the pride and honor that the people of America have come to expect from me.

Is there anyone you haven't wrestled yet that you'd like to wrestle?

I know I'm going to be wrestling Ric Flair in England soon. I've wrestled him before but only in tag matches, never one on one, so that will be interesting. He's very talented. The old American style, as done by Mr. Flair and Arn Anderson, is to me, great. I'm not into the crazy kind of bumps now. I wouldn't last two minutes trying to do things like that.

So we won't see you fighting Cactus Jack in the near future?

Well, you could. But you won't see me flying all over the place. I want to still be wrestling when I'm 40, and I know my body wouldn't handle that kind of abuse.

Your opinion of Hulk Hogan . . .

Obviously the greatest draw this business has ever seen. An old promoter said to me once, "You can always knock someone's talent as a wrestler, but it's how much money they draw." So if you look at him with that point of view, he is the greatest wrestler of all time. The wrestlers themselves judge each other by wrestling talent. The people who pay to watch wrestlers judge them by personality. Hulk Hogan has drawn more money maybe than anybody before him.

If you were given the opportunity to wrestle for Vince McMahon, would you go there?

Right now I'm quite happy in World Championship Wrestling. I think that whenever my time is up here, I shall go back to wrestling around the world. That's what I enjoy. I like traveling to different countries and facing different competition. Just last year alone I was in South Africa, India, Egypt, Germany, Austria. That's what I've done all my career. This is the longest I've been based anywhere. Last year in India, I wrestled a guy who won a silver medal in the Los Angeles Olympics and had never had a pro match before. There were 20,000 people in a soccer stadium, just me against this guy. It was near enough of a riot when I beat him. I had to have a police escort back to the hotel. And I wondered about that. I beat him quite easily. I wondered how he won his silver medal in the Olympics.

In a formal situation, is it proper to keep your napkin folded on your lap, or tucked into your collar?

Certainly not tucked into your collar. You'd look like a circus clown.

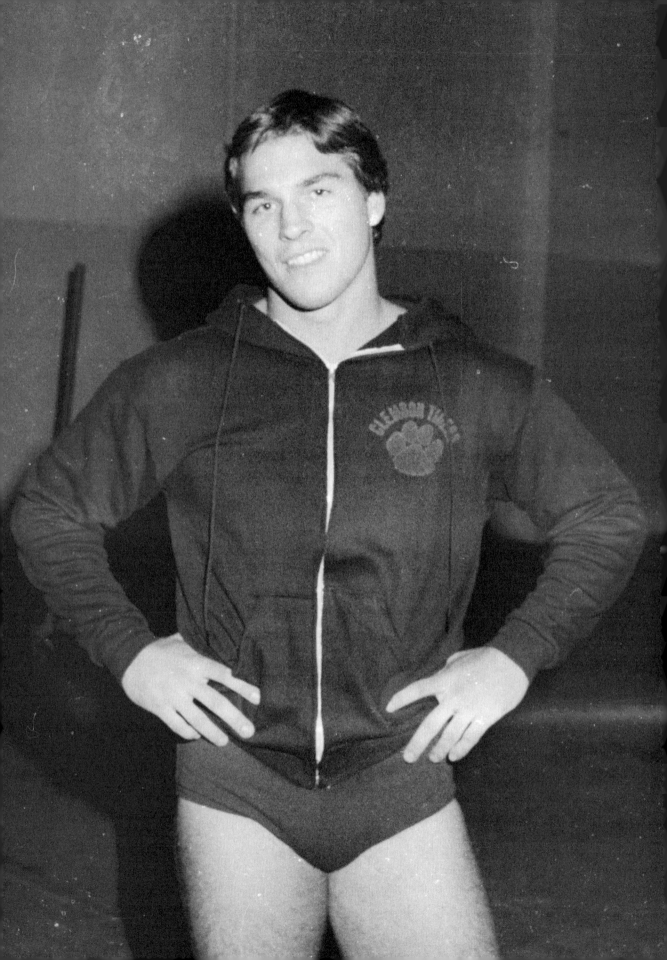

Terry Taylor

December 1993

It's hard to imagine which was more embarrassing for the talented Terry Taylor — playing the Red Rooster in the WWF or the Taylor-Made Man in WCW. But his in-ring skill was never doubted, and toward the end of that phase of his career, he was fun to listen to as a WCW commentator. Here he spoke about a right-time-right-place incident that got him into the game (Chick Donovan no-showed a TV taping), who his favorite promoter and promotion were (not what you might think), his relationship with Dusty Rhodes, and why he wasn't pushed as well as he could have been. He also shared a great inside story about a special meeting Ted Turner once held with the wrestlers. Taylor came across as a funny and insightful guy.

Let's welcome to Wrestle Radio USA the one and only Terry Taylor. Is it Terrible Terry Taylor or Terrific Terry Taylor?

It depends if you're talking to my wife. She thinks I'm terrible. Some people think I'm pretty terrific, me included.

Where are you today?

Vero Beach, Florida.

It is Vero Beach. We've been hearing that through the years.

3805 Indian River Drive.

We're on the air now . . .

That's OK. That's not my address, anyway.

Let's jump into a little bit of history. How did you get involved in the business?

I went to Gilford College in Greensboro, North Carolina, and a friend of mine, who was 300 pounds, his name was Steve Travis, he wrestled for a while and he had a tryout but didn't know what to do. My brother and I used to go to West Palm Beach and we were really big fans of WBTV in West Palm Beach, Florida. We used to go to the matches. I showed him what I knew just by watching. And he got a tryout and a job with the IWF in Greensboro. That was with Johnny Powers and Ernie Ladd. I don't know what happened to IWF — something happened. I didn't see him for three years and graduated from college and went to the matches in West Palm Beach and he was there. He said, "Come back to Tampa and we'll party and drink and I got to do TV tomorrow." I was working a regular job and said sure. Well, a guy named Chick Donovan no-showed for TV and they asked if I wanted to work. I didn't have any gear, so had to borrow it.

Right place, right time.

Yeah, timing. Pretty lucky.

Who trained you?

I didn't train. They liked me. I wrestled Bugsy McGraw and was basically a door-mat. But I made more money doing that than my regular job. I thought this was great.

That was in 1979?

That was 1979 and I won rookie of the year in 1980 for Georgia Championship Wrestling. I went from there to Kansas City, back to Georgia, to Charlotte, to Jerry Jarrett from '81–'84 and then to Bill Watts in Mid-South.

Who's been your favorite promoter to work for?

Probably Jerry Jarrett. I was making great money from '83–'84 and only had to drive from Nashville to Memphis, which was about 200 miles, and it was great. Bill Watts was a good promoter. He fired me when he came to wcw last year.

He fired you?

Yeah, he said that everyone comes in with a clean slate, but Terry Taylor, you're done. I was part of a package that made him a millionaire from '84–'87. That was kind of a down-point, but I went to Titan Sports [Vince McMahon Jr.'s wwf] and did alright this last time.

You did Titan twice. How did you get up in the broadcast booth with them?

It must be my James Earl Jones voice that I have. I have a degree in economics and I've been studying it for a long time and I like it. I like explaining to people what's going on through my experiences in the ring.

What would you prefer — the ring or announcing?

If I can be perfectly honest, after 14 glorious years I'd like to have an opportunity to do something that means something in the wrestling ring. If that means to be used as a preliminary wrestler, then I'm not interested. I feel there's my reputation, skill, and ability to talk. I'm drug free and can pass any test at any time, I'm a family man, so I'm pretty stable. I'd like to entertain people after intermission, and if wcw doesn't feel like doing that, I'd like to remain a broadcaster.

You're scheduled to fight Steven Regal soon. Is this a good direction?

I hope so. My biggest problem is my honesty, and nine times out of ten, the promotion keeps us in the dark.

Why?

I really don't know. I think they feel if we don't know what's going on that we're easier to deal with.

So you don't know where you're going with your part?

No, I've suggested some things, but they seem to have the same guys on top in wcw. They seem to have the ball and want to play with it the way they want. Well, I mean honestly. There's an influx of new talent and I haven't been on their TV in a while, so I'm almost new. But if they don't want to take a chance with me, I'll sit with Tony Schiavone and talk like crazy.

For Starrcade, you're facing the Equalizer. Does that mean you're being punished?

The first I saw of it was when I signed the one-year contract. When you come in here, they tell you that they'll promote you the best that they can. It's part of the contract. You have to take the good with the bad and don't mind wrestling this guy. It won't be a Ric Flair vs. Terry Funk type of match, but he's a big guy.

A little clumsy.

Not like ShockMaster. That was the most inauspicious debut I've ever seen.

It was also one of the funniest things we've seen.

I lost my mind. He crawled on his hands and knees looking for his head, then stands up and this horrible voice comes on.

Is Regal a better match for you?

Hell, yeah. He's 25 years old and has been wrestling for 10 years.

Well, if you had a job as booker and had to book yourself, who would you like to book yourself against to have a good series?

I'd like to wrestle Flair. I'd like to wrestle Steve Austin. I'd like to wrestle Steve Regal. I'd like to wrestle Scorpio.

How about all the federations?

Kenta Kobashi and Hiro Hase in Japan. He separated his shoulder, so he couldn't face me. I'd like to, if I had to choose, work for Giant Baba. It's fun in Japan. You are on a bus and they tell you where you are on the card. That's it. When I went for Baba two years ago, they treated me great.

What titles did you have?

All of them except the world title and anything in the wwf.

What happened in the WWF?

They were a good organization, and I mean that with the word "organization." No last-minute hairy decisions, everything was structured well, everyone knew what they're supposed to do. Just a great oiled machine. There's a wrench in there now with the legal problems, but they still didn't have to do with us. We got a stack of plane tickets at every television. They were always paid for. We made our towns and always got paid. It's a shame what's going on up there, and I don't want to say if he's guilty or innocent.

Is that the difference between Vince and WCW?

Well, I think what Vince did was to make it wholesome entertainment. No more blood, etc., and he said publicly that nobody got hurt. By doing so, it flushed our credibility down the toilet. Guys like me, who weren't freaks or geeks didn't fit in. He tried to make me into a freak as The Red Rooster and whether I could wrestle or not didn't matter because I was labeled a geek.

And they now have Tatanka with the red hair.

He has it! God bless him. He likes it. Everywhere he goes he has his hair like that.

How was merchandise sales for The Red Rooster?

They made 500 T-shirts of The Red Rooster and sold out in three weeks.

Sounds like a real collectable.

Yeah. I'm sure every pawnshop in the country is getting top dollar for them right now.

Where did you feel that you shined?

Jerry Jarrett from '81–'83 and Bill Watts in Mid-South and UWF. They went on talent and personalities and spotlighted me for three years and it was great.

Do you like working as a bad guy more than a good guy?

I think I'd be insulting people's intelligence if they thought we were really like that. Well, it's like playing baseball. If they need a pitcher, you pitch. Need a catcher, you catch. I like doing both and having the ability to do either. It's like a lost art with the advent of steroids and face paint; it became a bodybuilding contest and not an athletic contest. Think about it, when the Road Warriors came in, in 1985, and their peak in 1986–87. I'm not saying they're on steroids now, but everyone was then, to get like that, and the sport changed.

Yet, you made it through that.

Well, I had my family in wrestling. I wasn't the homosexual that somebody fell in love with. Let's be honest. I think every business has that. But I love what I do and I think that's helped carry me through. There have been a lot of times where I was down, wondering what in the hell I am doing in this.

What is your relationship with Dusty Rhodes? Did he job you out because you didn't get along?

Well you watch the television and you tell me.

That could be Bischoff calling the shots. It's a shame.

You think it's a shame? I won't say anything bad about Dusty. It's either he doesn't think I'm skilled or I'm not in his scheme of things. If that's not true, that's too bad because I feel I have something to offer this company and that's why I'm not in the ring.

Is there a big clique in WCW with Dusty and his friends?

I'd rather not say.

You were talking about steroids. What will happen five years from now?

Well, hopefully guys like Scorpio that can do some incredible stuff. . . . Mark Bagwell got mad at me the other day. He was wrestling Austin, and I said Austin outweighed him by 30 pounds, and he got mad at me. I said, "Who cares?" Some linebackers in the NFL are only 5'11" and 200 pounds. There are guys in Japan that aren't on steroids and are great wrestlers.

They'll train all day and have an athletic background, most of the time. They dedicate themselves.

I saw one kid who must have been 5'10", 210 and got back dropped 100 times in a row. How many guys here steroided up with face paint would come in and do that for an opportunity? They just want to look good and feel that this is enough, and it's chased off a lot of our fans.

We heard Ted Turner came down recently to meet with the boys. What did he have to say?

He is probably one of the most charismatic and funniest guys I've ever met. He was great. He shot the poop with us and talked and told stories and said that he's lost a lot more money with the Braves and Hawks than with us. "Don't worry, TV is doing OK, and now that Vince is having problems, we can go after the bigger venues that he had a monopoly on. I'm excited. I love wrestling."

So he does keep up with the promotion?

He doesn't know anything about it, but he's a fan. Somebody asked him about steroids and he said, "I heard they make you sterile and nothing's worth that. I watch a couple tapes of my wife and work out that way." It was nice to have a boss like that who has made a commitment to stand with us. We all took a deep breath after that and I wasn't worried about anything.

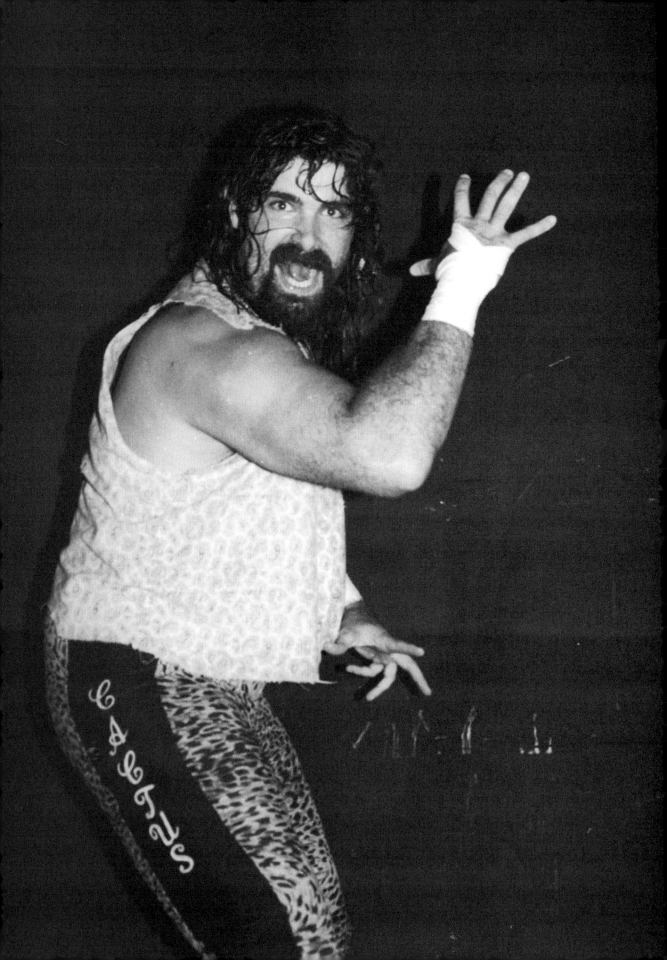

Cactus Jack
January 8, 1994

It was really a treat to talk with Cactus Jack, well before he was known as Mankind or even Mick Foley. And it was a coup to get such a popular guy on. The show was halfway into its second year, and Cactus was probably the first guest to be so open about how the business was run and so willing to talk about pretty much anything. He was already a major star, having come up through the ranks of UWF, Memphis, World Class, Tri-State, the NWA, World Championship Wrestling, and Global Championship Wrestling. His tenure in the WWF was still to come, but Cactus was already known for his reckless, flamboyant style and for being a genial character in and out of the ring. He was erudite and very talkative, responding to questions with true interest and long, thoughtful answers.

Tell us a little bit about your name. You used to be called Cactus Jack Manson . . .

Yeah, and you wanna know why I'm not that name anymore? I didn't like it. Understand something — it's like the John Cougar Mellencamp thing. He's given the name Cougar because they think that's the only way he's gonna be marketable. When I started wrestling, I was Cactus Jack Foley — my real last name. And when I was in Tennessee, guys would come down from Texas — at the time they were having a Tennessee-Texas war. And Eric Embry thought that I resembled Charles Manson. He told me that he wanted me to come to Texas, and somewhere down the line, they were gonna put that name on me. You see, when you were in Memphis or Dallas, you didn't ask too many questions. I didn't have such a foothold in wrestling that I could say, "No, I want my name and my name's Foley." As far as I was concerned, whatever they wanted was fine. But I was never told that I was going to be Cactus Jack Manson until I walked down the aisle for the first time at the Sportatorium. I heard the name over the loudspeaker and I said, "Well, I guess that's who I am now." Personally, I don't think that any good wrestler should have to rely on the heat that America's most famous mass murderer brings. It really bothered me to think that there might be a mother or father out there tuning in to wrestling and seeing this guy Manson walking around and saying, "Hey, I don't want my kids watching that." So when I went to World Championship Wrestling the first time I was just complying with what they wanted. I didn't want to take a chance. Whatever they wanted was fine. But as soon as I left World Championship Wrestling the first time, in 1990, I thought, "Hey, I've gotten to a point where I'm good enough, I don't need this thing hanging on me." And to tell you the truth, not too many people remember it. When I get a letter written to Cactus Jack Manson, I throw the thing out without reading it, because those are the dangerous ones.

Is it true that you and Maxx Payne recently signed a contract for one year for $37,000?

No, that's not true. I think that's an accurate figure for some people, but I think it's guys who don't have the stature in the business. Let's face it, up to a few years ago, a rookie in Major League Baseball got about $32,000. I know that Brian Pillman made $40,000 in the NFL his first year. So I think it's more for guys to get a chance to prove themselves. And WCW has cut back on their schedule a little bit. So it's more than guys can make working independently, because it's so hit or miss out there. I'm lucky, man, and I am thankful that I've proven myself enough to the point where I basically could laugh at that type of money. I'm doing all right.

How did you get into the game?

There's a story going around, that is true, that I got into the wrestling business by jumping off a neighbor's roof — diving onto a cardboard box. I showed the tape to a promoter in New York, where I was living at the time. And he thought he had a gold mine there. But what he didn't realize was that he was dealing with a guy who basically had no legitimate athletic talent, as far as running and jumping and that type of thing. So he kind of washed his hands of me, and Dominic Denucci took over. I'd go to this promoter's shows, and Dominic wouldn't so much wrestle with me as he'd beat me up and stretch me into different positions. You know, he's gotta test the guys' guts a little bit. And when he saw that I was coming back for more, I started going to his wrestling school in Pittsburgh. I think if you ask him, he'd say he's most proud of me because, like I said, I didn't really have any natural talent, but I did work hard. You know how I compensated for not being able to jump high? I jumped off high things . . . onto concrete floors.

Have you had any real, legitimate injuries?

Yeah. I've been in it eight years now, and I can seriously say not a place from head to toe hasn't been hurt. You want me to quickly — off the top of my head — list my injuries?

Talk about any replacement parts you have.

I have a new ligament in my knee — a cadaver ligament. For you people out there, that's a dead guy who no longer needs it. I've had my kneecap cracked, I've had my ankle sprained, I've had my big toe broken, I've had my groin torn, I've had my nose broken four times, I've had hundreds of stitches, six concussions, seven broken ribs, a broken wrist. And that's in addition to just that basic feeling terrible all the time. If I was to list my most serious injuries, it would just be that feeling of feeling bad all the time.

But do you love your work?

Yeah, but I used to love it a little more. You see, I just took it as a given that I'm Cactus Jack, and I'm destined to feel lousy my whole life. Then when I got hurt with Vader — because I was hurt, I couldn't wrestle — it kind of gave all these things that had hurt me for years a chance to heal up a little bit. So what you're looking at for the first time is Cactus Jack in comfort, and I'm not comfortable with that.

You once said in an interview that in order for you to succeed in this business, you would have to erase the notion that you're a funny performer. Have you accomplished that?

Well, actually, I think I went a little too far the other way. I think I lost the humor for a little bit. I was looking at an interview yesterday of me and Abdullah doing a birthday party for Sting. And there was a look [on me] that I hadn't seen in a long time, and I need to get it back. It was a look that I was having fun out there. It's just the joy of being out there and hurting people and being in front of a crowd. And then when I became a so-called good guy again, there were these personal issues, and I became so obsessed with Vader, I'd literally lie awake at night or daydream in the car for hours on end about all these things I was gonna do and all these things I was gonna say. And I think they were *too* serious. And I think people *like* this and I think it was good for me, but I think it's time for me to kinda rejuvenate myself.

When you were working in Memphis, you said you thought it would be better if you got hurt seriously, so you couldn't wrestle again. Was that said out of frustration?

Yeah, I remember saying that. Our boss at the time was a guy named Randy Hales. Randy literally wouldn't let me do anything. He'd say, "Cactus Jack, if you try doing any of that crazy stuff, we're gonna fire you." Because my stuff was so much better and so much more intense than their main event guys.

But Tennessee is known as a brawling state.

Yeah, but Tennessee has got their favorite sons. I mean, God forbid you start to steal the show. Do you really think that Jerry Lawler and Jeff Jarrett would still be on top there for so many years? Not to take anything away from them. As far as longevity, they've been great. But there've been shooting stars that have come in there that obviously could have main-evented over Jerry Lawler. But they just shoot them down and send them on their way. The secret in Memphis is not to be too good.

Right after you came into WCW, Ole Anderson was saying they might be using less of you because they were afraid you would expose the business.

I think Ole's line was that if people wanted to see my trampoline act, they'd be buying tickets to see Cathy Rigby. He just had a different view of what wrestling should be. Everyone was real high on Cactus Jack — the hard-core wrestling fans — but what they don't understand is if Ole Anderson hadn't gone in and said, "Hey, we don't really think that much of you," I wouldn't be where I am right now, because I probably would have already run my course. I hadn't really found myself in wrestling. The problem was that I was doing main event things, but I wasn't a main event wrestler. I wasn't ready to face a Vader or a Sting right then, but the stuff I was doing while I was in preliminaries was just too good to be in preliminaries. But I want to get back to what you were asking about Memphis. Randy Hales was a guy who thought he was better than everyone, but he got sick because he was such a dirty person. He chewed that Copenhagen and he never washed his hands. He got real sick, almost dead, just from being a dirty person. And it was strange that when the boss went on the shelf, that's when Cactus Jack started doing all his things. I got to do elbows off the side of the apron, clotheslines over the top rope.

Are you in pretty good shape right now?

Yeah, like I said, I feel better than I have in several years. I was thinking I might only have a couple of years left. At one point it looked like I had about two and a half weeks left. But now, I don't see any reason why I can't be wrestling for the next five years.

You have to pace yourself.

My first time in wcw when I came back in 1991, I was a much different wrestler — more serious, more focused. Like I said, there was just this look in my eye like, "Man, I *love* being out here." I guess they had a meeting and they were saying, "Hey, this Cactus Jack is pretty good. We've gotta do something with him." And one of the guys at wcw, in all his wisdom, raised his hand and said, "Well, if you're gonna do something with Cactus Jack, you'd better do it quick, because he's not gonna be around very long." And then six months later, the same guy kept saying, "Hey, Cactus, why don't you keep doing that elbow [on the cement] every night." I'd say I just couldn't physically keep doing it. And he looked at me almost like he'd been told there was no Santa Claus. But let's face it — there are limits, and I just about pushed them as far as I could go, even though this guy Sabu is pushing them a little further than I ever did.

You've been working solo for such a long time and now you're partnered in tag teams (with Maxx Payne). How has tag team wrestling been for you?

I've held four belts in wrestling. Three of them have been tag team championships and one, believe it or not, was the light heavyweight championship in Texas. But that was several Twinkies ago. I guess Gary Young was my first really good partner. We had a good team. We won the belts when he was the Super Zodiac. He was my partner in Tennessee and Texas. When I came into Continental, I had the Stud Stable with me, but my greatest partner was probably Abdullah the Butcher. Everybody that I've had a great partnership with — I'm talking about the modern-day Cactus Jack, from 1989 and up — has been just a little bit to the left or to the right of that straight line — like Kevin Sullivan and Abdullah the Butcher.

Do you have a preference?

Personally I like the solo thing better. It's like in organized sports — I was a tremendous basketball player at one time. I was shooting one on one, two on two. But when you got out there five on five, it was like I was just a little bit lost. Same thing with football. They'd get ready to choose up the sides in high school football, and I'd bend down to tie my shoelace because I didn't feel like being out there. But as long as the pressure's on *you*, and it's entirely up to you — you can't hide behind anyone — I tend to really rise to the occasion. Sometimes you reach certain plateaus in wrestling. I was in the main event of Halloween Havoc in maybe the best match of my life, with Vader. And how much higher can you get from there? I think the only reason they signed that match — and it wasn't a championship match — is that they hoped we'd kill each other, and they were hoping that people would buy the pay-per-view to see that happen. But once it came down to a title match, they didn't really want Cactus Jack in the picture. So I knew that I couldn't get any higher. Was I now going to go a step lower and a step lower and a step lower, and three months later I'd be opening up the show — or do I take somebody that I think has the potential to take me way up to that next level in tag team wrestling? And I think Maxx Payne does. The key word there is potential, because I think Maxx is maybe a little bit lazy as a single, whereas I'm lazy in a tag team. So you put the two together, and I inspire him and he inspires me.

Vader power bombed you on the cement during your match, and you got a concussion. Any thoughts about that?

The feeling of wrestling Vader was real strange. On one hand, before the match, I was more nervous, more frightened, and more anxious than I'd ever been with anyone else. There was no fun in preparing for it. But at the same time, when the match was over, there was more of a feeling of accomplishment. There was some incredible emotion. I was pumped up every time I wrestled him. And I only wrestled him seven or eight times last year. People think it was a tremendous feud, because the incidents where we did clash were so intense. For me, every time it was like Muhammad Ali and Joe Frazier. And I don't think you can afford to get that pumped up for an individual day in and day out. So at the same time, I was real disappointed once Halloween Havoc was over. I mean the high point of my career and the low point of my career were probably within that same match. There was a certain feeling when I looked up at the crowd in New Orleans. The people were in the palm of my hand, Vader was in the palm of my hand. But about 15 minutes later, when it was all over, there was a feeling like it's never gonna be this good again.

We have a few names to run by you for your opinions. Joel Goodheart.

Joel was real good for me. When I was an independent, if it weren't for him and, believe it or not, if it weren't for Herb Abrams, it would've been real hard for me to make a living. Plus, he was able to showcase me alongside a guy like Eddie Gilbert and put me in matches, like barbed wire and falls count anywhere, that really got me back in with wcw.

Dusty Rhodes.

Hey, I like him personally and I like him professionally. He took a chance on Cactus Jack and put me more in the forefront than anyone ever did.

Joe Pedicino.

I've got a good relationship with Joe. I thought we were gonna have a good thing there at Global, and he did too. It just didn't quite work out.

Jerry Jarrett.

I never had a bad word with him. If I went back there now and he tried paying me that kind of money, we might have a problem.

Dominic Denucci.

I'm not so good at staying in touch, but I wrote him a letter at Christmas. It said, "Hey, I've got it pretty good. I've got more than I ever thought I would." And really, if it wasn't for him, I wouldn't have any of this. And I know it.

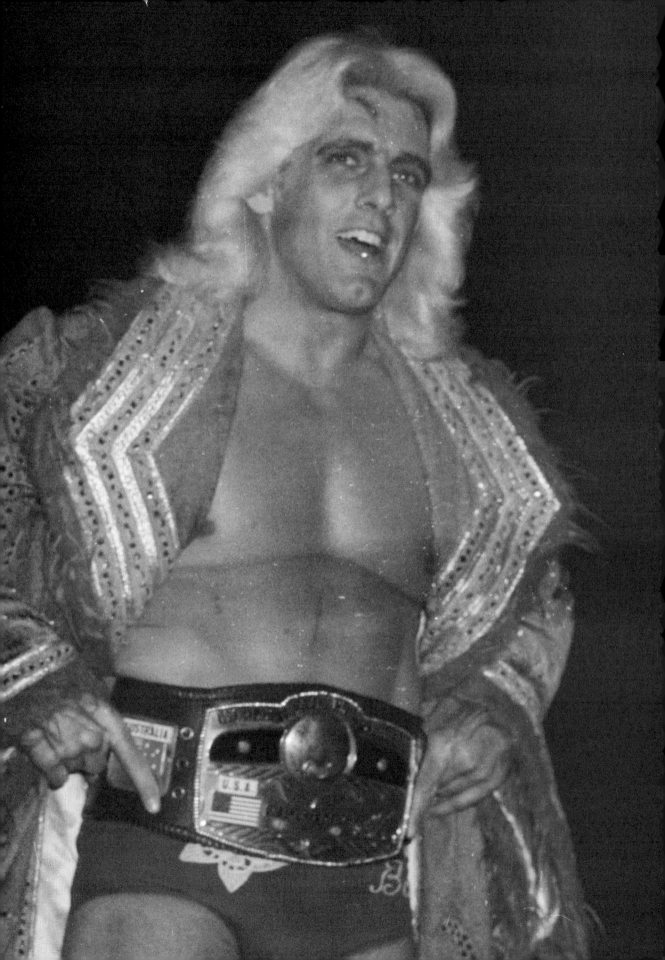

Ric Flair

February 3, 1994

Nature Boy Ric Flair, who was trained by Verne Gagne in Minneapolis, made the history books early on, when, after wrestling for just under three years, he broke his back in an airplane crash in North Carolina. Doctors told him he would never wrestle again, but that was well before he won his first championship. Starting in the AWA, he moved over to the NWA for a long run, sticking with the group when it became known as WCW. He switched over to the WWF in 1991, where he quickly nabbed the belt, but returned to WCW two years later. When WCW went under, Flair returned to the WWF. This brief interview was done in person, when Flair was a guest of honor at a special fund-raiser for youth sports at the Providence Civic Center, shortly after defeating Big Van Vader, to take the world heavyweight title for the 10th time. He was very protective about the business, but still very enthusiastic in talking about it.

How did you discover the sport, Ric? Tell us what you thought of it and how you broke in.

My earliest memories go back, of course, to Verne Gagne and Butch Levy and the Crusher, the Bruiser, Pampero Firpo, Larry Hennig — guys who were big-time mainstay professionals when I was growing up. I remember watching all of them on TV. Of course, I started in Minneapolis under the tutelage of Verne Gagne. He gave me the opportunity and I took advantage of it. And I've never looked back.

When you broke in to wrestling in 1973, did you develop a game plan that you've held to in your career?

No, I actually didn't really develop a game plan till after I crashed in the airplane in '75. When I was healing up and realized I was gonna be able to go on with my career, I started kind of deciding exactly who and what I wanted to be, and how I was gonna go about getting there.

Is there a big difference between the Ric Flair of today and before the plane crash?

No, not really. Not in terms of ability. But that did smarten me up to things going on in the world, and it probably made me get a little more focused than I was at the time.

Do you think wrestling has become a more dangerous sport, with everybody going after gimmicks?

It's only become more dangerous because the guys are just so much bigger and stronger than they were. There's always been big guys, but everybody's big now. I think every sport is experiencing that. Hockey players are 215, 220, 230 now. And 20 years ago they were 170 pounds.

What's your opinion on groups like the FMW, where they have exploding barbed wire matches?

I don't even know what that is. What's the FMW?

A Japanese group.

No, I don't know them. I don't bother with that.

How's your back feeling?

It's getting better. It's something I've had to live with. Wrestling a guy is very hard, physically. And any time he lands on top of me, I *feel* it.

You first took the heavyweight title from Dusty Rhodes in the summer of 1981. Did your life change radically?

Overnight. I became the world champion. If you can call yourself the best at whatever you do in life, that makes you number one. It gives you a whole new perspective on life.

How much longer do you think you would like to remain an active wrestler?

As long as I feel like I do right now, I'll keep wrestling.

I know you have some gyms. Any plans for something else within wrestling or in another business?

No, I really don't have any plans right now, except to go on and compete against — I know I've got at least five or six big matches this year. I've got Vader again when I'm healed up, I've got Steamboat and Sting, probably a unification with Rick Rude. I don't know. There's a bunch of guys out there.

A unification match with Rude?

I'd like to see that happen, and I think that's something that wcw will promote. I'm just taking a guess.

We'd like to get your reaction to a couple of names: Terry Funk.

Oh, tremendous. One of the greatest of all time.

Rick Steamboat.

The greatest wrestler I've ever competed against.

Lex Luger.

Luger is not a great technician, but he is in tremendous physical condition. You take that and add the size and the strength. Well, I guess I'm going backward. He's got tremendous strength and tremendous size and he's in the condition of a guy that weighs 220. So what he lacks in technical skills, he makes up for not only with strength, but strength with endurance behind it, which is a very hard thing to find in any athlete. Most guys who are that big and strong neglect the cardio, don't work it as hard. But he's in tremendous physical condition. I could never wear him down physically. I had to really pull it out of the hat to get the best of him.

You did a one-hour match with Bret Hart at the Boston Garden about a year ago. Your comments on that?

You can't say enough about a guy like Bret Hart. He comes from a great wrestling family, his dad's a great guy, and Bret grew up in the sport. He's incredible. He's wrestled in Europe, he's wrestled over here, he's wrestled a lot in Japan. He takes that fine combination of all the styles and puts it together. And he's my size so he's the kind of guy I like to wrestle. He's like a Steamboat. I don't think he is a Ricky Steamboat — but who is? — but he's right there. He's one of the top five guys in the sport.

How did you end up on the dais with George Bush (Senior) during the campaign?

Oh, the Spirit of America? Probably because he didn't know any other 10-time world heavyweight champions to put on the train with him. Actually, I've known him for about five years now. And I just jumped at the opportunity to get on the train. I was really pushing for him and hoping he would win the election. He's a quality guy. Not to take anything away from President Clinton — I don't know him personally, and he seems to be doing an adequate job — but George Bush is a quality person. He took us through some real trying times, and took us through with our heads held high. He was my kind of man.

Any major difference between the way you were treated in WCW and the WWF?

Well, there's been no difference since I've been back at wcw. I don't think my rapport with wcw before I left was very good. Certainly not with the personnel in the management end. But they have a whole new management team in there, they have new people heading up the organization that I get along fabulously with. And they are really, for the first time since I've been involved with wcw, totally committed to making this a successful wrestling company. And that's the difference. Turner Broadcasting is a huge conglomeration, and wcw is just a very small part of that big Turner empire. The other night Mr. Turner and Jane Fonda came down to the matches, and it was just glorious. The company is committed to making it the best product in the sport. And that's what makes me happy. As far as the WWF, I cannot say enough good things about Vince McMahon. He treated me like he *told* me he would. I'd never been around him until I went there, and he made my life whole, he gave me the respect and let me carry myself with the dignity that I felt I should in this sport, and he was great to me. I went there because I wanted to wrestle Hulk Hogan, I wanted to wrestle Curt Hennig, I wanted to wrestle Roddy Piper and Randy Savage, and then I got to wrestle Hart, too. So for me it couldn't have been better. I got to wrestle against three legends and two guys that will be legends. Piper, Savage and Hogan are legends in this sport. And both Curt and Bret someday will be legends in this sport. So it was an opportunity for me to wrestle the great guys. I was with Roddy Piper when he walked away. And I was with the Hulkster — who really *is* the man — when he walked away. So it all was a great moment for me and a great time for sports. If Hogan had stuck around and I'd been able to fight him at Wrestlemania, it would've been the biggest pay-per-view in the history of any athletic event ever. And it may still be.

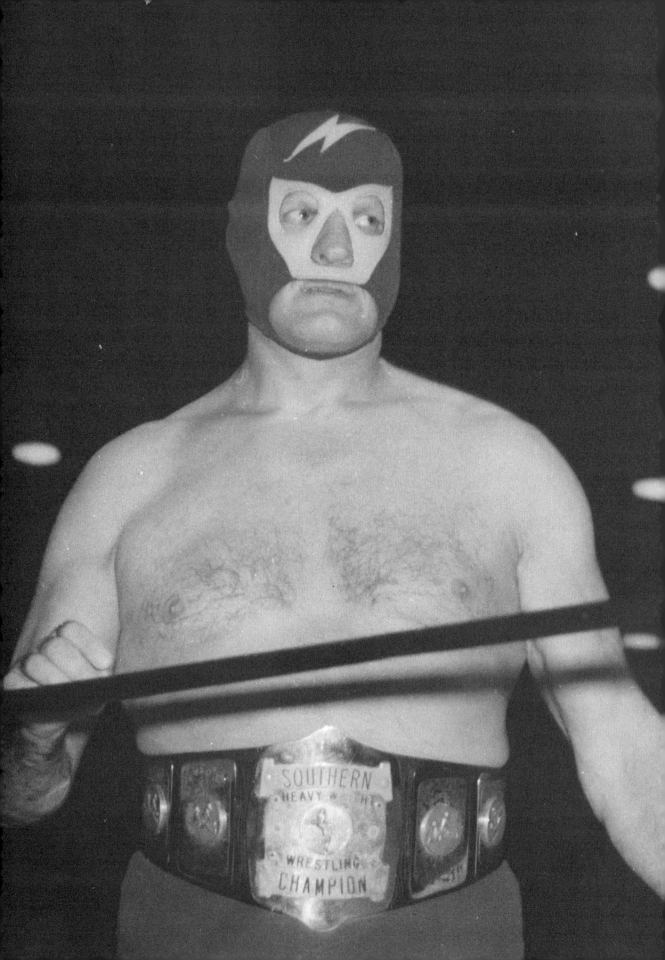

Walter "Killer" Kowalski
April 2, 1994

Walter "Killer" Kowalski was best known in the ring for his claw hold, which he would clamp on his opponent's stomach to make him submit, and for accidentally knocking the cauliflower ear off Yukon Eric's head in the middle of a match. Others might argue that his shining moment was when, after Pepper Gomez invited him to jump on his "cast-iron stomach" from the top rope, Kowalski instead jumped on his throat, starting a blood feud. He spent almost 30 years in the ring. At the height of his career, he stood 6'7" and weighed 270 pounds. He held belts in most of the federations, including the AWA, NWA, and WWWF. His last regular run was under a hood as half of The Executioners, in the mid-1970s, teaming with Big John Studd. Originally from Canada, he now lives on Boston's North Shore, where he ran the Killer Kowalski Institute of Professional Wrestling for a number of years. As he loves to talk, all it took for him to say yes to coming on the show was a quick phone call.

Welcome to the show Mr. Kowalski, and thanks for being with us. A few years ago when you were a guest on David Letterman's show, he introduced you as the most loathed wrestler in the business. And you said no, that was the most loved. Were you loathed?

Well, if I was loathed, it was by a lot of people who hated me. But the strange part about it is that people hated me when they saw me on television. But if they met me in person, if they saw me on the street, they stopped me and said hello and they wanted to talk to me. I was exciting to them. And I made things that worked differently in their life, so they didn't loathe me, they kind of loved me. I'm trying to change my image anyway.

When was your first wrestling match?

1948.

Did you win?

Are you kidding? I got the hell knocked out of me.

But you were known to be kind of a good guy at the beginning.

My first time wrestling they gave me the name of Tarzan Kowalski. I was a young kid, well built. They had me grow my hair long, which was unusual at the time. So they called me that because I looked like an athletic guy from the jungle to them. And I spoke half-ass English.

Why did you turn heel?

At that time there were not too many big guys around. Every time I stepped in the ring, people were going "Boo, boo." My opponents were much smaller than me, so people figured I had an advantage over my opponents, even if they were villains, because I'm so much bigger. So I'd go out there and pretty soon I took advantage of things. You now, if they were gonna boo me, I might as well take advantage. So I pulled their hair, I pulled their trunks, I put my hand on the ropes. The fans would say, "Why you dirty so and so. You don't have to do that. You could beat 'em up anyway." And I'd say, "Yeah, but I love doing it." So we kept on going like that, and pretty soon they dropped the name Tarzan and made it Wladek Kowalski, which is Walter in Polish. That made it sound more ethnic. Then people really started booing me, and I loved it.

Didn't you become a vegetarian at that time, too?

It was in April of 1953 — no meat, fish, or poultry. I was experimenting with it for a while. What does your body consist of? It's mostly oxygen. Your body is filled with oxygen. So when you come right down to it, how much oxygen is there in meat? Nothing. Zero. Decayed rotting flesh, including fish and poultry. The foods that have oxygen within them are fresh fruits and vegetables — almost pure oxygen. There were two runners that helped me make up my mind about it — Roger Bannister and John Landy — they were the first two men to break the four-minute mile barrier. It was at the British Empire Games in Vancouver, British Columbia. Roger Bannister beat John Landy, but only by about two inches. They both ran under four minutes. When they asked Roger Bannister what he attributed his endurance to, he said he was a vegetarian. And John Landy said the same thing. It took about three years for my body to become acclimated to the new regime of living. But then when I used to go in that ring, some of the wrestlers would dread meeting me there. They would blow up, jump out of the ring and walk around till they got their wind back again. But I would just keep on going. The one thing I made sure of was that I would make the people notice *me*. So when an opponent jumped out on the floor to walk around, I used to jump around, do the kangaroo hop, screaming and hollering. I would climb to the top ring buckle and threaten to jump down on my opponent — which I wouldn't do because I might kill myself — and the referee would be screaming and yelling and arguing at me — he thought I was a real nutball, too — to get down off that rope. In the meantime, the people would be looking at me and wondering, what's that crazy Pole doing. So people were noticing me. After the matches were over, I would take my time, take a shower, go real slow, because I wanted the people to get out of the building. I usually parked my car blocks away from the place. I wouldn't park it in the same parking lot because I was afraid the crazy fans might wreck my car. But one time I came out of the dressing room, and there was still a big mob waiting for me, telling me I was terrific and asking for my autograph. And they said, "You were great Mr. Kowalski. Who did you wrestle?" They remembered me, but not my opponent.

Who was your best opponent?

Oh, some old Italian geek by the name of Bruno Sammartino. I fought him quite a few times. In fact, when I was Grand Prix World Champion wrestling up in Montreal, Bruno came up there and challenged me. But I beat him. When I was the world's champion down in Australia and in Southeast Asia — I wrestled in Indonesia, Singapore, Hong Kong, Malaysia, Bangkok — he came down and challenged me, and I beat him again there. He had more to lose when I would come to New York. He got even with me there. He beat me to the ground and stomped me and wouldn't let me get up again. That was in Madison Square Garden, and he was the champ and it was a different story. He had more to gain by keeping his title than I had by taking it away from him. We respected one another. When someone asks Bruno who his toughest ever was, he says Killer Kowalski.

Is there a main difference in wrestling between 30 years ago and now?

You want to know the truth? I put the TV on one time and said, "Oh my God, that's what they're doing now?" I do not watch television at all now. I have a wrestling column in the *Boston Herald*, but I do it through phone calls. Friends call me and give me the latest dope and the details on what's happening in professional wrestling. I have friends in the WWF and in WCW. That's how I get the latest information.

What is your job in the wrestling business today? Are you just a teacher?

No, no, no. Besides teaching wrestling, I do fundraising for the Policemen's and Firemen's Associations.

At one of those recent shows, Perry Saturn and Terra Rizing were on the bill. Both of them are now showing up in bigger organizations.

In fact, Terra Rizing [Paul Levesque, now known as Triple H] is now done with me and is working with WCW full time.

Do you find these guys? Do they find you? How do you know who to push?

They contact me, and I show them all about wrestling. I teach them about amateur wrestling first. I explain to them how to protect themselves. In fact, when one of my guys, Perry Saturn, went to Japan, one of those guys went after him, and that other guy ended up with a busted shoulder. I show my wrestlers how to do these cute little things which are not allowed in amateur wrestling. But I went through it all myself in my heyday. To tell you the truth, I was challenged by an amateur wrestler one time, and I said, "Look, back off, leave me alone." He called me a faker and other things, and finally we went to the school gym. Well, the whole thing lasted about 30 seconds, and I broke his ankle. I apologized to him, and he said, "Oh, no, it's my fault, I'll know better next time." Another amateur wrestler challenged me, and I broke his leg, too.

Back when you were wrestling, what was your impression of Karl Gotch as a shoot fighter?

Mr. Gotch and I were very close friends. When he first came over from Europe, I was the world's champion up in Montreal. He came up and some people told me to go to the gym and look at this guy because he was good and really tough. I said no, I'll just go to the gym and work out with the weights a little bit, and that's enough. But we eventually became close friends. He was just starting out and I was trying to help him any way I could. Later we became very close friends. They took Karl Gotch to Japan, and had him train the Japanese in some really tough amateur wrestling called shooting. He trained them there. I had a reputation in Japan because one time I knocked the head off of Antonio Inoki. They sent a sumo wrestler out after me and I ended up crushing his nose. That was when I was in my heyday. When I went to Japan to wrestle, Karl Gotch was living there with his wife. But wrestlers always traveled separately there. One part of the train was for the Japanese, another part was for the Western wrestlers. When I went over, Karl Gotch started traveling with me. I asked him how he was doing and who the toughest person over there was. He said he was doing fine and the toughest person was Inoki. I asked him how tough he was and he said he figured Inoki could beat most of the guys in America. I asked him how long it would take him to beat me, and he said he could never do that. He said that Inoki talked about me and that I was the toughest guy that ever came to Japan. He told Inoki that I was the toughest guy in America, too. But we had one match, and Inoki tried to do a cutie on me. That's when I knocked him out.

You actually knocked him out?

That's true, yeah. He lay there, too.

What's your take on Lou Thesz?

Lou Thesz is a very dear friend of mine. In fact, when I went to wrestle in the St. Louis office, Lou Thesz was there — he was the world's champion. He took me to the gym and said, "Walter, you're going to meet guys in that ring that once in a while are gonna try to test you, just to see how tough you really are." So he started training me and showing me the stuff. I was challenged later on, and I would do one move, and the guy would back off. And pretty soon I had a reputation — don't mess with Kowalski, because if you get him mad, he'll get ya.

Could you share your thoughts on Gorgeous George?

He was before me, but we spanned each other, I did wrestle him in Fort Worth, Texas, one time back in the '50s. Gorgeous George utilized television for what it was worth — a form of advertising. That's exactly what it was. His real name was George Wagner. An ordinary, good wrestler. But when he started doing television, which was live, and black and white, he got this idea about all these fancy robes and the perfume and the valet, and spraying his opponent with the perfume. And he'd attract attention. And soon people recognized him as a big superstar because he stood out above everyone. Another guy who utilized the same thing and used television as advertising was Nature Boy Buddy Rogers. Everything you see on television, including the soap operas and all of that, is all a form of advertising for people who are sponsoring the show. You're sitting there and watching all this hype and baloney on television, and it's all for the advertisers who are paying for the time.

And you knew how to use it to advertise yourself.

That's right, because when I used to be on it, I would jump around, scream, holler, and make noise, and make the people notice me above my opponent.

Recently in your column, you mentioned that Brian Pillman signed with the WWF.

As soon as the WWF read that, they called me and said, "Walter, we didn't sign yet. There's something in his contract with WCW about a 40-day no-compete clause." They couldn't really admit or acknowledge anything, so I had to apologize to them. But on the q.t., he may be coming to WWF. Where else would he go? He's a pretty good man. He wants to make the bucks, so there's only one place to go. I know I couldn't pay him enough.

Walter, you retired from the ring in 1977, you came back out of retirement to fight John Tolos for Onita's group, FMW.

That's right. They called me up from Japan and asked if I would come there. I told them it depends on who I'm wrestling. They said John Tolos. I said, "John Tolos? He's my age, he stumbles and fumbles like I do. Sure, I'll wrestle him." And he was glad to hear the same thing — "Kowalski, wow. I'll go against him." And we had a ball. And they treated me really well.

If Onita asked you back to wrestle maybe The Sheik, would you go?

Sure I would.

So you still like it in the ring.

Well, after I came back I thought I was getting a little bigheaded. I wrestled Nikolai Volkoff a year ago, and I wrestled Honky Tonk Man, too. I got a call to do a special little wrestling deal in New Jersey, and I wrestled Baron Von Raschke. After that I said to myself, "Walter, who are you kidding? Knock it off." And I did. So now if somebody asks me I say forget it. I was just trying to prove to some young kids that the old geek still could move around.

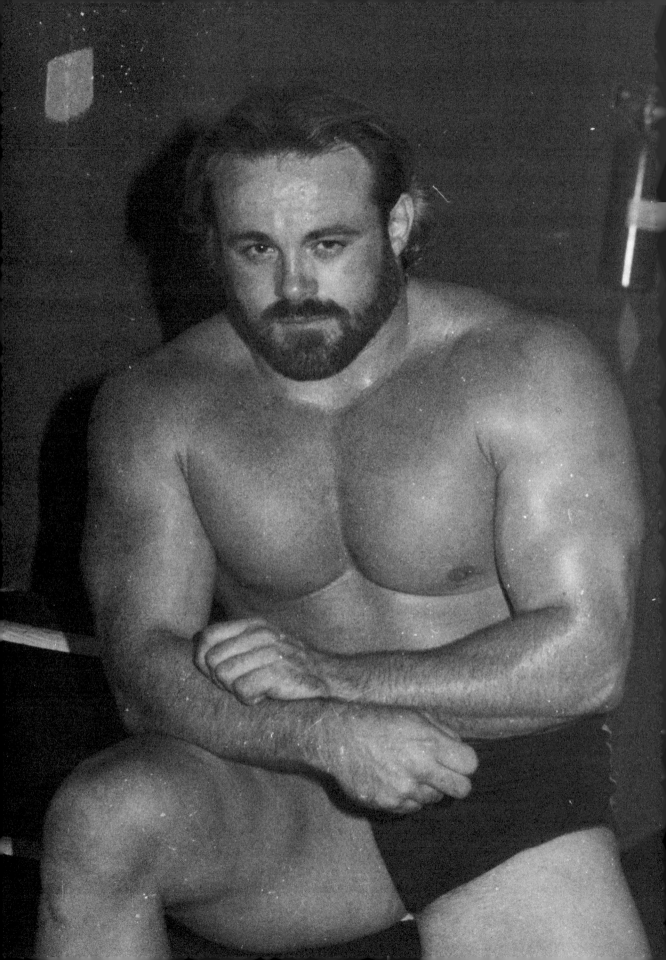

Kevin Sullivan
April 7, 1994

Kevin Sullivan was and still remains one of the toughest and funniest guys in the business. The interview was done from his home in Florida, where his wife Nancy (Woman) could be heard laughing at some of the questions and answers in the background. Sullivan had a ball throughout this interview, partly because he's from the Boston area and he knew he was talking with a couple of homies. He also seemed to really enjoy some of the obscure questions, such as the one about his days working with the bizarre Reverend Mr. Black. He was also quite clear about his love for the business and said that when his wrestling days were over, he hoped to continue working behind the scenes as a booker, a job he had already been doing for a while. It was interesting to hear him correctly predict how the addition of Mexican and Japanese wrestling would lead to some success for wcw, and that Terra Rizing would become a major star.

We want to introduce a local boy, born in Inman Square in Cambridge and raised in Lexington. During high school he did some wrestling, some baseball, football, some swimming and then went to college in California. If my memory serves, right after college he went into professional wrestling. First match was in Montreal in 1970 and before long he became known as the Boston Battler. And we've heard that he's bathed in the Ganges. We have with us today, Kevin Sullivan.

Absolutely right, I have bathed in the Ganges, and I noticed while I was bathing that I gazed off and you were there, too. And I don't want to bring this up to your listeners, but that goat you were with . . . I don't know why you had a goat with high heels and you were wearing a wig with sunglasses on.

Oh, this is going to be a tough interview. We have with us, Mr. Kevin Sullivan. Thanks for coming on the show, sir.

Thanks for having me.

Where are you speaking to us from?

From Daytona Beach, Florida, which is my hometown now.

Let's jump right into your wrestling history — was 1970 right?

Absolutely right.

So you've been around for a while doing this. You're stronger than ever. It's hard to believe you're still brawling like you are, but it looks like you keep in shape. How did you get into this business?

I was an amateur wrestler and I was working out at the Boston YMCU, which is a wrestling club, as most people know in Boston. And I was approached by a professional wrestler and thought of giving professional wrestling a try. I went up to Montreal and the rest is history.

It's quite a bit of history. You've been all over the world wrestling. You're currently in two federations right now — WCW and are you still working with ECW?

Yes I am. Smoky Mountain, too.

And they say that you find a little bit of time to go fishing once in a while.

Yes, fishing is my hobby. I live here in Daytona Beach, but we have a place in Key Largo, where I go fishing with some of the greatest fisherman in the world, really, seriously. One of my friends goes fishing with Ted Williams, my idol.

What's good right now?

Well, right now the dolphins are running. And it's not like the dolphin, Flipper.

You're talking about mahimahi.

Yeah, the dolphins are running pretty good. We've had pretty good tarpon run in the backwaters. I also skin-dive and the lobster season's been great.

Let's go back a few years. Did you watch wrestling as a kid?

Yes, I was very, very enthralled with wrestling as a kid.

Who were your idols? Wasn't The Sheik one?

He's my idol to this day. I've never been a guy that said, "Oh, this guy's my hero" in any [other] sports. And I think that's a problem sometimes in this day and age. There are people who people put up as heroes, and none of us are pure of heart all the time, let's say. But The Sheik was always my hero and still is my hero.

He's still working at an amazing rate, isn't he?

He's still a very mystical guy. I mean The Sheik's a personal friend of mine, and to me, he's the epitome of wrestling, in my style anyway.

Have you ever fought him?

Yes I have.

What was it like mixing it up with the likes of him? Was that tough stuff?

It was probably the only time that I've ever been nervous in a wrestling match.

Was there anybody else that you watched growing up as a kid?

Killer Kowalski.

We had him as a guest just a couple of weeks ago, as a matter of fact.

He's a terrific man. He was and probably still would be a great performer. I remember as a kid he was the big thing in Boston.

And did you know then that you wanted to grow up to be a pro wrestler?

I think I knew when I was six that I wanted to be a pro wrestler.

Looking back now, after all this time, what do you think determines who really makes it in the business?

I think it's like any other business. If you want it bad enough, you can make it. I mean, I'm sure that Ted Williams wasn't the greatest hitter of all time because he only batted during the game. He was the greatest hitter of all time in my estimation probably because he practiced more than anybody else. I'm talking mostly, I'm going to go with Boston — Boston athletes — Larry Bird certainly wasn't the most gifted basketball player of all time. Certainly wasn't the fastest. As most people know, white men can't jump. So, how did he become Larry the Legend? I'm sure [he practiced on] the court he had in French Lick and when he went home in the off-season he kept playing and playing and playing. And I'm not just saying it's in sports. I'm sure if a guy's a good car salesman, he goes out and does it and does it and does it. I think it's drive. It's in you. It's drive.

What does it take to win over the crowd, especially in a business where you've got to win them over?

In my opinion, when people pay their money, whether it's for wrestling, baseball, or hockey, they want to see the performer give 100 percent. I think intensity is the key. If you're not intense, then people feel that. Getting back to The Sheik, I remember as a kid seeing The Sheik wrestle and I couldn't believe the electricity in the building. I mean, I could actually feel a change in the building when he came out. So I think intensity is one of the keys; the people deserve to get their money's worth. And I hope that I've tried to give them Kevin Sullivan 100 percent of the time.

In the old World Wide Wrestling Federation days, you were a babyface. You've obviously had a bit of a heel turn since then. Is one role more fun or better to be a part of than the other?

You know, one thing I try to do is, like Satchel Paige says, "Don't look back." And people have asked what my fondest memories are or what match I like the best. And my standard answer is that I like the next one.

So you look toward the future.

I don't think you can look to the past in anything. I mean, the past is gone, so look at now and the future.

Are you really an honorary citizen of The Bahamas?

Yes I am.

And you were the Bahamian champ?

I am still the Bahamian champ.

Still? Have there been any others?

I was Jamaican champ, too.

What other belts have you had?

Well, I held the Florida title and Southern title. If people remember California as a territory, I held the U.S. belt there. Tag team champions numerous times with numerous partners and all of them great: Mike Graham, Ken Lucas, Steve Williams. I had the National TV championship in Georgia Championship Wrestling. I had the Georgia Championship title. Too numerous to remember.

That's a good little list. You've obviously spent a lot of time in Florida and we've noticed through cable the fans down there are rabid. When you first got down there and saw this kind of reception, did that do anything to your style?

It made me more intense, that's for sure, because I was lucky enough to be here when Eddie Graham was alive and active. And if you talk to anyone, from Steve Keirn to Dickie Slater to Paul Orndorff, they'll tell you that Eddie Graham was a genius of the wrestling business.

Was there one thing that put him above everyone else, as far as his operating style?

Yes. He was a student of the business and knew it better than anyone. Of course, this was in a day of territories, and I don't know in this day in age if he would be as tuned in.

You've mentioned territories a couple of times. Do you think that territories will ever come back?

I don't think you could go back in anything. Like, I'm a baseball purist. I think what they've done this year is deplorable with the Wild Card implementation. They've taken the very essence of the game away.

So you're still a Red Sox fan?

Oh, I'm a die-hard fan.

Let's go back to wrestling. Are crowd reactions different for you around the world?

In Japan, they know tradition. If you ask some of your listeners who Eddie Graham or Lou Thesz are, they might not know. In Japan, they know who they are because they're educated and they know tradition and take it very seriously.

Is wrestling big in Israel?

I remember when World Class Championship Wrestling went over there that the Von Erichs were like gods. There's great reaction. It was the first time World Class had come, and they had the tapes for years.

Tell us what injuries you're living with.

Fingers, ankles. My ulna nerve, elbow, like (Joe) Montana. I've injured that. That's the most serious.

Do you have one favorite feud?

There was Dusty and Black Jack Mulligan in Florida. At the time, it was the hottest thing, for like three years.

We don't see those anymore.

Well, now it's so MTV. Quick fixes. The reason why the NBA has been successful is making it faster. And look at the news. Most things are only on for 12 seconds. That's why it's an MTV generation. The one thing that's changed us is having the clicker in our hands. Sometimes I'll watch two basketball games and a baseball game at the same time.

Who do you like out there, as far as the future generation of wrestling?

The Harris Brothers, I think are phenomenal. I think that Cactus Jack and Maxx Payne are great. I think Arn Anderson and Steamboat are going to be great (as a team). I think Tazmaniac, Tommy Dreamer and Terra Rizing are going to be the future of this business.

Terra is one of Walter's boys.

Yeah, and all they need is just a little seasoning, that's all.

We're sure you'll be there to help them.

I hope so. The business is constantly changing and they need new faces, and I'm all for that.

Have you always had total control of your character and interviews?

Well, we used to drive from town to town, sometimes 150 miles and we'd use that downtime to do interviews.

Your character has evolved over the years . . .

Yeah and I've had control over it evolving.

That leads us to another area. The phase down in Florida with the whole "devil" thing, but I don't think the word "devil" was used. How do you handle the fans and character with this? Were there ever any confrontations with fans?

No, but you have to understand, I am and have been evil. We all can be, even you. We all have a yin and a yang. We have an evil side and a spiritual side. That's why there are wars. If it wasn't, we wouldn't have psychiatrists. We all have an animal side and a spiritual side. And if you think you don't, what about when you go to a Bruins game and Ray Bourque is checked into the boards and you start screaming?

You're a collector of oddities and we figured that we could play word association with a few names in the business.

OK.

Luna Vachon . . .

Luna Vachon. Woman (then his wife, now his ex-wife) cut her hair on live TV and Luna gave it to me. She's fabulous. I think she's one of the top five interviews in the business. I think she's total energy.

Bob Roop . . .

Bob Roop was a very talented amateur wrestler. He's had many identities in the business and I think he never reached his full potential.

King Curtis . . .

King Curtis — the greatest interview of all time. Dusty, Piper, Billy Graham couldn't hold a candle to this guy. I'd say they're up there, but they couldn't carry Curtis' jock. The best speaker in the business.

Gary Hart . . .

Gary Hart. A very smart guy, probably outsmarted himself a few times, but a smart guy. A very intense individual.

Yeah, you can see that in his eyes. Any idea where he is?

No I don't. I've lost track of Gary and I usually keep up on most when they leave the business. But I've lost track of Gary Hart. Maybe he's in the Isle of Misery or the Tree of Woe.

The Tree of Woe — hey, did you get that from the Conan movies?

Oh, you watched the movie, too. They stole that from me.

We're going on the record with that.

OK.

The Reverend Mr. Black. We've never seen him before, and don't know who he is. Can you educate us?

You know how I said that people make mistakes in the business? Don't blame that on me. That wasn't my idea.

What was that about?

Sometimes, when someone gets power, they think an idea will be good. I saw this and said, "Oh, boy. This isn't going to be good." We shot a film where the Reverend Mr. Black was digging through the earth and was brought to life by tannis leaves, like Boris Karloff. Well I ran out of tannis leaves the first night in Jacksonville, Florida, and he couldn't kick out of a dropkick by Scott McGhee. Someone at ringside said they expected better from me and I turned around and said, "Don't blame me, I think he's dead already." Just one match. Sometimes at night when my conscience is bothering me, he'll visit me.

The legendary Mr. Black made a name for himself.

Yes he did.

What else in the business would you like to do?

I'd like to do production. Stuff behind the scenes. When Carl Yastrzemski went down, he helped with the hitting. The younger boys are coming up and will need teaching. I made mistakes and still do and want to help the young kids. They're the future of the business — eventually it's going to be theirs.

Are you working on any booking committees right now?

No I'm not.

There are some problems with mismanagement. But who's doing it right, right now?

Well, you have to take into consideration that it's a cyclical business. There's starting to be a swing back up. The new talent and old talent mixing, and Japanese coming over here and possibly Mexican wrestlers. With all this blend, I think the business, when run right, runs itself; but when wrong, it's like a snowball, and hard to turn around. But I see a resurgence. There's a lot of good, young talent out there. There's Terra Rizing and Public Enemy and Brian Lee and Tommy Dreamer and Tazmaniac. Jungle Jim Steele. I think you'll see some of these guys turn things around in the next few years. They'll take the place of Sullivan, Anderson, Flair, Steamboat — but for now we need the veterans. With the imports, like I'd like to see Konnan from Mexico vs. Sabu. I'd like to see Kevin Sullivan vs. The Sheik. Sheik vs. anyone. Things are turning around and guys like you are helping, and maybe we should tip our hats more to guys like you for helping. I think in the next year you'll see the business back on track. I'll tell you what I tell everyone. I'm going to stick around and make everyone miserable, including you. And I won't tell people about when you were stuck to the Tree of Woe and the Princess of Uganda was plucking at your breast. It was very memorable. She told me to send the child support payments in care of me, anytime.

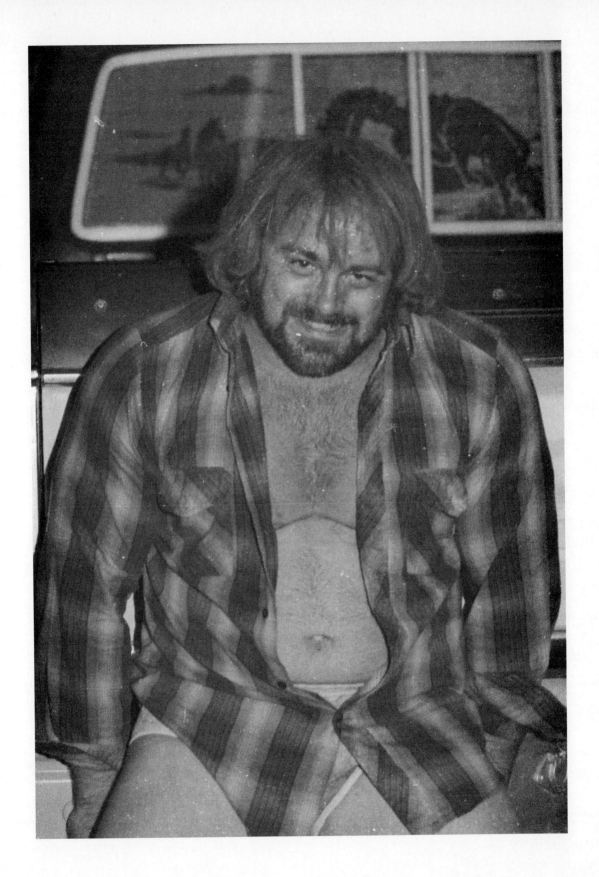

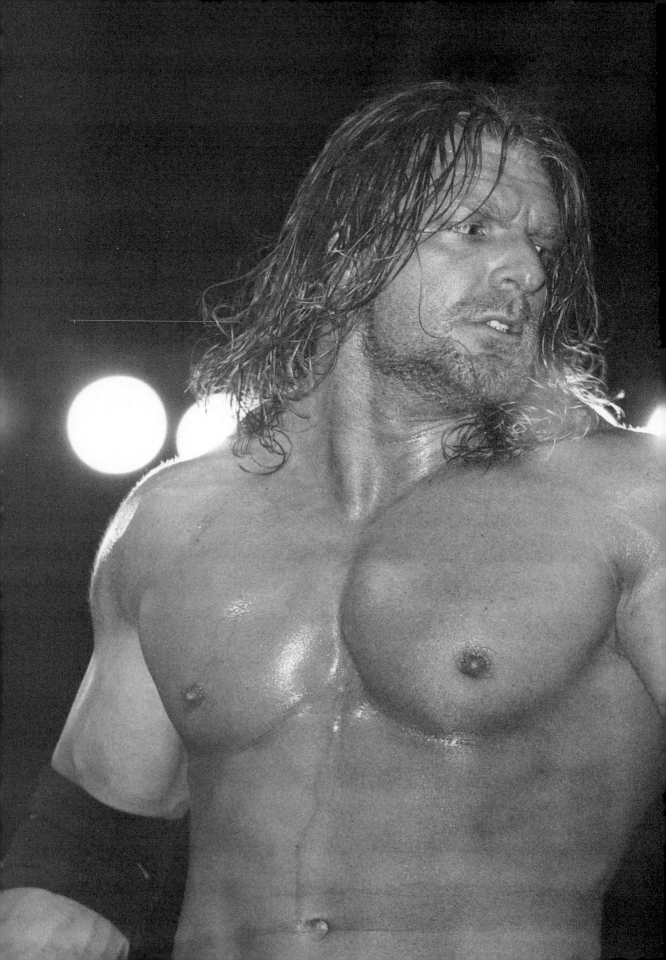

Triple H
April, 1994

There's no question that Triple H has become a Top 10 fixture within the world of wrestling, but who knew in 1994? The funny thing is that Paul Levesque wasn't even scheduled to be on our show that day. Dave Meltzer, the editor of the "Wrestling Observer Newsletter," was already scheduled for that afternoon. However, a few days prior to the broadcast, we checked in with the offices of WCW to schedule upcoming guests and realized that they had booked a newcomer on the program for that week! It seems that some new wrestler named Terra Rizing had started with the company a few months before and WCW was looking at promoting him for upcoming TV shows and possible pay-per-views. Of course we all know now that he left a few months later for the WWF and gained national fame as Hunter Hearst Helmsley (and then Triple H). But in this early interview, Levesque talks about signing with his first national promotion, the road he took to get there, and his thoughts on the business.

Is Walter Kowalski's school where you got hooked up in wrestling?

I met up with Kowalski a year or two ago and he basically saw some potential in me and asked if would be interested in going to his school. I accepted and we went from there.

What were you doing before that?

I was running a gym and was a competitive bodybuilder and had been interested in getting in the business for a long time. I was friends with a guy by the name of Ted Arcidi at the time . . . the World's Strongest Man.

Wasn't he a math teacher?

He used to be, he used to be — and almost became a dentist if you can imagine that. He's knocked a few teeth out, but I don't know about pulling them out. But he's a very good friend of mine and it just happened that I met up with Kowalski and took it from there.

Are you under contract with WCW?

Yes, I have a year contract that we're working with and now it's just a matter of what I can show them during the year.

Who recruited you from the independent scene?

It's really funny. I was in Columbus, Georgia, for a convention and I met one of their promoters who had approached me and apparently knew me from before and asked that I send him some promotional stuff. And within a few days, I got a call from Eric Bischoff and they brought me down there to work with Keith Cole and it went from there.

Did you have to do a tryout down there?

I wrestled with Keith Cole in the tryout and they made an offer the next day. I won my first match with a reverse Indian Deathlock that the Killer and I invented.

How long were you working with Killer before they made you champ?

I had only been with him for four months and then I beat his champ, Mad Dog Richard, who had been champ for four years, for the title. At about this time the wwf was looking at me as well.

What was that about?

Pat Patterson had shown some interest in me, um, wrestling-wise.

Thanks for clearing that up.

And they were interested in me doing a dark match for them on a tv taping. But I had more interest going to work for wcw. I think they're the future of this business. I think the day of the sideshow circus gimmicks are a thing of the past.

Now that Hulk Hogan is coming to WCW, how has the morale been since it appears that some wrestlers will have to take a pay cut to justify his salary?

I don't see a morale problem, but it does seem that guys are happy with a name like that coming in to help expand across the us. When Hogan comes to an arena, people will want to go see the event and then will be exposed to the product and then will think the product of wcw is tremendous. New faces will then come and, within a few years, they'll just overshadow the business.

Someone called earlier and said that you almost went to Memphis at one point. Any truth to that?

Perry Saturn, who was a Kowalski student, was trying to work out a deal where I'd come down and be a tag team with him. I never really considered it because I don't want to do tag team matches.

If Memphis offered you a deal, would you have gone down?

To tell you the truth, Lawler and Jarrett would have had to offer a lot of money to go down there after all the horror stories that I've heard. I'm in this business to make money, not lose money. And for me to spend my own money to survive is ridiculous.

Some will say you didn't pay your dues and got an immediate break. You went right into WCW with a nice contract. What would you say to people who might say that?

This is a business of opportunity and if it happened to anyone else they would've done it. Maybe it sounds cocky, but maybe I had more talent than they did.

What's it like being the new kid in town? Any good pranks pulled on you yet?

Not yet, although I probably shouldn't say that as someone might hear this. wcw is a very professional organization and I've had no problems with them compared with other groups. Although I shouldn't say that too loudly or some of my stuff will be missing.

How often do you go to Atlanta for tapings?

Quite frequently. I have an apartment down there.

Any roommates?

No, I don't know anyone well enough to have one, and most of the boys are into stuff that I'm not into. I'm at a point at learning the business and want to establish myself first.

Well, the Titan guys are in town tonight and will probably have a few beers at the Hojo's in Revere . . .

Right. Well, I'd go but I don't drink. I'll hang out and be a designated driver with them, but I'm not really into the scene that much where I'll get in trouble.

Do you have total control of your character?

Yeah, they tell me to go out there and establish myself.

What other sports did you do growing up?

Competitive bodybuilding — national level and small state shows. Some basketball and baseball, but wrestling was what I watched growing up.

Who were your heroes?

Dusty Rhodes, Barry Windham, and Ric Flair.

Who would you like to wrestle and think that you'd have a good match with?

I'd like to face Sting and Johnny B. Badd, but Flair has had classic matches against everyone. Today, I'd say Shawn Michaels is one of the best new talents out there.

What would you like to work as, face or heel?

I'd rather work as a heel.

Why?

It goes back to being trained by Kowalski. There's a sense of instinct in me to work aggressively, and it's not my job to decide if what I do is right or wrong in the ring. That's the fans' decision.

Walter had hands-on training with you?

Yes, he's the best trainer and motivator in the world. There are some people who may not like him but he does those things for a reason.

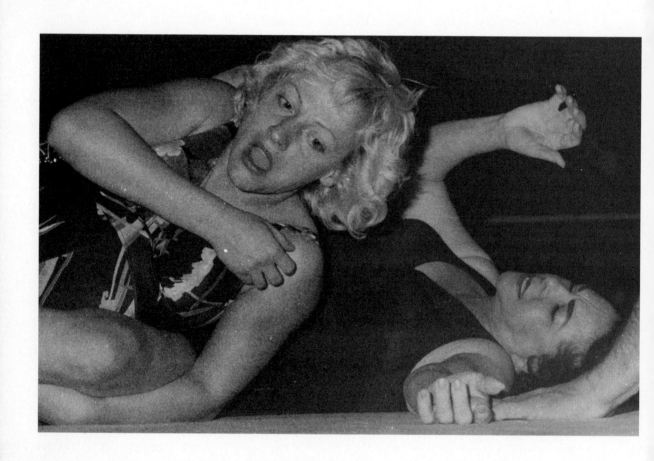

The Women

Unfortunately, women wrestlers in the United States will never be as popular or as appreciated as their counterparts in Japan, where they're regarded, in toughness and skill, as equals. Female stars have risen and fallen — just look at the history books for tales of Mildred Burke, Mae Young, and the Fabulous Moolah. But until recently, women in the ring were considered to be like the midgets — opening acts or side attractions for the big men.

Over the years, some promoters have tried to bring the gals into the spotlight. Vince McMahon put longtime champ Moolah's belt on a young and vibrant Wendy Richter in the early-1980s, and David McLane had some brief success with Gorgeous Ladies of Wrestling (GLOW) a few years later. But the whole concept was simply too gimmicky and soon burned out.

Today, Moolah and Mae Young still get involved (mostly for nostalgic laughs), but eager, talented performers like Trish Stratus have taken the reins from women such as Sherri Martel and Madusa Miceli. Now, female wrestlers have a new lease on life, and garner considerably more interest from fans.

Interviewing them was not all that different from talking with the men. The ladies' road might have been a little harder. But once they're in the ring, the name of the game is the same, and so are many of their stories.

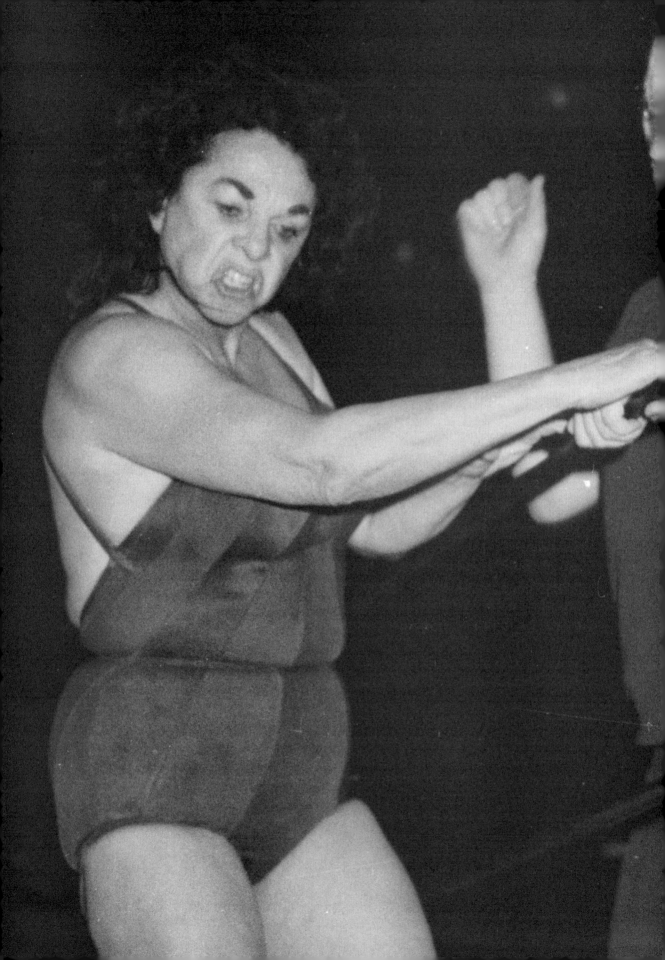

The Fabulous Moolah

May 1, 1993

Lillian Ellison was the first wrestler to be interviewed live on our show, and she pretty much set the pace for what was to come. She was obviously an old-school performer who was going to protect the business to a point, but she had no problem discussing a few behind-the-scenes stories. And considering that she was women's champ in the WWWF for close to three decades, she had a lot of stories to tell. Looking back on the interview now, after all the oddball hoopla she and her mentor, Mae Young, have been responsible for in recent years, it was quite eye-opening to find out how far back their professional and personal relationship went. Because we were still new at the game, the interview ran shorter than we would have liked, but we were worried about whether she was enjoying herself. She turned out to be one of our most charming guests.

Hello, Fabulous Moolah, you're in South Carolina, true?

Right. It's 85 degrees.

Thank you for coming on, especially since you told us the other day that you wanted to go to the beach today.

Yes I did.

You're a regular attendant of the beach?

Oh, yes. I have a condo down there.

Well we have a bunch of questions for you. We wanted to go back a few years. Tell us about working with the Elephant Boy. Was that how you started in the pro wrestling business?

No. I started when I was a valet for "Nature Boy" Buddy Rogers. And then I got the job of being with the Elephant Boy, which was better for me. And I made more money that way.

Were you called Slave Girl?

Yes, I was "Slave Girl Moolah."

What did you do?

Well, I managed him. And helped him win.

So you got in the way, back then?

Sometimes.

We're not really familiar with the Elephant Boy. Was he kind of a heel?

Yes, but he was a very, very nice man.

How long was it before you went off on your own to be a feature attraction?

Well, let's see. I was with the Elephant Boy I guess for about a year, year and a half. Then I started wrestling steady.

Now we're talking about the early 1950s?

Yes. And then in 1956 I won the world's championship in Baltimore, Maryland.

You defeated June Byers?

Yes.

Let's go back just a tiny bit because somebody mentioned to us that your first professional match was right here in Massachusetts. Is that true?

In the Boston Gardens.

Who did you fight?

Celia Blevins, a wild Indian.

Did you go under any different names?

Well, in that very first match I went in as Lillian Ellison.

That's your real name.

Yeah. And then my manager at the time changed my name to "Slave Girl Moolah" and I wrestled under that name until 1956 when I won the belt and world's championship in Baltimore. And the commissioners thought that the name was a little deceiving to the public saying "Slave Girl" because they expected someone to come out in a strange-looking outfit. So they changed my name to "the Fabulous Moolah." And that's been with me since 1956.

What are the changes that you've seen in the business in the last few decades?

Wrestling is my life. I think it's the greatest thing that's ever happened to me and I believe in real wrestling. I don't believe in all the paint and all the show and all the comedy and all that garbage. That to me has been a big downfall to lady wrestling, but the real downfall was when GLOW came in and called themselves lady wrestling. And a couple of other outfits, you know. But the LIWA is for lady wrestling — real lady wrestling.

Do you own this group?

Oh, no. This is a non-profit organization that was founded in 1985 by me, Mae Young, and Theresa Thyce. And our goal is to have a retirement center and a hall of fame for the wrestlers. And we're working very hard to do that. Every year in June we have a convention in Las Vegas. This year is going to be at the Union Plaza Hotel downtown, and on Friday, June 11, we're going to have wrestling called the "Golden Girls Extravaganza." We already have something like 23 girls signed up. This is the past, present, and future. We have girls like Mae Young wrestling. She's been wrestling for 53 years.

Mae Young. Wasn't she was your teacher at the beginning?

Mae Young taught me to wrestle. And I'm very proud of it. And I'll be wrestling on the card. Belle Starr will be there and we'll have different phases of girls like Candy Devine and Patty Franklin, Sabrina and Madusa may be there. Bambi may be there and some newer girls that have been in for only a few years. But it's real wrestling and it's ladylike professional wrestling. There's no G-string and there's nothing hanging out.

Who's the most inspirational wrestler you've encountered?

Well, I think Mae Young because she inspired and taught me. And I had a lot of respect for Mildred Burke, although I met her only one time when I started wrestling. But I can hardly remember that.

Now, when you parted ways with Vince McMahon and the WWF in the late '80s, was it on amicable terms?

Oh, yes. We've not parted by any chance and as far as I'm concerned, Vince McMahon is a wonderful man, and maybe he sees things differently than we do. Nobody sees everything the same way. And what I would like to say is he has certainly supported the LIWA and I must say that he is the only, and I want you to understand, the only promoter that has sent us donations or helped us with this LIWA, although it is for all of the wrestlers and not just us. I have to appreciate that, and even if he hadn't, he was very good to me and made me what I am today — him and his father, and I appreciate everything and we are on good terms.

Had you worked with Vince Sr. before the '80s?

Oh, yes. I worked for Vince Sr. I've been with the family for over 35 years.

Is it true that when you broke in you were wrestling in mixed tag matches with men?

Yeah, well that's how Mae Young taught me. The rougher it got the more I liked it. We wrestled in mixed tags and also we wrestled in singles matches versus the men as well.

You're involved with a group called M&M. M&M All-American, is that right?

Yes, Johnny Maye and I own this wrestling company. We train men and women. I know you've seen the Patriot wrestle, haven't you?

Del Wilkes. I've heard of him, but haven't seen him.

Del Wilkes, he's my special pupil and I'm really proud of him. We're promoting small shows to raise money for the LIWA. On Saturday night we'll have the banquet where we're honoring seven people and have a wonderful get-together with everyone.

What women wrestlers out there look to be a superstar in the next five years?

I can't say, there's a few good ones out there.

Especially in Japan, where the shows are excellent. Now you'll be attending the upcoming Slamboree pay-per-view. Who are you looking forward to meeting?

Well, Lou Thesz is going to be there. And a lot of the older ones like Johnny Valentine and about 40 other people.

What are your feelings on Sam Muchnick, one of the most revered promoters of all time?

Sam Muchnick is a wonderful person and he's always been very honest, and Paul Boesch is the same way. I really enjoyed knowing them.

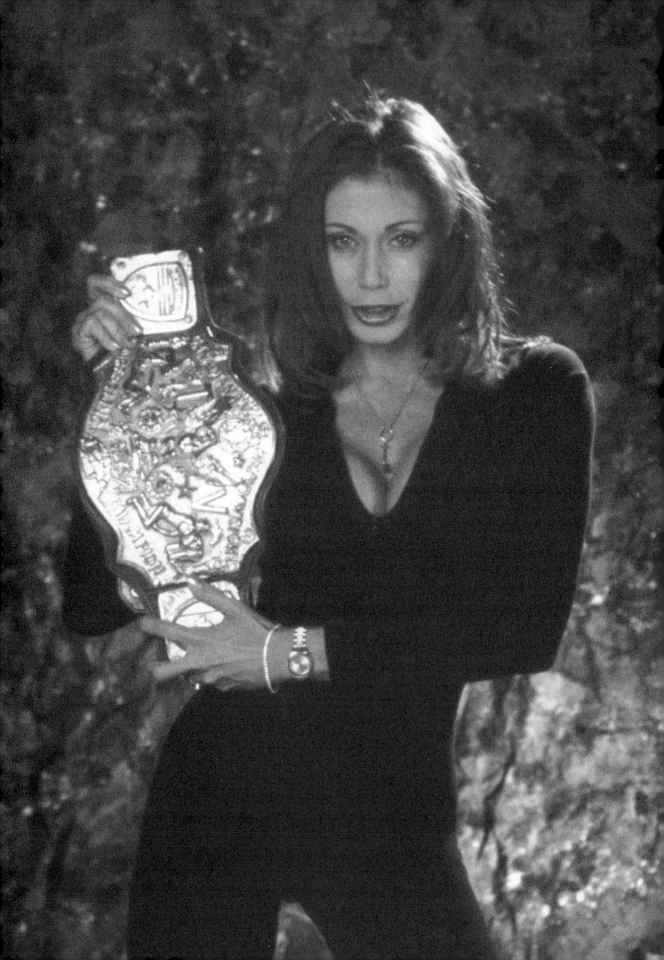

Missy Hyatt
April 23, 1994

While she wasn't the first woman to popularize the valet role in wrestling (Sunshine and Precious preceded her), she did become one of the most revered valets in all of wrestling by the mid-1980s. Even Vince McMahon brought her in for a tryout at one point. Here she talks about all things wrestling, and gives her public feelings perhaps for the last time about her ex-husband Eddie Gilbert before he passed away. She had been involved in a nasty legal battle a few years earlier with wcw, stemming from a photo she didn't approve of appearing in the offices of management. She also had trouble with Eric Bischoff that centered on her relationship with actor Jason Hervey around the same time. The interview turned a bit sad in that she had been in the business for almost 10 years at that point and didn't appear to have any friends left in it.

We have a very special guest with us today, a real coup. From the Big Apple, let's welcome Missy Hyatt. It's a great honor. You're one of our favorites. Well, there's a standard question that we ask people who get in the ring, even though you weren't in the ring much. Can you tell us your first memories of ever seeing pro wrestling?

I remember this very clearly. I was at home with my mom and dad and I was about 17 years old and I remember walking up the stairs and my dad was watching TV. I never grew up watching wrestling. And I remember seeing the Fabulous Freebirds on TV and it was Michael Hayes, Terry Gordy, and Buddy Roberts. It was back with Georgia Championship Wrestling on TBS. And I think they were putting a baby bonnet on Bam Bam's head. And I remember going, "Oh my gosh." I remember my dad flipping through the channels and I remember sitting down and going, "What is this? I mean, this stuff is great, what is this?" So I remember rushing downstairs, turning on my TV and watching it going, "I gotta watch this stuff. What is it? What is it? It's wrestling." I mean, I grew up in Florida so I always knew who Dusty Rhodes was. I remember seeing him. I thought this stuff was pretty cool.

So did you know at 17 that this was something you may want to get involved with at some point?

No, not really. I mean, I knew when I saw it that it was great, but I knew I didn't want to wrestle.

You never wanted to?

No.

So that explains the matches with you and Paul E. then, I guess.

What do you mean?

Actually we'll put the blame on him. Were you for that? Was that OK that you had to get into the ring and mess around a little bit?

I really didn't do anything. Usually the partner — it was like a mixed-tag — they did all the work and I'd come in for the glory.

Did you break into the business in 1984?

'85. You're trying to make me older than I am now?

Well, you're 31, right?

No! Boy, we're making me A LOT older than I am.

So how did you get involved, Missy?

I was with John Tatum. We were going out and David Manning and Rick Hazzard saw me one night and said, "Hey, do you want to be a manager?" And I said, "OK, cool. What do I have to do?" And they said, "Walk out to the ring with John." And I was like, "OK, I can do that."

That's it? No audition or anything?

Oh, no. I was in the right place at the right time.

Did you ever go under the guise of "Angel" for the Jarrett promotion?

I worked for them for a while.

Was that as Rick Rude's second?

No, that wasn't me.

We've seen a lot of female valets come and go like Baby Doll and Dark Journey. What women in the sport do you have a lot of respect for?

The only other woman that I really respect in this business is Boni Blackstone. And for a lot of people that don't know, she hosts a wrestling block (on TV). And she does a "Rhonda Shear's Up All Night" with wrestling in Atlanta, Georgia, and she's one of my best friends and she's survived in this business for a long time now.

That's right. She's married to Joe Pedicino.

And she's really great at what she does and I think being married to someone else in the same business is very hard because I was married to Eddie Gilbert and it's very hard having two people in the same business. I can understand actors and actresses being married — it's very hard. And she's done really well, even though her husband's in the same business. And they don't really have a lot of professional jealousy or anything, so it's really good.

It's interesting that you say that because there was an interview recently with Luna Vachon about her relationship with Dick Slater and how this business tears you apart. We saw that with Eddie Gilbert and Madusa as well, and it's a shame since you become so close, but at times work in different areas and drift apart.

Different things happen to you and it's competitive, and even if you love someone, you still have that competitiveness in you.

Well you brought up the name Eddie Gilbert a few seconds ago. We've always been so curious — obviously you're someone who's been pretty close to him. What is to become of Eddie Gilbert? Why is he not a superstar?

You know, it's always been because of his size. He can do great interviews and he's one of the best workers there is, but I think it's his size.

He's a great booker, too.

Oh, he's very smart.

He knows the business in and out, but he seems to keep vanishing.

Yeah, you know he does. He's running for election.

Oh, he's really doing it?

Yes, he's really doing it. I think it's next week and hopefully he's going to win.

Do you know what he's running for?

I think it's court clerk. All I know is everyone can get permits and tags — he can even marry people. That's a scary thought.

Do you still stay in contact with Eddie?

Every once in a while, yeah. I love his mother and he's got a really great family. I hope he wins.

We hope he wins, too. Well let's mention another name. Paul E.

Let me tell you something. Wrestling has been on TV since the beginning and has always changed with the times and how I thought that it changed with the times was that the old people should turn it over to the new, younger people. I think the Paul E. Dangerouslys and the Jim Cornettes are the future of wrestling. I mean they're the young guys and this is 1994. You can't do the things that you were doing in 1984. And I think that's a big problem with the bigger organizations. They don't have the young minds in there that really know what's going on. They keep going back to the old stuff that's just been done before. I think Paul E. is . . . I just saw his ECW tape a couple of days ago and thought it was some of the most exciting stuff I have seen in a long time.

But why does Paul E. Dangerously burn so many bridges in this business? A lot of people have trouble dealing with him. Is he a hard man to get along with?

No, I just think he knows what he wants and a lot of people can't, you know — they're in that old school or old mindset. He knows what he wants and if you can produce what he wants you to do — I mean all it is, is taking some direction and a lot of people don't like doing that. But I know of all the people who have ever worked with him, the people I know, they respect him highly. I do.

What is in store for Missy Hyatt and pro wrestling?

Well, right now I'm working with a friend of mine who's got a new concept for a television show that the Japanese have already bought. I really can't disclose that much about it but it's going to be a really exciting show.

And that's here in the States that you're talking about?

Yeah, it's going to be in syndication here in the States. And it's going to blow away anything. It's going to be a very exciting show.

Are you talking about like All-Japan Women's-type wrestling?

Nope.

OK, she's not going to tell us.

I can't tell.

Can you tell us about when we might see something?

I would say in a couple of months. We already have the pilot and we have Snapple and Revlon as the two major sponsors.

Now are you a major actress in this?

No, I'm going to be co-hosting the show. We're trying to get Mark Gastineau, as a matter of fact, to host the show, if he can talk. We know he can't box, but maybe he can talk.

If Jim Crockett's World Wrestling Network comes off and somebody buys his shows, will you go back to working for him?

Definitely. Him and Paul E. Dangerously — definitely.

What type of role would you like to play, heel or babyface? And what has been your favorite?

You know I really haven't thought about that.

It seems that you're more misplaced as a babyface. When you were with the Steiner Brothers . . .

Yeah, I definitely didn't like that. I like co-hosting a show. But doing it more professionally. I mean we're only typecast and the new show I'm going to be in will be something special. Now you're all up in Boston, right?

That's right.

A couple of my favorite hockey players are from Boston.

Don't say Cam Neely — he's married.

No, no — eewww. No, Brian Noonan, who plays for the Rangers, and Tony Amonte.

Are you a hockey fan?

Oh, definitely.

So Go Bruins, right?

Nah. I'm really rooting for the Rangers.

What was the deal with you and Vince McMahon several years ago?

The segment that I was doing wasn't that good, to be honest with you. I had only been in wrestling for a couple of years and I wasn't ready. It just didn't come off well.

Are you more at ease as an interviewer now, though?

Definitely.

What are your dreams? Any aspirations to act?

Well, I'd love to do a Broadway play with Anthony Hopkins. Sir Laurence Olivier's dead, so we can't dig him up. I'd like to do a soap or a film with Charlie Sheen. He's a babe. But I want to act. I've been going on some auditions.

For Broadway?

I'll do anything.

You should have a guest spot on "Thunder in Paradise."

That probably would be fun.

Since you don't work for WCW anymore, would you do work for Playboy?

No, not at this particular time. They had offered me and it kind of got ix-nayed, but no, not right now in my career. I would have done it then because it would have been the right time with the idea that they had.

Is there another step besides the TV show coming in Missy Hyatt's life?

The WWN and my new TV show and that's really about it.

Funny how Bischoff can impose a moral turpitude clause in WCW when some of the things they do are downright outrageous. We had also read that they wanted you to take voice lessons to drop part of your accent.

Oh, that was years ago. That was the first year that I worked for Turner and I did go to voice school and tried to get rid of some of my Southern accent.

Did they ever ask Jim Ross?

You know, sometimes I don't know what they're thinking.

Did a request like that upset you?

Hey, if they pay for it, I didn't mind. Anything to help. Anything that can help me do better in what I'm going to do. It's like taking acting classes. I've been doing that for the last couple of years.

Where are you taking these classes?

I'm starting up the new term here in New York. I'll be at the Actors' Studio. But before, when I was living in California, I worked with Ernie Lively and I did a Commercial Workshop at Tempo & Galego and did scene studies, one on one.

Now once we develop that singing voice, you're going to be a hit.

Oh, please. I couldn't carry a tune in a bucket.

Within the five years that you were at TBS, did you develop any friendships with anyone?

No.

No one?

No.

Who in this business besides Boni Blackstone would you consider a friend?

Um . . .

C'mon. Say Madusa.

She's a nice lady. I can't say anything bad about her. Road Warrior Hawk. Paul E. Dangerously.

Well you gave Hawk a pretty good slap on the face a few months back.

He deserved it. He dumped me.

Anyone in the WWF for the short time you were there?

No, I don't think so.

That's a shame. You've been in the business for a long time. Is there anything that you really learned — a good lesson out of all of this so far because we've got to wrap this up and want to end on a juicy quote.

Let's see. Well, the only thing that I learned at Turner is that working for Turner Broadcasting is a great place to be a tree but not a woman.

I've never heard that one before. Did you by any chance ever meet Ted Turner?

I sure did.

Was he nice?

No comment.

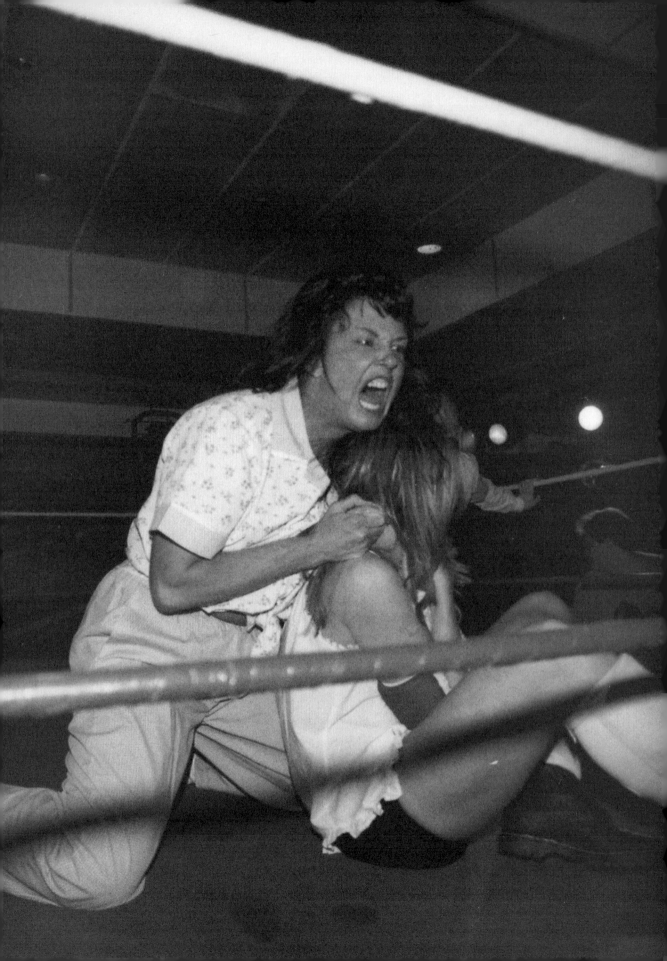

Sherri Martel
June 18, 1994

As a wrestler, Sherri Martel was fearless, learning whatever she could from the training camp of the Fabulous Moolah, wrestling throughout the South, and eventually wearing belts in the AWA and the WWF. As a manager — her charges included Ric Flair, Shawn Michaels, Randy Savage, and Harlem Heat — she was seemingly able to flick a switch and become a raving lunatic. Both in and out of the ring, the bad blood between her and Madusa Miceli became infamous. Her reputation for being a tough character preceded her, and an interviewer never knew what kind of mood would be waiting at the other end of the phone. Interestingly, Sherri made two appearances on the show. On her second, she was a firebrand, playing a nasty character. On this, her first, she was friendly and charming, and much more open to talking about herself and the business.

We have with us, the lovely, the sensuous, Sherri. How are you doing down there?

I'm just lovely. I'm cleaning out my aquarium. You have to do maintenance on them too, you know.

Well, now we know what your hobby is at home. All right. Have you been tending to fish for as long as you've been in the wrestling business?

Well, I started my hobby with fish probably about two years ago. I've been in the wrestling business for 14 years.

Fourteen glorious years. We're both longtime fans up here. You come from New Orleans, is this true?

Yeah.

Could you lead us up to just before you got into wrestling and tell us about what you were doing?

I was mama's little girl.

We can't picture that at all.

Well, I was. My mother gave birth to me out in the woods and my grandfather had to elevate her feet to slow the blood flow, so we were both kind of fighting from the day I was born. She started going to wrestling long before I did. So my sister and I would usually go roller-skating on the night that she went. She would go to the TV tapings the next morning, which was in a little bitsy studio-type thing. So she finally got me to go with her and then I went with her. I'm like, "I don't want to go," but I wound up going and fell in love with it.

Probably right away, didn't you?

No, it wasn't right away. It was after she took me 10, 15 times.

And did you know then that this was something you wanted to do?

Well, I wanted to get into some type of entertainment. I've always been a tomboy. My sister and I both are. I went to a wrestling school in Memphis, Tennessee. I'd probably say that was in 1979. Then I went to the Fabulous Moolah school to be, how would you say . . .

Groomed?

Groomed. Thank you. Yeah, I was there for about a year.

You took lessons from Moolah herself?

Yeah.

And then you kind of took off. Did you hit early on?

No, it actually took me about six years. I went to her in like September of 1980 and January and February of 1981. I did a two-month tour of Japan. Then I came back to the States and I worked for about a year, and one of my knees dislocated and then I quit for a while. Then I started back up in Memphis, Tennessee, and I started managing there. It's where I first started managing. As a matter of fact, one of the guys that's in the Heavenly Bodies, Tom Pritchard, he and Pat Rose were my first Heavenly Bodies. That is where I was first a manager.

Before coming to WCW, you were working for a hot organization in Mexico called AAA. What did you think of working for that organization?

Well, I think they're doing really good. The only thing is that our shows usually start at 7 and are over at 10 p.m. Well, their shows start about 8 p.m. and go until midnight. They're very slow people when putting things together, but when they eventually put things together they have to go according to time sequence.

It must have been strange seeing these rabid fans in Mexico throwing things at the bad guys.

It was terrible. I can understand people releasing a little bit of energy, because that's what I do. I never argue with anyone at home because I would save everything and take my aggressions out at work. Some of the guys hate me for that.

Looking back from this point, have you had a preference in working as a manager, valet, or wrestler? What do you like to do most in the business?

Well, when I was wrestling at a particular time, then it was wrestling. When I started managing, the thing that scared me was that I didn't know how to talk on TV. And you know yourself when that red light goes on, there's no turning back. It's true that you can do the interviews over, but you just have to get comfortable with the storyline. Greg Gagne was the worst in the world when I worked in the AWA. But I thank him to this day — he's in WCW now — but he used to make us do two-and-a-half-minute interviews and we'd have 60 markets to do, and it would take all day.

Man, that's a long interview.

He wanted it perfect. You couldn't say, "damn" or "hell" or "bitch" or all these kinds of things that you're not supposed to.

Aren't you glad that you can say it now?

I've been known to cross a few lines, guys. So I apologize. Y'all caught me on a good day! It's really hard on the women today, because most of the women who have been able to last a long length of time in this business have been able to do interviews. A lot had to do with the interviews, then my love was managing. I still got to put my two cents in.

You mentioned Japan. What do you think of the WWF crossing over to promote with All-Japan Women's?

Well, hey that's fine. I have nothing against Mr. McMahon. I've nothing but respect for him because he treated me good for six years. They've got Alundra Blayze and she lived in Japan, so it'd make sense to me to have her there since Japanese is her best style.

By the way, we call her Madusa up here.

Whatever. I never did like that name. It reminds me of "Clash of the Titans," with the snake in the hair.

What was your working relationship with Debbie Miceli (Madusa)?

I worked a little bit with her in the AWA, and after I left there I haven't seen her very much. You know, she keeps trying to shoot her mouth off. She's the one that has something to prove — I don't have a damn thing to prove to anybody. I've whipped her ass on more than one occasion.

But is there legitimate animosity with you and Madusa?

You can formulate your own opinion on that.

Because you did an interview with John Clark of the "Wrestling Flyer" newsletter where Vince McMahon asked you if you could get back into the ring and, of course, you knew that there was a lady wrestler that would be going into the WWF, perhaps to replace you. And he said that it'd be Luna and you said that it wasn't a problem. If it were to have been Madusa instead, would there have been a problem?

Well, it was coming close to my time to leave there anyway, so I didn't really give a damn one way or the other. The way I figure it, there's enough work out there for everybody, but if someone's going to take my spot, they're going to have to back that up, too.

A few years back, a whole new thing started in wrestling. This has nothing to do with you, but we'd like your take on it. What was your first reaction, Sherri, to GLOW?

Some of the girls were very talented. I don't know where half of them got their names from, but I had heard that they watched a bunch of Japanese women's tapes and that none of them had actually trained and knew how to wrestle. And in this business I believe that if you can't go out and back up what you're saying about what you can do, you're only going to wind up degrading other people in the sport. Now those ladies out there, they wore some stuff — you know Vince got onto me for wearing this revealing chap outfit in England, and there are people wearing less on the street. Besides we were in England and I know it's legal over there. And then Luna got him on that one and started to wear thong outfits, so I called him on that one.

But let's talk about the idea of GLOW. Did it degrade the sport or women in the sport, as you don't see much of it now?

Don't bother me any. I figure there's enough for everybody. The federations out there now have women that will wrestle.

Are there good ones?

Working full-time, I only know of Alundra Blayze, Luna Vachon, and myself.

Have you been a fan of women wrestlers in the past? Have there been any bright spots that you look back on?

That'd have to be Moolah, because number one, she's my teacher. She taught me so many lessons in the ring that went over into my life and everything. Penny Banner is a wonderful lady. Kay Noble, remember her?

Know the name, never saw her work.

Yeah, well the last time I saw her was in Kansas City. Oh, God, Maria Benardi. I go to the Cauliflower Alley convention and I always see the ladies out there.

Yeah, there was a photo of you from the Cauliflower banquet. You had the biggest smile I've ever seen.

Oh, I was having a great time!

If Tonya Harding wanted to become a wrestler and asked you to train her, would you do it?

No. Number one, I don't want to train anyone because I don't want to wrestle anymore. My body's beat up enough. And they've got schools out there for that. And it's hard for a guy to get into the business today, much less a woman starting out. And to me, seems she needs an attitude adjustment, anyway. I might just do it just for the fun of it.

You mentioned injuries. Any serious injuries throughout the career?

Just about a year and a half ago, Shawn Michaels busted a mirror over my head and got glass — he didn't mean to — but got glass in my eye. Things happen. It took me out for a while.

Do you think women will ever sit on the booking committees?

No.

Why not?

Because it's a male-dominated business and it's always gonna be.

Have you ever tried to crack into it?

No. I wouldn't ever want the headaches. It'd be nothing but a headache. Moolah would do that, book them into other promotions, but it's a pain in the ass.

So she booked them into other federations?

Yeah, but when I first started out in the business, if you weren't working for Moolah, you weren't working anywhere.

Would you be blackballed from the business?

You just wouldn't get booked because people knew if you worked for Moolah that you were top quality.

Well, let's talk about your current role. What brought you back to WCW? How did you get into your current position?

Well, I left New York last July. And I was just working on the weekends and stuff because I was going back to beauty school so I could get my license. And I called my friend Cassidy in Philadelphia and she said she had seen [wcw promoter] Gary Juster and that I should call and say, "Hi," as Missy Hyatt's contract was coming up. And I said, "I'm not looking for a job, Cat." And she said, "No, just call him and say hello." So I did, and he said, "Sherri, if you're looking for a job . . ." And I said, "I didn't call looking for a job. I just called to say hello." I said, "What's the deal with all you people? Can't anybody even be nice or what?" So two weeks later, he calls me and wants to talk to me about a contract.

This was Gary Juster?

Yeah.

Who is your immediate boss at WCW these days?

Eric Bischoff.

It looks like you're being programmed into a manager's spot again. True?

Yeah, oh gosh I hope so. I've had so much fun.

Yeah, well you sound like you do, and look like you do when you're on camera, too.

Well, when people watch it, I want them to feel satisfied. When they come away from the arenas with ticket prices and souvenirs, I like for them to feel like they've gotten their money's worth.

That's nice to hear.

Well, if I don't feel like I've given it all I've got, then I'm unhappy with myself, and I don't like to feel unhappy.

Well, we've seen what you can do in the ring and know what you can do. When was the last time you appeared in the Boston Garden?

Oh, about two years. I used to love that place.

Okay, so you're coming in as a manager now. We've seen you out there scouting.

Looking for a man.

Looking for a man. We've seen you specifically looking at the likes of, oh, I don't know, someone named Brian Pillman.

Well . . . so?

So, what do you think of him?

Well, number one, he's very handsome.

He's also one of the hottest wrestlers out there.

He's hot all right.

Who else are you thinking of?

Well, if you watch the Clash, you'll find out who my guy's going to be.

Shameless plug number one. What color hair does he have?

We're not telling.

I think it might be Ric Flair.

That would be good. Curt Hennig would be good, too. He can sing, too. Put him on the piano and he can go.

Sherri, a serious question. July looks like it'll be a heated month for Vince McMahon (on trial for steroid distribution). Personally, do you think something will happen to him as far as seeing time?

To be perfectly honest, I don't know what's going on up there because I'm not in the dressing room with the guys and I don't know what they do. I'm not in the office. I will say this. I hope the very best for him, because when something like this happens, it affects the business and fans.

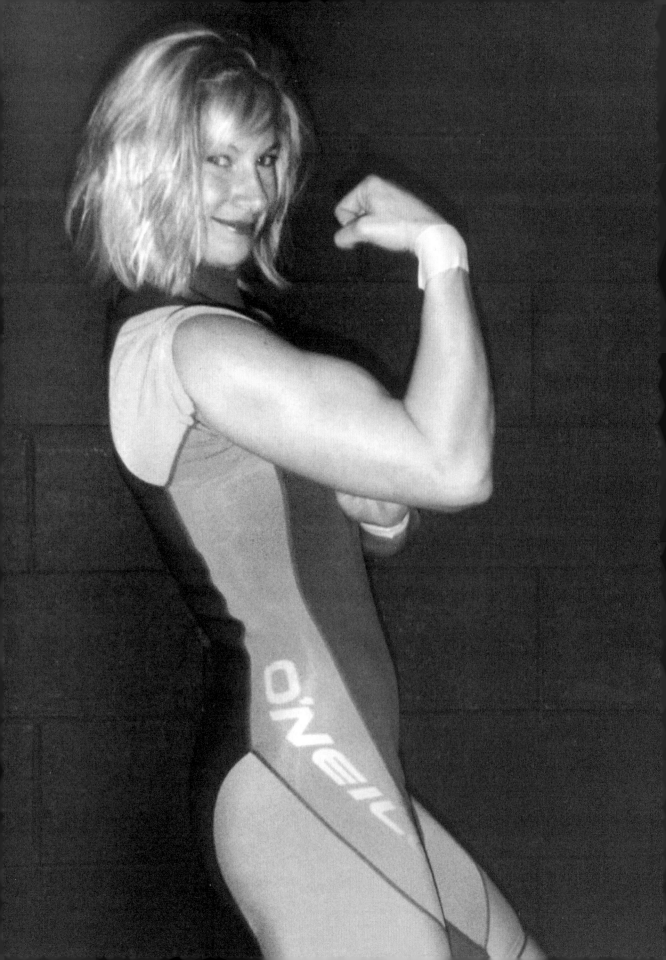

Madusa Miceli
March 2, 1996

Debra Miceli worked in and out of all the major US promotions during her wrestling career, as well as making a big splash in the Far East, eventually wearing title belts in the AWA, All-Japan Women's Wrestling, and the WWF, where she was known as Alundra Blayze. One of her strangest moments was when she left the WWF, took the belt with her to WCW, and threw it in a trashcan during a live broadcast of "Nitro." After agreeing to come on the show to discuss her accomplishments in the sport, she opened up to talk about her own previous careers, other women and men she's worked with in wrestling, and the differences between the American and Japanese promotions, and to share some thoughts on success and failure in the business, and what else she'd like to do besides wrestle.

Madusa, we'd like to get a little bit on your background. The first job you had was at an Arby's and then you became a model, and then a nurse, before getting into wrestling. Is that right?

All of that is correct. Let's see, I started when I was about 14, that's when I was on my own.

At that Arby's?

Yeah. Fourteen, living on my own, had my own apartment and a very poor family. I'm an only child. My mother and father divorced when I was 7, so I mean it was survival.

So you grew up to become a wrestler?

I wasn't really watching on TV, it's something that I didn't plan, that I didn't have big hopes or dreams to be. What happened was with all my athleticism, gymnastics, with all that athletic background I just fell into it. And it was probably my best career move yet.

Do you remember the first time you actually saw it on TV and had even a flicker of an interest?

Oh, I remember the first time I did see it on TV. It was the AWA, because I was living in Minnesota at the time, and I remember these two guys doing an interview and they were just spitting and hollering and everything at each other. And I thought: God, what two goofs could sit there on TV and holler like that? And make a living at it.

Wasn't Eddie Sharkey one of the first people you worked with?

Yeah, that's correct. Eddie Sharkey's pretty cool. He used to wear big, long trench coats and had watches under his jacket selling door-to-door to people. That's how Eddie used to make his bucks. And a friend of mine, Ky Michaelson, introduced me to Eddie Sharkey and he said that I'd be really good at it, in entertainment. I thought mud wrestling or something like that. So I said, "Take a hike." He said, "No, professional wrestling." So he introduced me to Eddie and he brought me to this wrestling camp, which was the size of a bedroom. It was a mat, with guys doing these rolls and stuff in the middle of the floor.

Didn't Brad Rheingans train you?

Brad, he came after, when I went into the AWA. I did a lot of independents in Minnesota first. I had to drive 300 miles each way, 600 total just for one shot. And I remember Eddie paying me $15.

And then he probably took his piece of it, right?

He still took his $5. I look back at those days and the days that I slept in my car and got my car repo'd. I lost everything. I got kicked out of my apartment. And then I had to sit down and have a "come to Jesus" talk with myself and say, "What the heck am I doing?" But I never quit!

Then what brought you to your first big break with Verne Gagne and the AWA?

Well, again it was my friend, Ky. He said that if I want to get anywhere that I better start putting together a portfolio and start sending it out. I remember way back in '84, I had my own business card. No one had their own business cards in the business back then.

What did it say on it?

It said, "Madusa Miceli — Professional Wrestler in Entertainment." I still have one of them. It was in blue and gold foil. And I just handed them out. I'd hand out a portfolio and everything that I'd done in my background and I submitted it to Verne. I remember Wahoo McDaniel called me at home. He's the one that really pushed for me in the AWA and I've got to say that Verne Gagne probably is the only one that really gave women a big push way back then. I mean, nobody else was.

Was Sherri the champ then?

Sherri was champ at the time, right. I remember she would kick my butt around the ring from post to post and I would wake up in the middle of the night hurting and bruised and all broken up and she'd never talk to me. She hated me. She hated me I think for 10 years.

You're talking out of the ring?

Oh, yeah.

That's got to be tough to work with someone that way.

Yeah, well you just go in the ring and business is business and you've gotta do what you've gotta do.

Was it because you were the new kid in town?

Probably. I think that wherever Sherri went, she had this apparition of me following her, you know? Maybe she was scared to death.

That happened for a while, too, didn't it?

It did. She was in AWA and I came in. She went to the WWF and I went and enhanced my skills and went to Japan and lived there for three years. And I came back and went to WCW and then WWF. She left. I left and went to WCW, where my home is and "where the big girls play." And I come here and she comes in.

You were AWA champion when the organization was falling apart, right?

Yeah, Verne had a good thing going but just didn't change with the times. He was stagnant. If you lived in a log cabin and traveled with a horse and buggy, nowadays you just wouldn't survive. That was kind of how Verne Gagne was. But he was a great guy and he promoted me well and he paid me well and I have nothing bad to say about that organization at all.

Was there anything different about how Verne ran things versus the other groups you worked for?

Everything changes and gets better. Verne was good at the time but he wasn't changing, nor was he getting better. So that's just bad. The TV wasn't enhancing. It was the same boring blue backdrop with no excitement.

So how did you get involved in Japan?

I remember the Japanese girls came to the AWA. Verne was so into it, so right with the times right about then. I mean way back then he was bringing over the Japanese, and there was something established that he could have gone far with. But after that the company starting crumbling and after my match with Chigusa, the Japanese were so surprised an American could keep up with the Japanese. So they spoke to me after the match and asked if I'd be interested in coming over, probably intermittently back and forth. And I did that, and when I went over the first four weeks I did really well. I did so well that they asked me to come back another six. And then I came back for another four. And then after that, they just offered me a contract. The first time an American woman ever got a contract over there.

What was the training like over there?

It's so hard, like boot camp. They get 3-4-5,000 girls once every two years for try-outs to become a wrestler and they start at the age of 16. And these poor girls — 3,000 girls are trying to become a wrestler and only five make it. So you can imagine. I remember that we would go once or twice a year and that they'd bring us to the mountains and they'd make us run mountains, go through swamps, climb these trees, run these rocks. I mean we'd literally have to do a workout without any weights. We'd have to pick up bodies and put them over our head for endurance and stuff and it was unbelievable. I was so beat up. I'll never forget it. I'll never, ever. But I don't regret anything that I've ever done in my wrestling career. It's all been a step forward. I never had to do anything that I felt bad about. And I wouldn't change anything. I think I really made a difference for women in wrestling. I made a mark wherever I've gone, kind of like a male dog does. I feel good about it because I've opened up doors and made people realize what they have to do and what the need is to have women and to keep women. Just like with the previous federation I was with. I mean I was there, I spoke my word on what they needed to do and now you see that they're finally doing it. And there are more opportunities for women. I was glad that I was able to do that.

A lot of difficult things have happened in this country over the years. Why hasn't women's wrestling gotten over with the audience here?

I think mainly it's because you are who you are in this business because of who's behind you, promoting you. Anybody can take you and make you a star overnight. It's the promotion, it's the marketing, it's what's behind you. I mean there's a lot of things that go on behind closed doors that I have seen and heard that is not the public's business. But it's just that there are other things that really make people who they are and a star or pop idol. A lot of people say it's who you know. Well, they're right. Nowadays, it isn't just talent. We have wrestlers that cannot wrestle worth poop. It's not talent anymore. You've got to have a lot of charisma.

What was GLOW about? Was it a disgrace to women's wrestling?

Well, GLOW or POWW or any organization, it's just they probably felt, well . . . I mean think about it. It was a genius idea, OK? As a businesswoman myself, I thought it was an absolute brilliant idea. It's just about promoting it correctly. I mean why is *Baywatch* so hot?

Maybe they were trying to do what GLOW was and have women in skimpy outfits.

Exactly. It's not always T&A. If you have a great package, they could be worth a lot of money. Some of those characters on GLOW were funnier than . . . and some of them were real good but I think the direction got lost. It could have been good intermittently, but something full-time won't cut it.

Do you know whatever happened to Wendi Richter?

Wendi is married and a real estate agent.

Was Bull Nakano easy to work with?

Bull is phenomenal. A good-hearted person. An incredible talent. I had my best matches with her. And to be voted best match at a pay-per-view with her and stuff like that makes me feel good inside, and that I've accomplished what I've wanted to accomplish.

Have you sustained many injuries?

Throughout my career, I ripped my ACL, busted all my fingers, blah, blah, blah.

Who was your first pro fight against?

"Wrestling Rose."

Did you win?

Of course.

Were you still in nursing at the time and was wrestling part time?

Right, correct.

Did anyone recognize you in your whites?

Yeah. It was kind of cute. I was working in the nursing homes first and then I was working in home health aid. And that was nice. You'd be surprised when a lot of the elderly people watch the wrestling. And I went to a few homes and stuff and then they'd kind of be staring at me, and they weren't sure and they'd start asking questions. It was great.

Have you ever thought about getting into a booking position in this business?

There's a lot of ideas and feelings that I have. There's a lot of directions and paths that I can beat down. But there's a few things that I have in the works that I plan on doing that I cannot do right now. I'm still active in the sport. And I still will be at the time, but I need to finish a few things, accomplish a few things. In life I kind of sit down and re-evaluate things and see how things are going. I mean overall we have adversities that we all have to overcome in life. Boy, I've had my share.

But you've had some ups, too.

Oh, yeah. The ups have been great. And the downs actually have been great because they've made me what I am today. I sit down and make my yearly plans and five-year goals. It's kind of where I'd like to be in five years and these are my steps to make it there. And I kind of learned that by listening to these motivational speakers and reading these books. Tony Robbins and Vic Zigler are a big part of my life.

Have you had any movie offers?

I have done a few motion pictures.

What have you done that I might see in the video store?

Well, there's some B movies on video, such as *Streetfighter 2*. I choreographed and did my own fight scenes. It was a cage match against this one martial arts girl and she was incredible and the fight scene was phenomenal. And I killed her at the end.

What about your music in Japan?

Isn't it funny that I had to go to Japan to be a bigger star than here? I had one CD and I sang in Japanese as well and I had my own picture book and videos and posters.

What was the name of your CD?

"Who's Madusa?"

How did the whole WWF thing come about? Did you get a call from Vince one day?

No. I was speaking to J.J. Dillon, in fact. And then I had a meeting with Vince McMahon.

Initially, it seemed like you were getting a big, big push there. Was the initial stuff what you were hoping it was going to be when you first got there?

Oh, yeah, it's just like anything. I think there's a big picture painted for anybody wherever they go and a big hoo-ha. But then I think it just fizzled out. I have a lot of talent. I was stagnant there. I don't think I have that bad of a body. I think I can speak eloquently when needed. I think I can carry myself well and I think I can wrestle probably better than a lot of men.

Well there's no confidence problem in Madusa.

No. Absolutely. Confidence is what makes you. If I don't have confidence, I'm not going to be successful. I'm not going to make the kids laugh.

So what was the deal with the wild speech you gave when you came back to WCW, when you threw the belt in the trash?

Well, I had a contract with the wwf, and it expired in the middle of December. And I was still the wwf champ when it expired and I think I'm still ladies champ. They couldn't meet what I needed, being in the wwf. They wanted me to sign and continue, and if I went elsewhere, to come back when they wanted me. But I wasn't for that. You know, they've gotta do what they've gotta do and I've gotta do what I've gotta do. This is business, and they're not gonna be there tying my shoes when I'm 80 years old.

Where did the name Alundra Blayze come from?

I liked the name.

Did you make it up?

It was Vince and me. We both worked on the idea

It was just so odd not to see the name Madusa. Did somebody else own that name?

Yes, I had the name trademarked. I had it done a long time ago, being the businesswoman that I am.

So why then Alundra Blayze instead of Madusa in the WWF?

Because I said if he wanted to use Madusa he'd have to buy it from me. So he chose not to.

Do you see yourself going back to Japan to work?

Absolutely.

What does one do to prepare to go back over there?

You've got to program yourself to their ways, their training especially. You've got to put yourself back in the groove and program yourself to wrestling every day and training every day. It's pretty intense. You've got to be fit, definitely.

You are fit. What do you do in downtime? Any hobbies?

I have two cats, a dog, a Macaw.

What are their names?

The dog's name is Kiska. And the bird's name is Parador. He's huge. I got the name from the big Godzilla movie. And then there's Ewok and Phantom. And it's just like having four kids. I was polishing my Harley earlier. I ride my motorcycle a lot. Water-skiing, a lot of scuba diving. I love to read books. I have books everywhere. And I like to write creatively, and numbers and computers and, I don't know.

Do you know where things are going with you and WCW at this point?

Oh, yeah. I know exactly where it's going. And I like where it's gonna go and the longevity of it. I think that everything's going to be geared towards TV and PPVs.

Once in a while, just house shows. I think wcw's ahead there and I think the biggest step is that they're at Universal Studios. They have the settings throughout the day and it's good exposure to all kinds of fans.

Are you still dating wrestlers?

I've dated others outside of the business. I live, eat, and breathe the business and if I communicate with my loved one about my work and they don't have a clue, it's like talking to a wall. My past relationship with a wrestler was great, but we grew apart. I was doing 90 and he was doing 10.

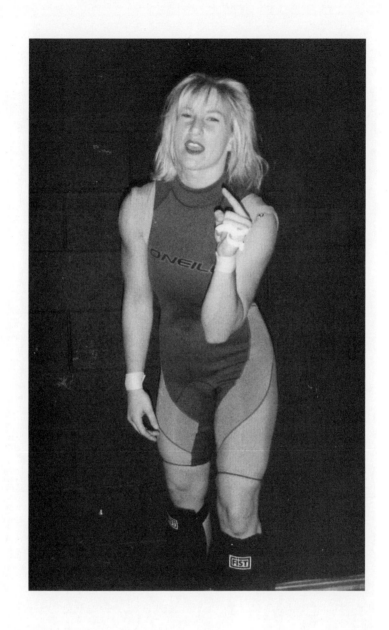

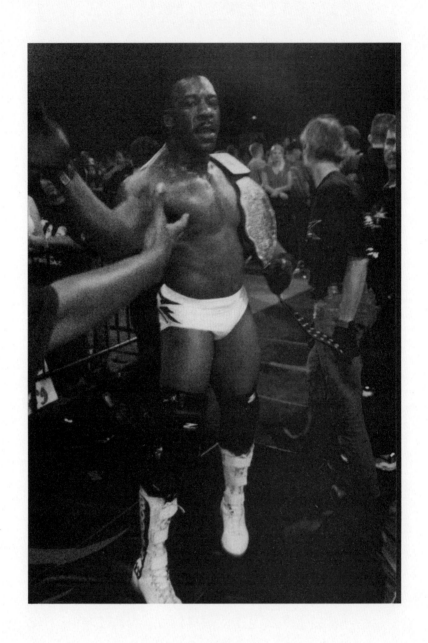

The Wrestlers Part 2:
May 1994–November 1995

This was a point where the show really hit its stride. Both of us had become very comfortable behind the microphone, whether we were talking to a wrestling hero, someone we didn't know much about, or a fan. Actually, the fans were never difficult to talk with, since both of us were fans, too. The biggest change was that we were both doing more pre-interview research on our subjects. And the whole atmosphere of the show changed — for the better — when wrestling journalists such as Bruce Mitchell and Mark Madden started making regular appearances with us and sharing even more background information than we had before.

On top of that, there was a lot more diversity in the offers of guests — or in some cases, in the guests we went after — from legends to young upstarts. A few of the following interviews were among our longest and most informative — we could've stayed on the phone with Ricky Steamboat and Lou Thesz for the entire two hours.

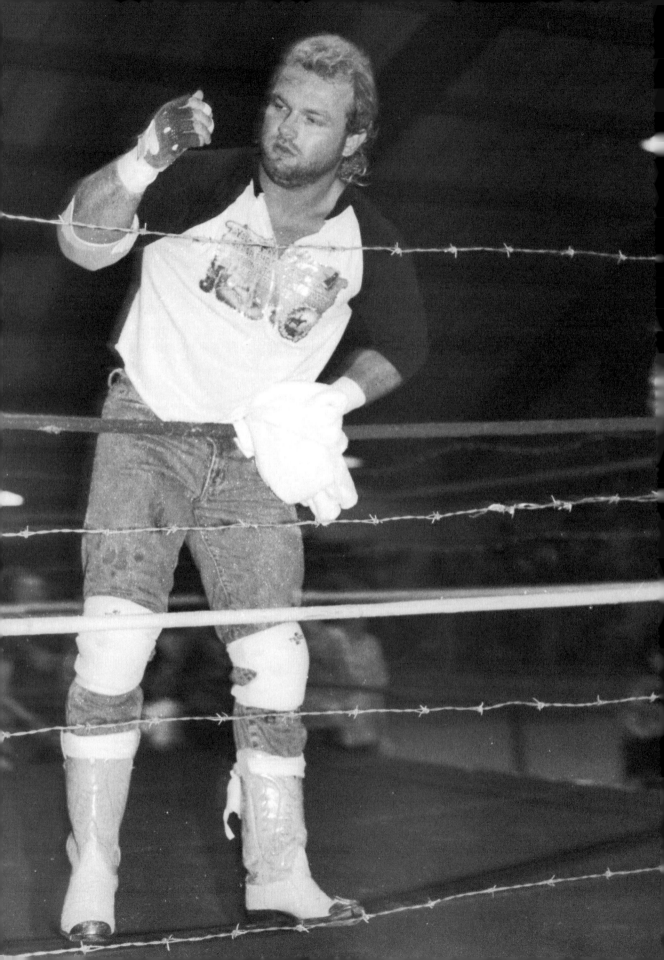

Eddie Gilbert

May 21, 1994

This was a really cool interview with Hot Stuff. He revealed a lot about himself here, had a down-to-earth charm, and had no problem talking openly about his history. He certainly had his problems in and out of the ring, both as a wrestler and as a booker. But he had one of the greatest minds in wrestling, and many of his accomplishments went unnoticed. A week before this interview, The Dream Machine was scheduled to be on the show, but when we called to confirm Gilbert picked up the phone at the WMC-TV studios instead, chatted for a while, and agreed to come on the next week. He talked up a storm about anything thrown at him.

"Hotstuff" Eddie Gilbert, do you work with Vince at all now?

No, I don't. I haven't had any contact with Vince McMahon since I was there 12 years ago.

There was some talk a few years ago that you might have been the successor to Pat Patterson for the head booking job. Was there serious talk about the job?

Yeah, there was a lot of speculation, there was talk at different levels. There was never a Vince McMahon – Eddie Gilbert conversation. There were other conversations with Titan Sports. But, heck, whatever. Someday. Someday.

We played a sound bite a few moments ago of you from the Great American Bash (1989), when you were a part of that committee with Jim Ross, Flair, and Sullivan. How did it feel working with all those people?

Well, it was tremendous. There were seven of us in all, with Jim Barnett, who was one of the first promoters to be on television back in the '50s, Jim Herd — whatever you want to say about him, he at least had an open mind, enough to bring different people in to listen to their ideas — Kevin Sullivan, Ric Flair, Jim Ross, myself, and whoever else. We had a great time in there, but what happened really was me being as young as I was [27] and being in there with some great minds and people that I look up to. You know, like Ric Flair and Kevin Sullivan. Kevin Sullivan helped me out a lot when I first started in the business. I remember selling pictures of him when I was 8 and 9 years old, when he was wrestling in the first and second matches in Union City, Tennessee, and Lexington, Tennessee, my hometown. You know, I'm like Jim Cornette in a way. I'm still a fan now and it was a great feeling to sit there. But I didn't realize at the time that what was going on was that each person in that room wanted to be the booker. And me being naive and young, I was thinking, "Well, we'll go in there with our best ideas and we'll all come together and we'll leave the room and the best ideas will just get put on the table, that's what we'll use and we'll all work together in a team effort." But I didn't realize when we left the room that everyone went in their own directions and began stabbing each other in the back or whatever, to try and get ahead and become the booker. That was the only disappointment that I had. But I also learned a lot.

What was your favorite promotion to work for as far as being the booker behind the scenes?

Continental was great and so was the UWF. But Continental was great because I went there and everyone said that there was no way that I was going to be able to bring the place back. It's dead. It's written off. I remember Dothan, Alabama, on Saturday nights drawing $1,200 houses. After a month and a half there, we had it up to $10,000 houses. We went in there and overhauled the place, cleaned it out. They had three different titles and we took them and had just one. And we tried to change everything. New background, new announcers, new everything. And there was the feeling of knowing that you went in and took an organization over and changed it with a new facelift, bringing some rear ends into the arenas to sit down and watch the matches, knowing that you accomplished something. My brother Doug finally told me, "Don't you realize that you've finally turned this place around?" I was working so hard, 24 hours a day, I didn't realize it.

What were some of the problems behind-the-scenes with David Woods? You wanted to expand, he didn't. What was the situation?

I wanted to expand, so did David. The wrestling business is a cutthroat business. In the wrestling business, if [someone] sees someone else getting ahead, then the wrestler's into the owner's ears saying, "Don't trust this guy. Be careful. He's trying to take over." And that happened in a lot of different places I've been in. We started making headway, Ron West was the general manager of the company, I started taking that slot over and he didn't like it and he led a group of guys kind of against me. And when I saw there was no more that I could do and it was just arguing after arguing, I just threw up my hands and said that it's not worth it anymore.

Did you get along with David Woods though?

Oh, yes. Yes I did and I'll tell you that David Woods and Tod Gordon and these people like that I've still remained friends with and have close relationships with.

What about Randy Hales?

Randy Hales, too. Randy Hales and I are working together. No one calls me up and asks my opinion. No one says, "Eddie are you mad at this guy or are you working with this guy?" All you read is that Eddie Gilbert quit here or he's disappeared or done this or done that. And I'm not talking about myself on an ego trip here. I'm just saying that no one ever, ever takes the time out to see what I'm thinking or what I've got to say, and I'd like for everyone to know that I'm working very, very hard and close with the USWA office. I guess you would say that I'm involved in it. And I don't want to go any farther than that but I'm working very close to Jerry Lawler and Randy Hales right now.

Please tell us and the listeners about the attraction of wrestling. Why do we keep watching?

I don't know. My father didn't start wrestling until I was in the third grade. My grandfather had wrestled at fairs in Tennessee. But I grew up watching every Saturday on TV, and I remember going to school and I would sit there and daydream about something I'd seen on TV. There was something about the high from the applause and boos and the ability to manipulate the people whether they liked you or not. I think when you really get down to the bottom line, everyone loves our interviews. When I was a kid, I was doing Jerry Lawler. I'd walk around school saying, "I'm the king, I'm going to be the king." And I was doing the smirk and I was doing the strut and everyone thought I was crazy. Well, then I graduated from high school and what do I do? Well, right now I'm going on TV doing Jerry Lawler, and Terry Funk and so forth. But every wrestling fan that I know of, they have this inner thing that they want to do an interview. They get in front of the mirror and when no one's around and no one can hear you and the door's shut and you get in front of that mirror and say, "This week I'm going to kick your butt." You know everyone does that and it's a great feeling and everyone wants to do that and know the people are behind you.

So when you got into the professional ranks, was it what you thought it'd be?

Tremendous, yes it was.

How is switching roles and going from on-camera to behind-the-scenes?

You never take the time to think about that. If you stop for a second, that's where you'll mess up.

Tell us a little bit about some of these interesting marriages that you've been in.

They are interesting.

Were there only two?

Well, there was someone I lived with beforehand and if we want to go back, there was someone I was supposed to marry in high school and didn't.

So what's the rumor with you and Debbie Combs.

Oh, my God. No, no, no, no. Debbie Combs and I — that is just rumor. I'm dating someone right now that I went to high school with. Believe it or not, I'm actually helping coach a Little League team. I played on one when I was a kid and I'm having a great time with that. But Debbie and I sold pictures together when I was 9 or 10 at the matches when Cora and my dad would wrestle. I remember Debbie and I selling pictures of our mom and dad. Debbie came to me about four months ago and said something about, "Who's next?" after Missy and Madusa. And I, kidding, said, "Oh, you are." And she said, "Boy, wouldn't that be something. Let's get that going." And I said alright and agreed to it. But the thing was we let her mom know it and Cora loves that. She calls me "son" and I call her "mom." But we're just real close friends and that's just total rumor. I'll say this, though. There will never be another in-the-business type relationship.

What are your thoughts on John Tatum?

What's funny about him — as weird as this may sound — is that we have a very special bond. I don't know if it's because of our relationship with Missy. I'm sure it is. But when I was booking Global, I made sure that I took care of John. He's a great talent. I think he's someone that if he gets his head on straight is a credit to our business. And he is a talent. I have nothing against him at all.

Was there legitimate heat in the beginning, though?

Oh, in the beginning, of course there was.

Because it was turned into a wrestling angle . . .

Yes it was, but I've got to say this, anytime he and I worked in the ring, nothing transpired in the ring.

There had to have been real feelings there.

Oh yeah. But can I point this out now: she left him for me. I did not take her. Her words were, "Eddie, if you want me, you can have me." And I did.

Do you know where Gary Hart is?

No, I don't, and he's another man with a great mind for the business. He was very good to me. There might be some out there with different opinions of him. But I don't know what's happened to him.

Are you working full time now?

Yes I am.

What's the next big thing that we're going to see out of Eddie Gilbert?

Anything's possible. I don't know. Anything. I'm open to any suggestions right now, but I will think them through. And I've got to say this though, it's summertime and I'm very, very happy at home.

So we shouldn't expect to see you up in the New York offices of the World Wrestling Federation with this trading back and forth at all — or should we?

I wouldn't think so.

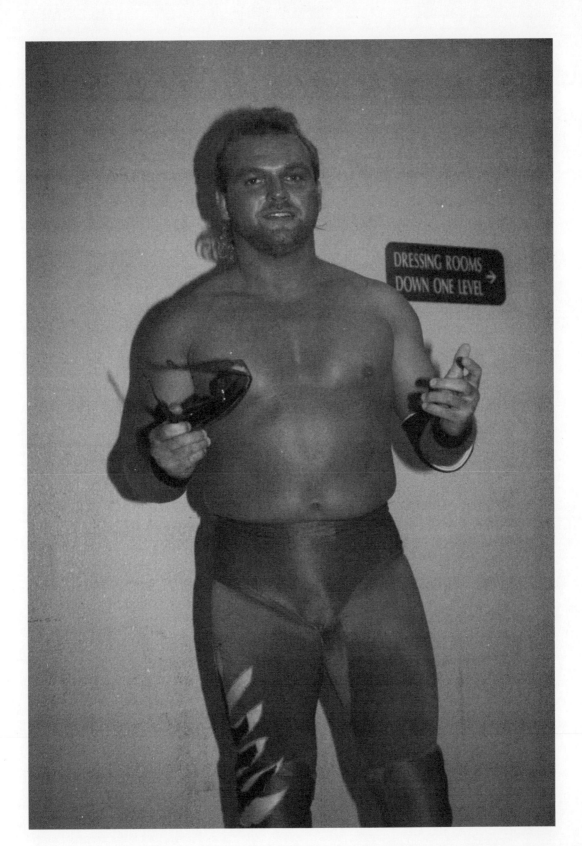

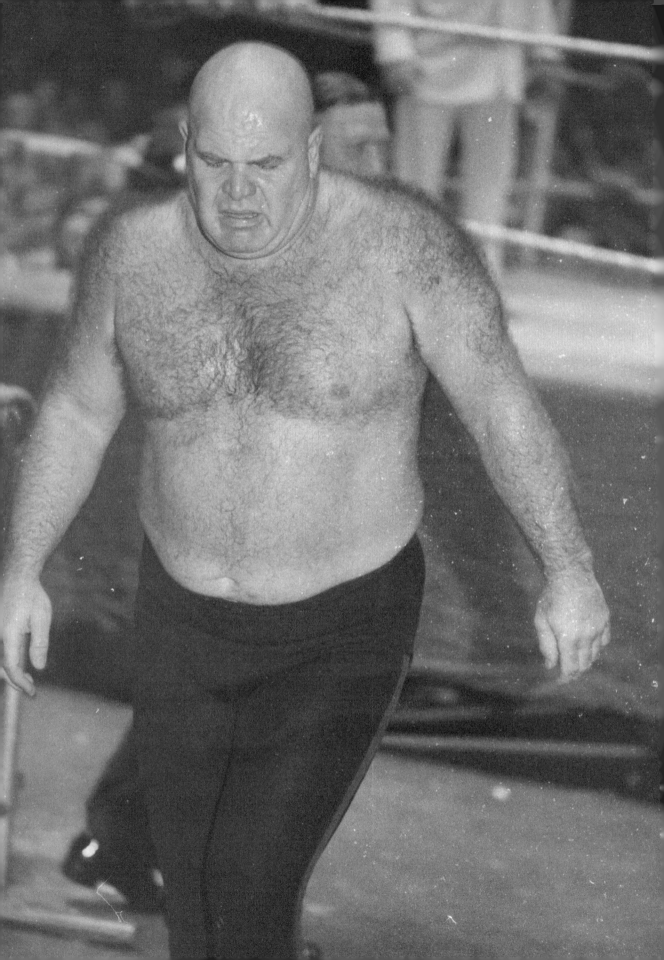

George Steele
October 4, 1994

Because we were still having trouble getting the WWF to provide guests on the show, we went through Buena Vista Pictures — distributor of the movie *Ed Wood*, which featured Steele as the Swedish actor Tor Johnson — to land the interview. Steele — real name Jim Myers — had retired from fighting a few years earlier, and still worked part time as a road agent for the WWF whenever they came through Florida. He had gone through a variety of changes in his character, from a fast-talking hipster who kept saying "Hey, daddy," to a monstrous heel to a simple, very friendly buffoonish guy with a green tongue. The last incarnation gave him his biggest surge in popularity. Throughout the interview, Steele was soft-spoken and friendly, every once in a while breaking into a chuckle. He protected the wrestling business to some degree, but was also quite open about his own involvement in it, and wasn't afraid to share his future acting dreams.

George, was it difficult for you to retire from the ring?

No, I had a lot of happy moments and good memories, but it was time to get out, as the guys were getting bigger, stronger, and faster.

How long were you an active wrestler?

About 28 years. I started in 1962.

I had heard you were a teacher in the Detroit area. Could you talk about that?

I taught for 25 years, and not nuclear science, that's for sure. I taught phys ed and coached football and wrestling. But I didn't teach driver's training in the summertime. I wrestled. Other teachers taught that or had some other employment to supplement their income.

Did you finally get out of teaching to go full time into wrestling?

I probably did my whole life backward. I retired from teaching in '85, then went full time into wrestling. Prior to that I just wrestled in the summer, which was quite unusual. I think I'm the only fellow who ever did anything like that.

Your character changed quite a bit over the years. There was the beatnik that said, "Hey, daddy-o." Then the big monster heel. Then kind of a goofy babyface. Who called the shots for those changes over the years?

I changed it each year when I came back. Because I was gone for eight or nine months, I could sit back and see what was happening in the business, and make my changes so I didn't get obsolete or boring from doing the same thing all the time.

Was it hard for you to adjust from being a heel to all of a sudden being adored by the fans?

I didn't change anything really, in my persona. I did the same thing. I guess society probably changed. And I enjoyed it. I enjoyed the acceptance of the crowd.

Did you have a preference for being the good guy or the bad guy?

Oh, certainly. I enjoyed most of my career because I was not accepted.

Where did the name George "the Animal" Steele come from?

The people named me the Animal because of the hair on my back and the appearance. George Steele was adopted because when I first broke into wrestling in the Detroit area, I taught there. And I didn't feel that the two would mix. I knew that the kids would be on my case big time. So I wore a mask and called myself "The Student." I wrestled maybe two years like that. I wore a cap and gown — a "student" of the business.

Were you a heel back then?

Oh, certainly.

Now you're a road agent for the WWF. What exactly is that job?

You observe the matches. You set up the order of the matches. And that's pretty much it. If there are any problems on the road, you handle them. You know, you've got young kids working out there and there's always the potential of a problem or two.

Do you still travel around quite a bit?

I was traveling all over. But for the last couple of years I haven't been doing too much traveling. I stay in the Florida area.

Early on did you work for anyone else besides the WWWF?

I was very fortunate. I started with Bert Ruby in the Detroit area and I stayed there for two years. Bruno Sammartino came in there to wrestle with an entourage of his people and they spotted me and before long I was in New York. It was just perfect because there was a two-month-out-of-the-year deal for me anyhow, and it was a great market to be in.

Did you watch wrestling as a kid?

No, I wasn't really a fan of wrestling. The first live event match I ever went to was one I was in.

How were you approached to work for the first time?

I had two children, I had just graduated from college and had signed a football contract with the Buffalo Bills. But I had a knee problem. So I became a teacher and I was making $4,300 a year in 1961. I definitely needed a supplement to my income and I was looking for a job as a bouncer at a bar. A friend of mine who was a big-time wrestling fan was always telling me I should get into wrestling. I never really considered it, but on the night I was looking for the job as a bouncer, he was with me and I called a promoter about 2:30 in the morning — that made him real excited about me — and I told him I wanted to be a wrestler. He invited me over to his house the next day. I went over and when I knocked on the door, he opened it and said, "Beautiful." Now I knew there was something not quite jibing there because I'm certainly not beautiful. Then he took me in and introduced me to his family and I relaxed a little bit because I figured he was at least straight. Then he took me into his parlor and asked me to take my shirt off, which I didn't understand. When he saw the hair on my body he went absolutely bananas. Later he took me over to the gym and started breaking me in. Usually it's a year or a year-and-a-half process.

So you actually did have some formal training?

Well, I had wrestled a little bit in college, and I had trained with some people on the wrestling team at Michigan State. So I had a little background there. And I was from Detroit so I had a little bit of a street background. What they used to do [at the gym] was take you in and beat you up three or four times, and if you kept coming back, then they would start breaking you in a little bit and start teaching you. Well, they had a problem with the first part. So they started training me pretty quickly and showing me a few things. And they told me not to tell the promoter. Then I was in the ring after six or seven weeks.

Do you remember who your first opponent was?

Yes I do. Klondike Bill.

And what did you do to him?

God, what did we do to each other! I mean the endurance part of it is tough anyhow. I was in pretty good shape and so was he, but the nerves take over. This was something I had never been involved with before, with the crowd watching and everything. It was the nerves and the excitement. I call it blooming up. I could hardly breathe.

Did you win?

Yeah, I did.

How has the World Wrestling Federation changed since the days of Vince, Sr.?

Well, I think there's been a drastic change. What I'm going to say has no disrespect toward our business for the way it was. But looking at it the way it was — the old locker room, cigar smoking by some of the promoters, but certainly not Vince. He was always a real gentleman. But I think we've gone from sleaze to high tech. And that's great.

What kind of shape do you think the business is in today across the world?

I think one of the major problems is that the World Wrestling Federation has become a major industry, and in this country that only leaves room for one or two other promotions. And there are a couple of really tiny ones that are struggling to make it. I broke in in Detroit. That's where I learned to wrestle before I went big time in New York. But today there's no place for the fellows to go in and learn the ring. There are no more territories.

Do you think that will come back?

Oh I don't know. I think it's going to have to.

Is there anyone out there in the business who you really respect today?

Oh I respect all of them.

But does anyone stick out as having major talent?

I think this young kid we have — Diesel — has a potential of being a super, super, super star in any organization.

Anyone in the business end of it who's doing a great job?

I think Vince.

He came through the whole court thing pretty well.

That was one of the worst things I've ever seen. They had a two-year probe into a man's life that's a multi-millionaire. They looked at his books trying to get him for income tax evasion. They looked at everything and they could find nothing. And then they did the steroid thing which I think every NFL team and basketball team at that time was involved in because it was legal.

And the wrestling people, too.

And us, too. A hundred percent. We never denied that. But what bothered me was the money we had to spend to defend ourselves. Then down the road when the court case finally came up, the prosecution had absolutely no case and our lawyers never called a witness. They rested and gave their final statements and he was found innocent. I think it was horrendously wrong that the government could do that to you.

Let's talk about the movies. How were you first approached to play Tor Johnson?

They told me the Tor Johnson part was the hardest part to find. First they were looking at actors, then wrestlers, bald-headed wrestlers, naturally. They were having a hard time with it because they wanted someone who could wrestle a little bit in the film and still play the role of Tor. Tor was kind of a strange character, to say the least. They finally chose me because I was a look-alike, and we do look an awful lot alike. When I first went out there they all told me, "You look just like Tor." Then as I started researching a little bit I found out that Tor was the first guy to do monster movies without makeup. It wasn't a hell of a compliment I was getting. But that's backhanded Hollywood, right? But the way I actually got it was that [the film's director] Tim Burton had contacted the WWF and asked me to send a tape. Just to stand up and say my name and list my height and weight, and so on. And I felt silly doing that. So I called a production company friend of mine in Detroit and asked him what he could do. And he said he'd do a skit. We had great facilities at the WWF, so I got in front of their camera and started saying "My name is . . ." And as I was doing that, I had Harvey Whippleman come in with a box and say, "Federal Express! Federal Express!" And I'd say, "Excuse me, I'm busy." But he kept sticking it in my face. So I took the box, with a disgusted look on my face, and threw it over to the side, and started doing my thing again, "My name is . . ." And he'd go, "No, you gotta sign here, Federal Express, you gotta sign here," just like they do. And finally I picked him up by the throat and threw him off the set and started again. Then this hand hit me on the back, but I didn't look back there, I just kind of waved it off and said I was busy. But the third time it hit me kind of hard and I turned around and it was this big giant we had at the time — Gonzalez — so I turned around back to the camera, and one of the lines I had to do [in the script] was "You take charge!" with a little bit of an accent. So I turned around and said, "Tim Burton, you take charge. I'm outta here."

So it worked.

Well, it got their attention.

It sounds like you wanted the part.

Sure, it was a different experience. I thought it would be fun, and it was. It was great. I was out there three months and it was just fantastic. The cast and the crew were great to work with. In fact, I didn't know because I had never been there before, but everybody told me that you don't expect this all the time. It was a very unique situation where everything just came together. It was almost like a family.

Had you ever actually heard of Tor from his wrestling days?

No, I hadn't. What did happen to me was, probably in the early '70s, I had a match in the Gardens and I was walking down Broadway that day. And there was a mask of Tor Johnson in a window. But underneath it didn't say "Tor," it said "George Steele." I went in and asked him about it and he said, "Oh no, no, that's Tor Johnson. But because you're so hot right now in wrestling we put your name under it. No one knew who Tor was." I forgot about that really. But over the years people would come up to me and ask me if I had made a movie where I was coming out of a grave, and I didn't know what they were talking about. Then it all came together when I finally started looking into the Ed Wood series.

When you were doing research for this did you actually sit down and study Tor's acting technique?

I'm not sure he had a technique. But I did have a film he was in — *Plan Nine From Outer Space* — and the thing that was most helpful was a tape of when he was on Groucho Marx's "You Bet Your Life" show. That gave me the home character. What was neat about it, and unfortunate, too, was, well you know you hear everybody say my best stuff ended up on the cutting room floor. In this case I thought it did because I did Tor from a family side, too. It was all in the movie, but it didn't work out to be in there.

Did he have a wife and children?

Yeah, he had a wife, Greta, and two kids, Carl and Connie.

Looking back on the whole experience now, is acting in the movies different from working in a wrestling ring?

Oh certainly, a hundred percent different. You do one small scene, then you go sit back for an hour and a half while they set the cameras up. It's a totally different thing.

You have to be an actor in the ring, though, to get your character across.

I think a lot of people misconstrue that. Your character is something that's very important in wrestling. And people look at it and say that's not real. But it is real. The difference in the NFL or in basketball or hockey is that you have good guys and bad guys there, but only when they're away from home. So we develop the same character, but it's home and away really.

How did you feel about seeing yourself on the screen?

Well, I saw it in New York at the film festival, and it was quite an experience. But the funny thing is, anything I've ever done, you know, I'd get a little excited about it. You know, there's a nerve factor. When I got on the set of "Ed Wood," that never happened. I felt like I had been there before. I was totally relaxed. It was unbelievable. No butterflies at all.

Did you have butterflies in the wrestling ring?

Oh, sure.

What's next then? Would you like an acting career?

Well, when we went out there I told my wife that we'd just go out and have some fun and enjoy it, but not get hooked on this because it could be really dangerous. So we were out there about two and a half months and had two more weeks to go, and I enjoyed it so much I was looking for an agent, which I found. And now I'm going to acting class. Tim told me at the beginning to just relax. He said, "This'll be your best one because you don't know what you're doing." He said the best film he ever did was his first one because he wasn't sure what he was doing.

And it worked.

And it worked. But I don't know. It was fun, so if it happens, it happens.

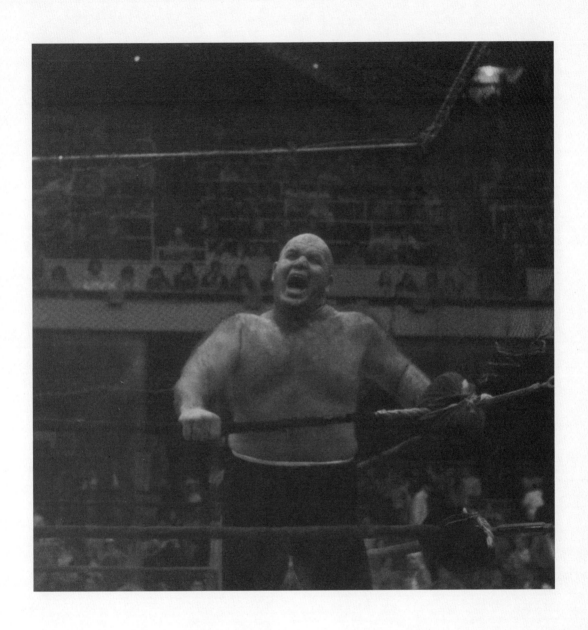

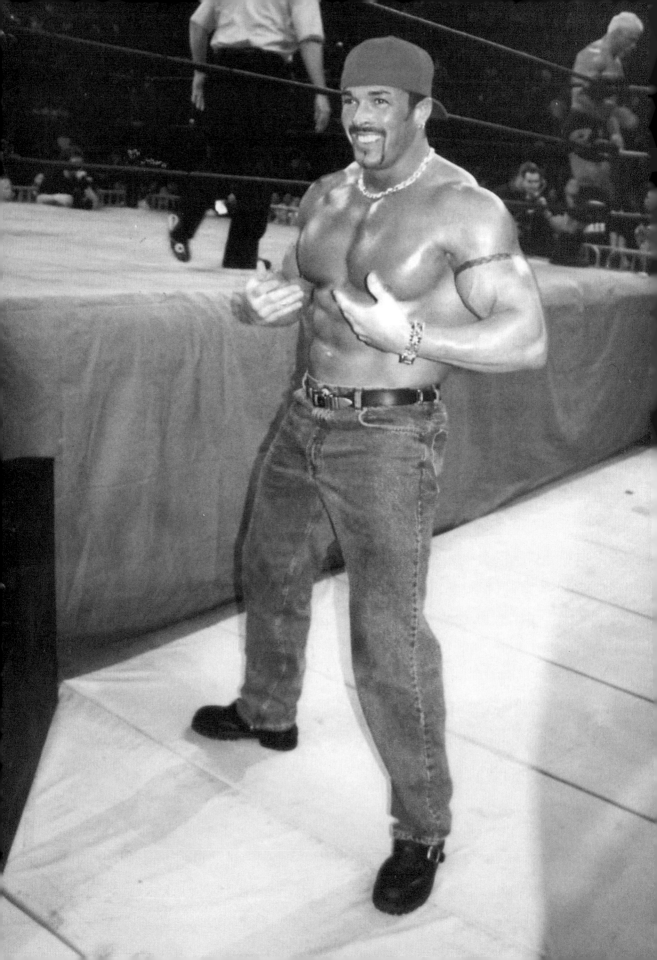

Marcus Bagwell

October 8, 1994

Marcus Bagwell remains one of the more controversial performers in the business, jumping from promotion to promotion apparently because of attitude problems. At the time of this interview, he was working for wcw as a successful mid-card babyface. He was just as eager to talk about how he got his big break — a memorable phone call from Magnum T.A. — as he was about his less-than-amicable break-up with his former tag team partner 2-Cold Scorpio. Unfortunately there was a time constraint that cut the interview short just as he was warming up to us.

Marcus Bagwell, where are you today?

I'm in Atlanta, Georgia, my hometown.

How long have you been a wrestler?

Oh, yeah. It goes back to [when I was] Fabian in North Georgia Wrestling. Joe Pedicino was the promoter who came up with that. He said I reminded him of Fabian.

Are you even old enough to remember Fabian?

No I'm not. I'm 24. And from there I went to [being called] Handsome Stranger.

How long ago did you start?

I started when I was 20 years old. I've been in the business 3 1/2 years.

Who was your first fight?

My first professional fight was with Steve "The Brawler" Lawler. I actually won the TV title on my first professional match. So it's been a long road to WCW, but I made it.

Did you wrestle in Baltimore as Scott Stevens?

Scott Stevens, wow you're bringing back memories that even I forgot about. I actually wrestled as Scott Stevens in one match. And the company didn't come through with the money, so I was out the door. Actually, it was Shawn Stevens, so you didn't get your sources right.

Somewhere there was a stop in Global?

Yeah, that was a big learning experience for me. The Patriot was there, Bill Irwin, Eddie Gilbert. It was a big stepping-stone for a 21-year-old kid on ESPN.

What went wrong with Global?

Personally, I think they tried to swallow too much at once. They had the right idea, they had plenty of talent to start. They started flying us out there first class. They tried to redo the Sportatorium out in Dallas and maybe bit off too much. Everyone was pulling for it to work.

How did you get into WCW?

Funny story. Magnum was still in the office at wcw. We were at home and Global had called and said they were cutting back on shows. I was like, "Oh, God, you're kidding." I was sitting at home depressed and I swear it wasn't more than 30 minutes and my phone rang and it was wcw. They called and asked for Marcus Bagwell and I said that this was him. He said, "This is Magnum" and I said, "Magnum who?" "Magnum T.A." I was like, "Oh my God, what's up?" He said, "Listen, we want to give you a tryout." They said they liked me and wanted to send me to school and learn some more. They signed me to a weekly deal and at the same time, Barry Windham got hurt. So I went on the road to replace him. And, like a lot of athletes, if they get a chance to show their stuff, they do. And someone liked me and signed me to a two-year deal. I just signed for another year, so I've been there for almost three years.

How did the tag team thing come about?

I couldn't get into a big match, so when Chris Benoit came in, I had a helluva match with him. I lost, though. Scorpio came in and saw what I did with Benoit and it impressed him. He thought we could make an impression as a tag team.

Do you and Scorpio still talk?

We don't. I don't miss our team at all. He browbeat me. I thought we had a good thing going. We had words in Germany and cleared it up at home. I think he was listening to the wrong people. I told him to quit listening to the other people who were jealous. I called him about it because I had heard that he wanted to go singles. I said, "It's totally up to you, but I want to know because I'm not begging to be partners with you. If that's what you want to do, you go." After the conversation, he got fired for smoking dope.

It seemed that the heat was between him and the company, not you.

Well see, Scorpio told me of that same conversation, but that I was getting fired. And I said, "Scorpio, I just signed for one year. What are you talking about?" And he was like, "Well, that's what I heard." Needless to say, in less than a week, he was the one that got fired for smoking dope.

Did you guys hang out?

No, we were friends in the ring but we didn't really travel together.

Do you want to do singles or tag team?

I love being in a tag team. It gets to me personally. It seems more impressive to have a good partner and make it work for the both of you. Being tag team champion feels like being a world champion.

Wrestling right now is in tough times between small crowds and drug abuse. Where do you see the business in five years?

What I see in five years is bigger than life. Ted Turner isn't going anywhere and we can't get anything but better. I see overseas becoming very, very big and still running house shows in the States. I see Australia and Europe skyrocketing and the States stabilizing and mainly doing TVs over here.

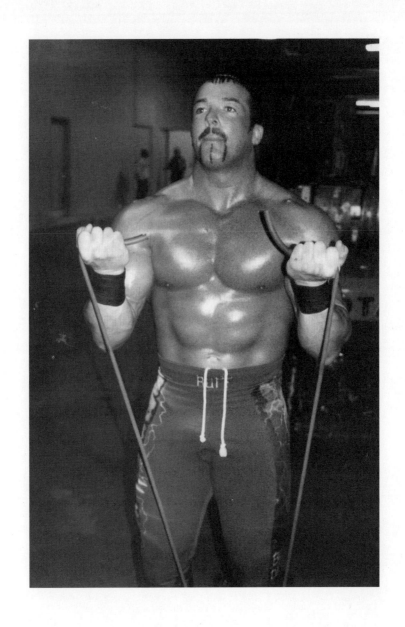

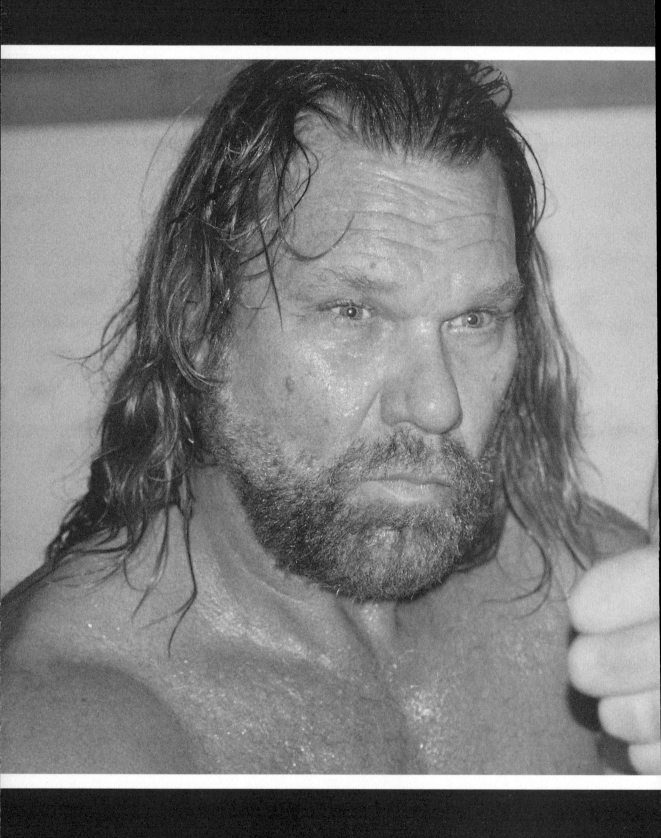

Jim Duggan

October 22, 1994

Although he remained low-key throughout this interview, 180 degrees away from his goofy onscreen persona, Duggan opened up quite a bit, discussing how he broke in to the business, his football career, his relationship with Bill Watts and Mid-South Wrestling, why he left the WWF the first time — he was with WCW at this point — and how he almost got into the shoot fighting world with Gary Albright. This interview was done before Duggan discovered that he had life-threatening cancer that almost ended his career.

How are you today, Jim?

Well, before we start, I first have to give a quick "hooooooo" to all my fans out there.

Where are we talking to you from?

I'm calling from Orlando, Florida. I moved down here and have been here for the past five years and live on the east coast right outside of Orlando.

We've heard that you are the son of the chief of police in Glens Falls, New York. Is this true?

That's right, my dad was a policeman up in Glens Falls for about 43 years and he recently retired. Everyone up there still calls him "Chief."

So you were brought up straight and proper, right?

Yeah, I went to a Catholic school in my high school days and I have three older sisters, so I had a strict upbringing, I'd guess you'd say.

A friend of yours, Gary Albright, has said in interviews that you were quite the amateur wrestler before you got into the professional ranks. Can you talk about those days of being an amateur?

In Glens Falls, I was in my sophomore year and playing on the varsity basketball team. Of course my basketball skills weren't quite where I wanted them to be, but I still played on the team. I saw the wrestling team and thought that would be a good transition. My first year was quite successful as I made it to the state tournament, winning the Intersectionals, but didn't do well after. But in my senior year, I won the New York State Championship.

You got a little bit better at it, did you?

Well I didn't realize that there was as much to amateur wrestling as there is. You learn a few moves and the training and some of the guys were doing amateur since the 8th grade, so it was challenge. It was also a thrill for me to come out of a small town like little Glens Falls to go to a big three-day tournament in Syracuse, New York, and wrestle all these kids from New York City schools and Buffalo high schools and to come out a winner. I was the first one from our section, section two in upstate New York, to ever win the New York State Championship. More and more people were coming from my hometown when word got out as to how well I was doing. And during the last day, there was quite a crew from Glens Falls.

You still like working in front of crowds, don't you?

Yeah, it's quite a thrill to be in front of people. I enjoy it quite a bit.

How did you make the transition from the amateur ranks to professional? We know there's some football in the middle, but if we can just stick with wrestling, how did you get into that game?

Well, I'll have to go through football.

Go ahead through football.

I was highly recruited out of Glens Falls by many different universities. Ohio State, Penn State, Syracuse, Kentucky. But I ended up signing a letter-of-intent with Southern Methodist University in Dallas, Texas. And while I was down there on a recruiting trip, I met Fritz Von Erich. He suggested I try professional wrestling. Back then, I was so focused on football that I didn't give it much thought. And after four years of starting with SMU, I made the move to the Atlanta Falcons; they picked me up in '77–'78, and during the off-season I would go back to Dallas. That's when I gave Fritz a call and started to do a little ring time and understand a little about the ring.

So you actually worked for Fritz?

I sure did. I broke in there as Big Jim Duggan. I was clean-shaven with short hair and a real straight young man and started to learn the ropes, as they say.

OK, so you were "Big" Jim Duggan. Now, somebody also told us that either in the late '70s or early '80s you were known as "Moose" Duggan. Is that true?

"Moose" Duggan was a high school nickname and even now when someone yells out, "Hey, Moose," I know they're someone I knew back in high school.

So that was never a ring name?

Never a ring name. I've changed ring personas a couple of times until I felt comfortable with "The Hacksaw."

Can you tell us where "Hacksaw" came from?

Well, actually, "Hacksaw" was back to my football days. My main deal was to be a special teams player, punt returner, kick returner. And my deal was to run down and break the wedge up on the kickoff, so I would cut through the wedge like a hacksaw. Well, I carried it over to wrestling.

Well it works.

Yeah, it works good for me. You know, people will say that I'm much different in person than I am in the ring and I say, "My persona in the ring is just an extension of my personality." I can't function in everyday society going around, going "hoooooo" and trying to catch flights that way.

No, you'd be locked up.

Yeah, I'd have to be much more low key.

You hit the big time working for Bill Watts in the Mid-South.

Yeah, that was my first big break in the business, as they say. I was down there in Mid-South for about four years in the Louisiana, Texas, Oklahoma area.

Now how did you actually break into that game? Because that was pretty much flourishing then.

That was a very hot area at that time. But I broke in with Fritz in Dallas. I moved from territory to territory, which is unheard of nowadays.

They don't exist anymore.

Right. But I went through Hawaii with Peter Maivia, and I wrestled in Tampa with the Grahams, Pensacola with the Fullers and before in Georgia Championship Wrestling in all the stages of learning the business, learned how to talk on the microphone, learned how to wrestle in front of people. And then I was in San Antonio with the booker Buck Robley, who was picked up by Bill Watts. He suggested that Bill bring me in and that's where I got my first big break.

Was Bill much different in the way he ran business from the other promoters you worked with?

Bill was a little more hard-core than a lot of other promoters, I'd say.

Did you find it any different with your personal relationship working for him?

I got along OK with Bill because he was an ex-ballplayer. It's like being from the same university. In professional wrestling, you have guys from many different backgrounds. Amateur wrestlers, boxers, bodybuilders, football players. And the football players always seem to stick together.

Have you ever worked as a heel in the territories or were you always the good guy?

In my early career I switched back and forth, but since I've been successful, I've always been the good guy.

Did you ever want to go the other way, though? Is it more fun?

No, I really think that the way I act and the way I feel and the way I relate to people, I enjoy being the good guy. I like to get out there with the folks. I love interacting with the people, signing autographs and stuff like that. So I really enjoy being the good guy.

What titles have you had?

I've never been much of a belt guy. Well, my deal was that I may not win the match, but I'll win the fight. And so, a lot of times I'd get DQ'd for having the two-by-four and I was kind of a rogue good guy and liked to mix it up with foreign objects, as they say.

You worked for Vince McMahon for a while in the WWF and in between. Can you talk about that at all? Was that a good time for you? Was it a different style of working?

Yeah, it sure was.

How did it change from Mid-South?

Vince McMahon took professional wrestling mainstream. Back in Mid-South, it was very bloody, very violent, a rough atmosphere. The crowds were made up mostly of men. You had a lot of cigar smoke, a lot of swearing. McMahon changed that whole deal and made it sports family entertainment. You know, it's not just the wrestling, it's the whole packaging. It's the costumes, the music, it's the fireworks, it's a light show — and he made it so popular. Now you're not just competing on a wrestling level.

You're competing for the entertainment dollar with the people, which means you're competing with the NFL, the NBA, and folks like that. If you look at them, they have these elaborate half-time shows. They have all the cheerleaders. They have the mascots. So to be competitive in today's society, you have to offer people more than just pro wrestling. That's what the WCW does, also. And now, actually, the WCW is kind of taking a lead and really gaining momentum and I think in the next year or so that we'll be the largest wrestling organization in the world.

What were the circumstances of you leaving the World Wrestling Federation?

Well, I had a good run up there. I was there seven years with Vince McMahon. I left on good terms. He offered me to stick around, but I just thought that I had run my course there. My wife had just recently had a baby and everyone knows McMahon's schedule is 25, 26, 27 days a month on the road. And after seven years of straight wrestling, I took a year off and spent it with my family here in Florida. And then when I decided to get back into wrestling, I renegotiated with both organizations and I took a look at who I thought was the place of the future and I made the move to WCW.

You did some independent work in between, right?

I sure did.

Is that good? Do you have a preference?

The independent circuit is pretty good. It's quite an experience. You can book yourself when you want to. If you just want to work weekends, you can work weekends. It's just very inconsistent. There's a lot of cancellations, that makes it hard, but the independent scene, it gives people in smaller towns a chance to see you. The high schools and armories get shows that the bigger groups would never go to and gives them exposure there.

But now you're inside again. Was there any connection with Hogan? Did he bring you into WCW in any way?

I discussed WCW with the Hulkster because I think WCW's future coincides with Hulk Hogan's future. He's bigger than life and is a friend of mine and we talked it over and when he said he'd be here, then my stance with WCW got a little stronger.

Any idea who you'll be working with after your program with Steve Austin?

No, I really don't. Things here are in transition with wcw.

Anyone you would like to work with?

I look forward to working with Vader. I've watched him for a couple years on TV and he's one of the most agile big-men in the business. I think that he'd be a challenge to work with.

Is there anything that you can tell us about this transition going on down there? Are we going to see a new kind of product coming?

I think you may just see a better product coming. I don't think a new kind of product, probably just a different packaging, but basically the same thing. You'll just upgrade it a little bit.

Are you going to be working with Gary Albright on the shoot fighting shows coming up?

Well, I've talked to those folks a little bit and we're still trying to negotiate that now. I did the commercial with Gary and he's a nice guy. I may be involved. Never say never in this business.

There are problems right now with low attendance and drug problems. Do you see any kind of cure, or something to revive it?

Wrestling is definitely in a downswing, but the economy is in a downswing. I'd say that it will pick back up. Maybe wcw is the shot in the arm that professional wrestling needs. Bring in guys like Honky Tonk Man, Earthquake, myself, some of the established stars that were disenchanted with the wwf and who got out of professional wrestling, that a lot of people enjoyed watching, and now are coming back into wcw. So there's going to be an influx of established talent coming back in that hasn't been in the last few years.

Hopefully mixing well with the new talent, too.

There's so few places for guys to learn the business. As I said earlier, I traveled from territory to territory and learned how to wrestle, learned how to talk on a microphone, learned my profession. Nowadays, guys get an opportunity and then they're on nationwide TV. True wrestling fans can tell who the established pros are from someone just breaking in.

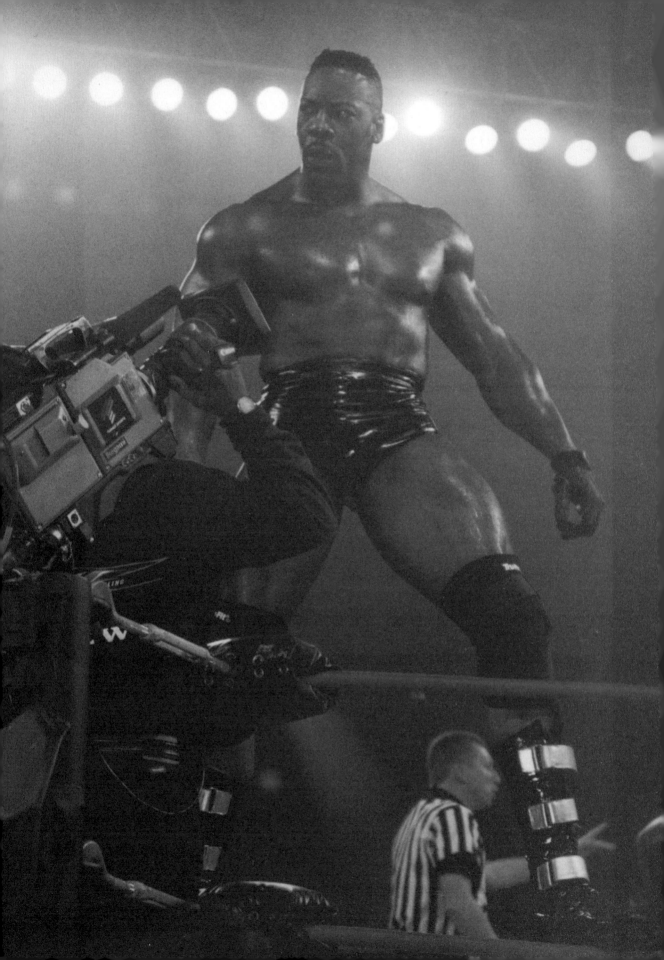

Booker T
December, 1994

Booker Huffman was a guest on the show just as he started to catch on fire in WCW with his brother Lane (Stevie Ray) as the team Harlem Heat. Though he wasn't yet a major star, he had some good stories about his early days with Global Wrestling and about how his relationship with Sid Vicious helped to further his career. He spoke candidly about working with his brother, and wasn't afraid to heap praise on Eric Bischoff, and scorn on Hulk Hogan. In all, he provided an interesting glimpse at his own frame of mind at that point in his career.

Booker T, you're taking on the Nasty Boys at Starrcade in a few weeks. What's going to happen?

We will be the champs soon in wcw.

The first time we saw you was in Global on ESPN. Did you work anywhere before Global?

Me and my brother started out as a tag team in Global and before that, we wrestled on our own. We came together but we worked in Texas for some small organization that I can't even remember the name of. We did some small things, but wrestled out on the bottom and we worked our way up. We're not second generation wrestlers, we have no ties in the wrestling business. We came from the streets and we're at the top of the wrestling business right now.

What do you think about what's going on in Texas right now with Jim Crockett bringing back the NWA?

To be honest, I think it's a good thing and I think there should be more companies opening up like that to bring back wrestling the way it used to be. Nowadays, guys are struggling because there's not a lot of places to go. Places like that are letting guys come through like me and my brother. If it wasn't for a place like Global, there's no telling where me and my brother would be.

Was it Joe Pedicino or Max Andrews that you were working for there?

We were working for a guy named Grey Pierson.

He put on the Kerry von Erich Memorial show.

Right, he did a really good thing and a lot of good talent has come out of that place like Stunning Steve Austin, and me and my brother.

Who did you hang out with in Global?

We pretty much kept to ourselves.

Let's set the stage. You're in Global and get a phone call from WCW. Who was it that brought you up there?

Well, we were working in Global and Sid Vicious — everyone knows that he's a good friend of ours — Sid called us and invited us to come down and talk with them. One thing about Sid — one thing he liked was we were good workers and saw talent in us and, like I said, we had no ties in the business, but people like Sid have helped us. I give him all the credit for where we are right now.

There were some rumors originally, and correct us if we're wrong, that at the very beginning of WCW when Sid was going to bring you guys out, that you were going to be in chains and represented as slaves, until somebody nixed that. Is that true?

No, that wasn't true. It wasn't anything like that. It was kind of blown totally out of context before it got started. It could have been something good, but it really never got a chance to develop, so they killed it before it started.

Didn't you have your debut at Fall Brawl '93 in a tag match? The ShockMaster was involved in that as well.

Right, right. And Ice Train and Charlie Norris.

What did you think of your first match on television?

Well, in this business there's a lot of ups and there's a lot of downs. You look at where we are now and look at where those guys are now. That's the way I look at it right there.

Can you compare working with Bischoff and Grey Pierson?

There's no comparison. Grey is a great guy and helped us a lot, but hasn't been in that long, and came in, and was running it. Bischoff was in the AWA and got his feet wet and you can't compare the two. Bischoff's the better businessman.

It's no secret that WCW is following the formula of WWF in 1988 by bringing in Duggan and Savage and so forth. It seems behind-the-scenes that there's some heat with some of the guys that have been there longer. Do you sense anything going on?

I haven't seen any, personally, but when you have egos clashing in this business, when everyone wants to be the biggest star, you might see it. Not of people going over others, but just male egos clashing.

Do you agree with the direction that Bischoff seems to be going in bringing in ex-WWF wrestlers?

I do, and I think it's a positive thing and the most positive step in two years. Someone like Hogan, people want to see those guys. And people might talk about it being an older generation, but I think it's a good thing.

You've been in the dressing room. Do people get along with Hogan? Does he act as a leader for the wrestlers?

I'm not a big fan of Hulk Hogan. But as a man, he's one of the greatest people in the world and I have nothing but the highest respect for him.

Is he an egomaniac behind-the-scenes? Is he a nice guy?

I mean, like I say, I don't like him personally, but Hulk Hogan is truly behind-the-scenes the person that you see on the scene, also.

What is Ric Flair's role right now? Is he just a booker and getting everything straightened out?

Ric Flair's behind-the-scenes right now and hopefully one day he can manipulate his way back in the business, too, because a person like that can't hurt the business, but can only help and enhance it and hopefully one day he'll return.

I would imagine at some point there'll be a Vader and Hogan vs. Savage and Flair match.

You can't leave Sting out of that.

His contract expires in January. Are you friends with Sting? Do you think the WWF would make a play for him sooner or later?

He's the only player that they haven't made a play for and he seems loyal to the company and I don't think Sting will be going anywhere.

Right. He has a great traveling schedule. I believe he has a contract for $750,000 annually.

You really don't need to go anywhere when you're getting treated like that. I don't think he's going anywhere. He's a franchise player and a part of the company.

Does he seem happy now that Hogan's getting the spotlight and not him?

Well, like I said, it doesn't look like he's unhappy. The thing with Hogan is that it can only help everybody. It can't hurt anybody. If he can sit back and have Hogan do the work and he makes his money, I'm sure he'll be glad about that, too. In this business, you don't want to be unhappy. When you do the things we do, there's really no reason to be unhappy.

Recently the World Wrestling Federation recruited Brian Armstrong and Shanghai Pierce. Has Vince McMahon and the World Wrestling Federation had any contact recently with Harlem Heat?

I don't want to make any comment on that question, but as far as going to the WWF at this time, me and my brother, we're really not interested and want to stay with WCW for quite some time.

Both of you are under contract, right?

We are under contract and we're in negotiations to renew our contract.

Would you like to see some Japanese competition?

Harlem Heat has a destiny. I don't want to wrestle any singles matches and be without my brother. Our destiny is to win every major title in every major organization. Here, New York, Japan, we want to win every major title while we're here in existence on this earth and in this business.

What tag teams out there would you like to wrestle?

To be honest with you, there's really no tag team in the same category at this point in time. There have been some great tag teams like the Road Warriors, Steiners, Head Shrinkers, Axe and Smash. When you talk about tag teams, I want our name within that realm of people.

What are your impressions of the Steiners?

One of the greatest tag teams. They seem to be underexposed right now and in this business, if people don't see you, they'll forget you.

How about the Fantastics?

They should have retired 10 years ago.

Heavenly Bodies?

That was one of Vince McMahon's worst brainstorms bringing in those two guys.

Would you like to go to Japan?

I've been there and it's very stiff. I went once — and once with my brother. Great Muta is one of the greatest workers I've ever seen. He and Hase, you've got to realize would get beat to a pulp. Me and my brother grew up together, we slept in the same bed together, and we are blood brothers. We are not a gimmick. Same mother, same father. You can look it up and no other tag team has that type of continuity.

How long is Sherri going to be with you?

We have great continuity with her and she's the best thing that's ever happened to us since we've been in the business.

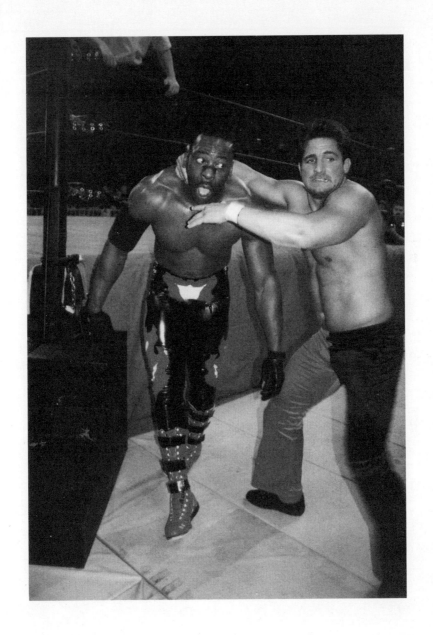

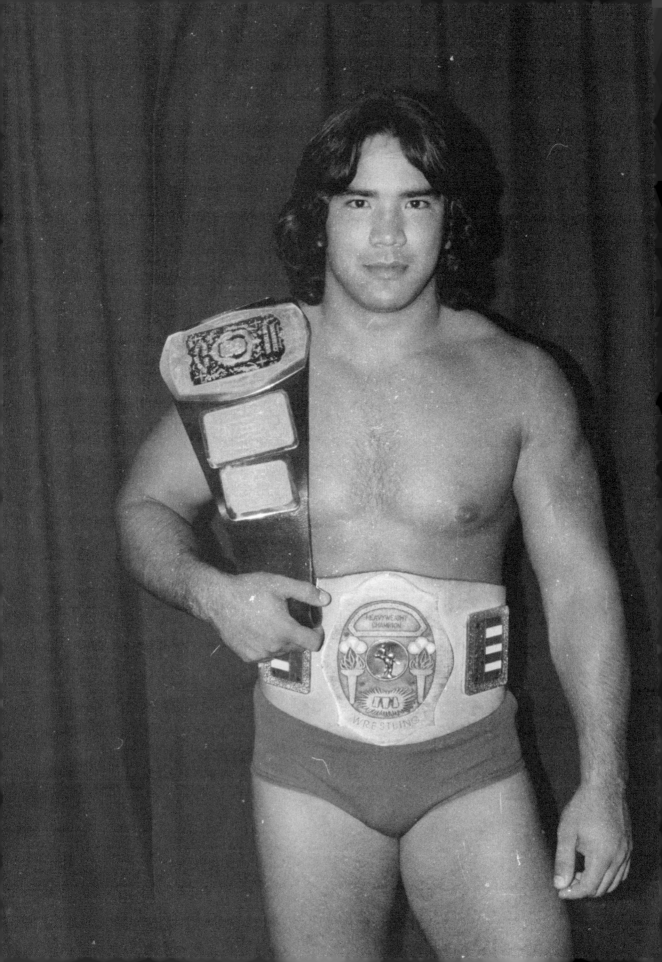

Ricky Steamboat
February 4, 1995

Richard Blood, the consummate, highly respected wrestler, spoke to us from the gym he had started in his hometown of Charlotte, N.C. He answered the phone himself when we called him cold there, and was initially nervous about doing the interview. But he decided to go through with it when he realized our questions were going to be thoughtful and somewhat serious. Though he had been in the business for a long time, Steamboat only won his first heavyweight championship, from Ric Flair, in 1989, even though he had turned pro in 1976, winning several lesser belts along the way. He started out in the AWA under the tutelage of Verne Gagne, and had major runs in both the WCW and WWF (where he wore a rather silly "Dragon" outfit). At the time of the interview, he had retired from the sport due to injuries. This was a long, very candid conversation.

Thanks for everything you've done in the business, Rick. What are you doing right now in wrestling?

To be honest with you, not too much. In late August I hurt my back in the area they call the L3, L4, in the lower back. And my day-to-day life is dealing with lower back pain. It goes left down my hip and into my thigh. A herniated disc is what's causing all the pain. I went through a couple of months of rehab here in Charlotte. They taught me to do some exercises to help strengthen that area, and it has relieved some of the pain and pressure. Until last week, I've been to four doctors, and they all have told me that it would be wise for me to retire, that another bad incident with my back would probably require surgery.

Will there be some kind of celebration for you at the upcoming Slamboree?

That's all tentative at this point. You know, guys call me and ask how I'm doing. I hear rumors. They drop me a line saying they're gonna do this and that with you at Slamboree. But what's funny is that the wcw has yet to call me. Not even a letter or a phone call.

What's your relationship with them right now?

Personally, I'm not on too great of terms. Having about 10 weeks left on my contract, which would have finished out 1994, once they found out what the doctors were saying about my back, they terminated me. I know a number of wrestlers that have been under contract with wcw and maybe wrestled three or four times a year, and they continue to get their paychecks.

Let's go back to a match in March of 1983 at the Greensboro Coliseum. You and Jay Youngblood were in a cage taking on Sergeant Slaughter and Don Kernodle for the tag team titles.

Youngblood was coming off an injury prior to this match. Kernodle had been a collegiate wrestler, and hadn't done too much with his career. Slaughter took him under his wing and taught Don the ropes of what it would take to win in our profession. You have your good guy/bad guy scenarios. Kernodle at the time had always been a real clean-cut type of wrestler. But Slaughter taught him how to go the extra mile, and do the underhanded things that would make you a winner, and Kernodle wanted to be a winner. After getting with Slaughter he started winning matches and working his way up the scale and becoming a main eventer. A number of things were building up to this match, and the Crockett promotion did a wonderful job promoting it. We had a contract signing which was aired on TV. This was one of the first times this was done in the southeastern part of the country. Stipulations were put in, last minute stuff was put in. One was that if Youngblood and I didn't win, we could no longer wrestle as a tag team. We were that hot as an item in the southeast and in Japan. Sergeant Slaughter and Don Kernodle knew this, and I guess they put our backs up against the wall. We weren't the biggest of guys. Jay weighed in under 220. And I was hanging around the 230-pound mark. But there was something between the two of us. As tag team partners, a friendship developed, and we were almost like brothers. This would be the icing on the cake of becoming a real good tag team. We could trust each other in the ring no matter what the consequences were. Slaughter at the time was around 280 pounds and Kernodle close to 260, and both were consummate wrestlers. But with stipulations on our backs and the fact that it was a cage match and with all the build-up, it was a very exciting night for us. And we did win the championship belts, then went on to later wrestle against Jack and Jerry Brisco. Very exciting time in my career.

Let's go back a little earlier. Watching wrestling as a kid, was there anybody you looked up to who made you say: "Hey, that's what I want to do?"

I went to school in St. Pete, Florida. Florida Championship Wrestling with Gordon Solie was very popular. I admired guys like Eddie Graham, for his brashness. He was always considered older than your average wrestler, but he was tough as nails. This would have been in the late '60s. I also admired the young Jack Brisco — collegiate national champion and a consummate technician in the ring. So watching both styles, they were my two real favorites.

Did anyone take you under their wing once you broke in?

I went through Verne Gagne's school of wrestling up in Minneapolis when he had the AWA. It was a tough school. We had about 16 guys come up, and four of us finished. Some great athletes graduated from that school, Ric Flair being one of them — Ken Patera, Jumpin' Jim Brunzell, and of course, Greg Gagne. The Iron Sheik is a graduate from that school. In the first several weeks of training, if you weren't tough enough, you were weeded out. They made sure that guys who made it through would have pretty successful careers.

Shane Douglas was recently saying that you have a great reputation with bringing young wrestlers into the business. Is there anyone you're particularly proud of who you've worked with?

I can't single out any one guy. Currently, Johnny B. Badd. More so on ring psychology as opposed to technical work. I think Johnny can probably do it all. But when it comes to tactics, timing, and psychology, a lot of the younger guys may be lacking. Learning it comes with being in the ring time and time again. You can learn all the moves and holds and be a good technician, but there's also when to apply this or when to apply that, and when to go forward or to back off and catch a breath. In my wars with Flair over the years I don't know how many times we went to a 60-minute draw. And doing that would teach you how to pace yourself, and when to do what at certain times of a match. Or else there are times when at the 30-minute mark you're gonna run out of gas, and there ain't a gas station in sight.

Tell us about your memories of your match with Randy Savage at Wrestle-mania.

You know, you had two guys in there that physically balanced out pretty well — both in height and weight, and strength and speed. It was almost the kind of match where two wrestlers almost complement each other's styles. And there was a great promotional build-up the wwf had done leading up to it. It was two guys who could go hold for hold, and move for move. If we were running a hundred-yard dash, we'd probably cross the finish line at the same time.

That was the same Wrestlemania that had Hogan vs. Andre. That was the match that sold the show, but yours was the match that stole the show.

Well, that was on my mind. The Savage-Steamboat match had gotten a fair amount of PR, but nowhere near the build-up of Hogan and Andre, which was understandable at that time. I guess the biggest mistake the promotion made was putting us on before them. It was an all-out situation in terms of burning up the gas. It was classic match and a highlight in my career. It was unbelievable to hear 93,000 people pop underneath a closed dome. The sound was just unbelievable. I get many remarks on that match comparing it to my matches with Ric Flair.

What about on November 27, 1984, at the second Starrcade in Greensboro. You were taking on Tully Blanchard in a great grudge feud.

It wasn't too long after that that I ventured to the wwf.

Were there internal problems between you and booker Dusty Rhodes at the time?

Yes. Dusty was still active in the ring. And being in that position in the office while being active in the ring, and being a babyface type tough guy, like myself, you can understand the slot positionings that were coming forth. Also, I had a good talk with Jim Crockett Promotions and had a fairly decent employee-employer relationship with him. I had been in the area for a number of years. And knowing the situation in the office, I really wanted to make a move. George Scott, who was booking at the time with the wwf, was a booker with Crockett Promotions before he went up north. I had an excellent relationship with him. So it was a number of things. I wanted a change. I wanted to venture out of the Mid-Atlantic, southeastern area, wanted to see if I could do in other parts of the country what I had done here in terms of popularity, and being able to carry my weight as a main event guy, and not having to deal so much with the politics at the time.

You've had your share of turmoil with both groups. Who's been better for you to work with, the NWA or the WWF?

God, if you drew a list up and had your pluses and minuses, I think each side had both, but one of the main reasons I decided to leave the wwf and venture to Atlanta and the wcw is because it was closer to my home. Their base was closer to Charlotte, and after a number of years with the wwf, the traveling . . . the money was great, the glory was fine. But there comes a time in your life when you put all the monetary things to the side and start thinking about family. The family unit will be there a long time after the career is gone. If you jeopardize that now, what will you have after the career? So that probably played a 50 percent value on me making a decision of coming back to the southeastern area.

Let's talk about your brother Vic Steamboat. He's been in the business for about seven years now. There are reports that you initially tried to discourage him from getting into pro wrestling. Is there any substance to that?

Yes. But it was just one sit-down conversation. It wasn't something that I was persistent about. I drew up the pros and cons of the business, and laid everything on the line. I gave examples of a number of guys that were consummate wrestlers, but were always stuck in that preliminary slot and never given the chance. That was about it. I let him make the decision from there, and he did. He's currently living up in Massachusetts and has a full-time job. So he just does wrestling as a little sideline. In the last couple of years he seems to have found that more pleasing.

Was there any thought of having the Steamboat brothers?

Yeah, that conversation took place. But for each of us, and our careers, and in respect to our family units, at that time it just wasn't gonna work out.

When we spoke to Ric Flair last year, we gave him a few names and asked for a response. When we mentioned you, he simply said the best all-round wrestler in the business. Was there much difference between the fights you had with him here and the fights you two had in Japan? Was there another level you reached over there?

No. If you wanted to compare the matches here and in Japan, they would be on equal terms. Flair and I have not only developed a respect for each other over the years — a very competitive type of respect — but because of the times we've wrestled each other, there's been an almost inside feud between us. It wasn't anything the promotion would capitalize on, it was just a personal, inside feud that had a lot to do with conditioning and pushing each other to the limits. Several times during a match it would be like, "Well, you're not gonna blow *me* up." And this developed over the years. So whenever we met it would be like, "How long is it gonna take me to blow your butt up?" And that's why we had those 60-minute matches. But getting back to Japan, we had a lot of pride going over there, knowing how hard the Japanese wrestlers work. The Japanese promotion and the boys there had heard so much about Steamboat and Flair, this and that, so we went over there and just gave 'em one hell of a match. As far as the personal stuff between Flair and myself, none of it is negative. In the long term, it helped our careers because we would just go out there and work so hard. When we were with Crockett, they knew that putting us in a main event match in Greensboro Coliseum or Charlotte Coliseum would just boost the company. They didn't really have to do a whole lot. People were coming to the matches time and time again, I guess because they knew they'd get their money's worth.

There was a great match at the Landover Arena in Maryland, where you two had a tremendous match-up.

That went about 40 or 42 minutes. Arnold Skaaland and Gorilla Monsoon came back in the locker room after the match — and they were WWF guys — and said, "My God, is this what you guys have been doing down south?" Actually, that match, late in '84 when I decided to leave Crockett and go to the WWF, made it almost like a cakewalk to come in to the WWF. Skaaland and Monsoon and guys like that would put a good word into McMahon's ear before I even knew Vince McMahon. It was a good move.

Back in '89 when you and Flair had the match, the great thing was that people knew they would get a good match and a tremendous angle. It was set up with Barry Windham and Flair doubling on Eddie Gilbert. He needed a mystery partner. This was in late 1988, right around the time Turner took

over WCW. You came out as his partner, probably had the best match of that year on TBS. When you finally pinned Flair, did you have a good feeling about what was going to happen in 1989?

I did. That was the second time I'd beaten Flair on television. And here I am, starting in the business in '76, beat him in the latter part of the '70s, in the Mid-Atlantic area, which really helped my career. And then here we are, the second time — and I couldn't tell you how many hundreds of times we'd wrestled each other in between — but it's a big plug for your career. You've got a main event guy, especially as well known as Ric Flair — able to put *his* shoulders down on national television. At that time, the promotion was real high on me, and I knew that coming up in '89, things were gonna start looking really good. I had a good feeling about myself and my career at that time.

Who was your first professional match against and how did that go for you?

That was against the late Scott Irwin, in Chicago, with the AWA. I can't remember the name of the building.

Did you win?

Yes.

At that point did you feel you made the right decision to get into this business?

No, not really. It probably wasn't until about six months later that I said this was gonna be my thing. But I was only gonna give myself five years. Five years to make it to the main events. During the first six months, it was just talking to guys like Ric Flair and Randy Savage and Sergeant Slaughter. I feel fortunate that we all came along in an era when it was the end of guys like Verne Gagne, Bruno Sammartino, those hardcore old-timers. We were coming along just as they were finishing up, so to speak. And I feel very fortunate to have been brought into this business during that era. It taught you a lot of respect for the business. And learning from the guys from the school of hard knocks, paying the price, and so forth. They just sort of passed the torch to us. "OK, you guys. Now it's your turn. You're gonna have *your* run." So for the 19 years that I've been wrestling, now we've had our run. Now, coming into this age of wrestling, I don't know who should be passed the torch.

What prospects are out there?

Johnny B. Badd, Steve Austin, Shane Douglas. I think he's got a lot of promise, he's just having some political office difficulties here with the wcw. He was very much underpaid at the time he and I were tag team partners. Big-time underpaid, and that was a major problem. Being promised things and then reneging on 'em when it comes to the pay, I think was the straw that broke the camel's back for him to finally bow out of this area.

Is that why you think he's so angry with Ric Flair during his interviews now?

It's a possibility. Flair's got a lot of political pull. I didn't hear of it when Shane and I were partners. Flair never expressed himself to me about it, but there are a lot of things that happened in the office that we don't ever find out about.

I believe Flair is the sole booker right now. So he shouldn't be having the headaches that would happen when there was a committee making decisions.

That does make it difficult. If you've got four or five guys on a committee, each guy is gonna have his friends, buddies, pals, favorites, and they're gonna express their desire to give that person the green light. It's a difficult time.

You've always come across as a team player, sometimes probably doing things for the company you didn't want to. Is that just part of the game that you learn to deal with?

I learned to deal with it in this fashion. I knew that in most cases, whoever I was wrestling with, whether I got the thumbs up or the thumbs down, the fans were going to go home with a hell of a match. So that's the way I felt. In both companies they found out that I wasn't the kind of guy that would go storming into the office, ranting and raving about this or that, even though there are guys that do it. But I never worried about all of that because I knew that the fans were gonna go away with a hell of a match and say they got their money's worth. I had some great matches with Lex Luger. And I had Randy Savage and Ric Flair and Don Muraco and Jake "the Snake" Roberts . . . I think [Dave] Meltzer made a comment one time that I just seem to be the common denominator. I took it as a compliment. Whoever I was working with, I would adjust to their kind of wrestling. I had one-hour matches with Black Jack Mulligan toward the end of his career. And the action was *there*. But it does get kind of hard on the back when you're pulling a 340-pound man around the ring.

1989 was your year. There was a great angle at the St. Valentine's Massacre Clash of the Champions, where you and Flair had the infamous BVD bumping angle. That was reminiscent of an angle that happened years before. One of the women with Flair then was named Bonnie, who went on to become Bonnie Steamboat.

That was in 1979. Crockett Promotions at the time had hired two models. Flair was doing his normal thing of projecting himself as the flamboyant wrestler, per se, always having baby dolls and girlfriends and flying all over the country. Crockett Promotions spiced it up by hiring two models, and one of them happened to be Bonnie. We had our thing in the ring where I ran out and jumped on Flair and tore his clothes off. The models, not knowing what would happen were going, "Oh my God, what's happening here?" About five years later, Bonnie and I met. She was working at a modeling agency at the time, and a friend of mine was also working there, who brought me some pictures. I looked at the one of Bonnie and said, "I have seen this girl somewhere," but I couldn't remember where. It was really hard for me to get my first date with her because she remembered back in '79 about that thing. She was telling her friends that she didn't want anything to do with wrestlers. But I played it safe. We had lunch, and it turned out to be a three-hour lunch. You know, everybody has their wrestling face, and then you have your personal side. And you try to leave one at work, and you have one at home. Just don't bring your work home with you.

So how old is Ricky Jr. now?

He's 7, and he's in his second year of amateur wrestling. I started him out last year and he was the North Carolina State Championship his first year. And he's doing real well this year. We're at the time of the season to where the tournaments are starting to come up. We're really excited and I'm hoping he can return and win the state championship the second year in a row

Is there a second-generation wrestler in the making here?

You should have seen him last year, when I took him to wrestling practice. He was out there wanting to pile drive and figure four leglock all these kids. So I had to explain to him, no, no, this is like high school wrestling.

We have a few questions from listeners. Is it true you used to wrestle as Sammy Steamboat Jr. when you first broke in.

No, I was his "nephew."

Did Verne Gagne give you the name?

No, it was Eddie Graham. When I first broke in with the AWA under Verne, I was wrestling as Richard Blood. After a few months, they sent me down to Florida. I walked in the office and Eddie Graham said to me, "God, you don't look like no Richard Blood. Blood would be a heel." In the '60s, Sammy Steamboat was pretty popular in Florida. So looking at me and my physical features, and with Sammy being Hawaiian, Eddie said, "Well, let's just call you Ricky Steamboat and you'll be like a nephew." At my first match in Florida as Ricky Steamboat, I was the opening match in West Palm Beach. I walked in the ring, the announcer says, "Ladies and gentlemen, we have a substitute this evening. Richard Blood is unable to make it. But standing in for him, and I'm sure you'll recognize the name, is the nephew of Sam Steamboat, Ricky Steamboat." While the announcer is saying all of this, that Richard Blood was unable to make it, I lost all sense of what was taking place. I was grabbing at the announcer's shoulder and saying, "No, I'm *here*." And he was shrugging me off and saying, "Get back in your corner, kid." Then it hit me. I was so green and awestruck, I had forgotten.

Is there anyone out there you're envious or jealous of?

Well, Hogan has done a lot for the business, both pro and con. You've gotta pat a guy on the back that's able to sit down with a promoter and negotiate a salary and contract as he's been able to. When you're in the driver's seat, as he has been over the years, and you're able to carry that kind of clout when you walk into the office . . . being in the right place at the right time has a lot to do with it also. He's got a lot of charisma and does great interviews. His wrestling work is sort of average. I've never had a match with him beyond being tag team partners a couple of times in the WWF. But to answer your question about being jealous or envious, I often thought back, and would have discussions with close friends — not with people in the office. But I would think, "What would happen if they gave me the same amount of airtime and promotion as Hogan? What would the course of careers and the history of wrestling have been back in the '80s?" It's hard to say, but it's something that wanders in your mind. When I first went up to the WWF in '85, I thought my popularity at the time was almost on par with the Hulkster's, but I wasn't given half the airtime. But I'm not the one to go bucking the system or knocking down doors to the office. And I never believed in doing a lot of brown-nosing. I believed that my ability in the ring and my work ethic was enough to carry me through. I guess that sort of commanded my pay scale.

It's too bad more people in the sport don't have the same outlook as you.

Well, I think what we're having here in the young kids coming into the profession today, is that they didn't have the opportunity like I had and others like me had — being brought up in the time I was brought into the business. That doesn't really exist anymore. I've told people that I wish wrestling would go back to what it was 10 or 15 years ago.

So what do you do from here?

Currently I'm working my gym in Charlotte. I'm going on my 11th year there. Bonnie and I live about 30 miles north of Charlotte, up on Lake Norman. This area is growing a lot and we're thinking about opening another club up here. And we've got a few business ideas. She's talked a number of times over the years about opening up a little coffee shop — just something for her. People have asked me the golden question — Have you missed it? and I say, "I can't." I'd be a fool to try with my situation, I just don't want to go under the knife with my back.

You've done so many things throughout your career. What do you consider your greatest personal moment?

Bottom line, I'd have to say Feb. 20, 1989, Chicago. That year Flair and I had three classic matches — Chicago, New Orleans, and Nashville. Out of the three, I'd have to say the match in New Orleans gets the nod. Although career-wise and as far as personal feelings, winning the world championship, without a doubt.

For that match, Jim Ross was doing the commentary, and it was possibly the best work on commentary for any match.

I've heard that from other people. I've seen the tape, and it gives you goosebumps just listening to him. There was the match itself, but he did a great job.

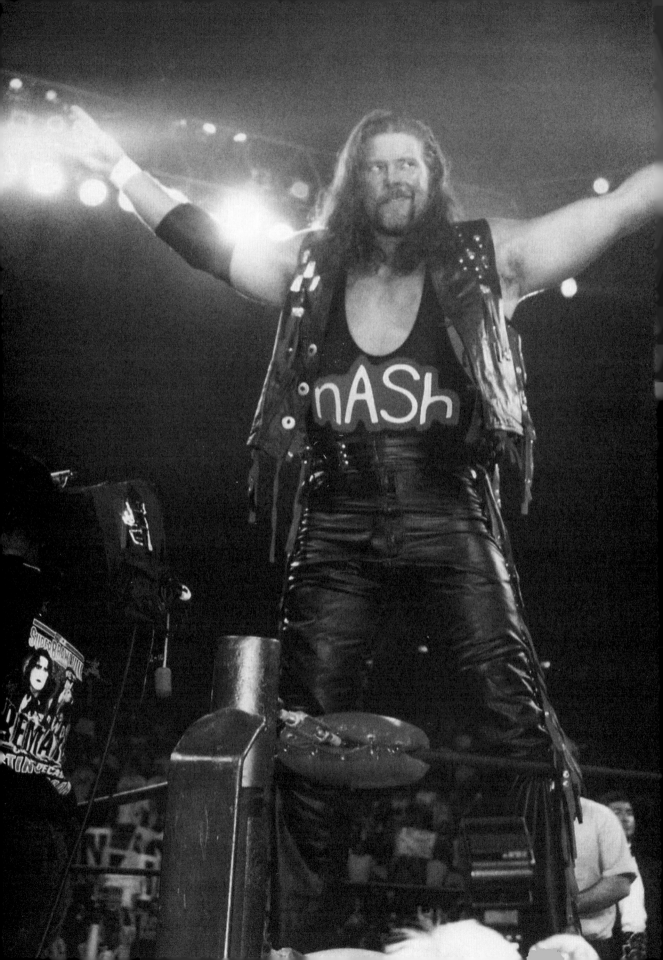

Kevin Nash

March 20, 1995

Nash wasn't yet going by his real name at the time of this interview, which was conducted in person at a press junket held at the Boston Garden to promote Wrestlemania 11. It was one of the first times the WWF allowed us access to their performers, and interviews were limited to about 10 minutes. And Diesel, as he was then known, was about halfway through his reign as WWF champ — he had defeated Bob Backlund and was later beaten by Bret Hart. He came across as low-key and cordial during the interview, but was perfectly willing to answer all questions, especially since Vince McMahon had uncharacteristically used his real name on TV a couple of weeks earlier. Nash had been in the business for about 13 years and wrestled as Master Blaster Steele, Oz, and Vinnie Vegas with WCW before making it big as Diesel in the WWF. He came across here with a sort of "aw shucks" attitude.

We're talking to Diesel, and it's just a couple of weeks until Wrestlemania. Is there anything that you're seriously nervous about for the upcoming fight?

It's my first title defense at a Wrestlemania and without a doubt, I've got to be concerned about Shawn Michaels because he's a great wrestler. I've also got to be concerned about Sid Vicious, so there are a few intangibles.

Yeah but Sid could run away and be one of those replacement players we were talking about off air. He does have an affinity for softball they tell me.

I hope he does.

During *Raw* a few weeks ago, Vince called you by your real name. Is this the first time that happened and did it catch you off guard?

Yeah I guess it did. But, I mean my friends call me Kevin. They don't call me Diesel, so I don't think it was that big of a shock. I am Kevin Nash.

It was just kind of unprecedented for Vince to do something like that. He never lets the cover go, so I was kind of surprised.

I guess they're making me more human.

Could you go back just a little bit and tell us how you got into this game?

I was working at a club in Atlanta that a lot of wrestlers frequented. I got to talking with them and they told me what I could make in professional wrestling. I had been a fan as a kid growing up in Detroit. The Sheik had the promotion at that time. And I pursued it through Jody Hamilton, who was one of the Assassins. He taught me for nine months, and I broke in down in wcw.

Were there any other heroes you could remember when you were a kid watching saying, "Hey, I want to grow up and be like that guy?"

Like most kids, I liked gimmick guys when I was real young. I remember Moose Cholak, who used to come out with a moose head. I thought that he was pretty cool. I liked Bobo Brazil. I liked the Bruiser. I liked the Kangaroos.

Is there anybody now, and it doesn't have to be just the World Wrestling Federation, but the whole wrestling business that you'd like to test?

That seems loaded. Maybe you're trying to point to a balding, blond-haired guy. I don't know.

No, we're talking about the new generation here.

I guess the people would really like to see me wrestle the Undertaker. Somewhere down the line I'm sure he and I will have a contest.

Yeah, how do you think that will go?

I don't know. He's awfully tough. I don't think he's had too many losses in his career.

One last serious question. There seems to be fewer and fewer people around the rings these days. What can be done to bring the crowds back?

I don't think it's really up to the wrestlers. I don't think it's up to the promoters. I think it's more up to the economy. I think the economy is down. I think the entertainment dollar is down everywhere. People who used to run the Van Halens and bands like that that used to run arenas now are running a lot smaller venues. There's not that much entertainment dollar out there and I think, you know, you still get the same piece of the pie, I think the pie is just a lot smaller.

So you don't see any change in the near future?

I think the World Wrestling Federation is giving them a different degree of athleticism than some of the other promotions. I think the quality of our promotion is unparalleled in the business but by the same point, I think this company is turning the corner. I think the crowds have been coming up in our major markets. And it's just a matter of time. I think wrestling goes in cycles, we've had a down cycle and I think we're on our way back up.

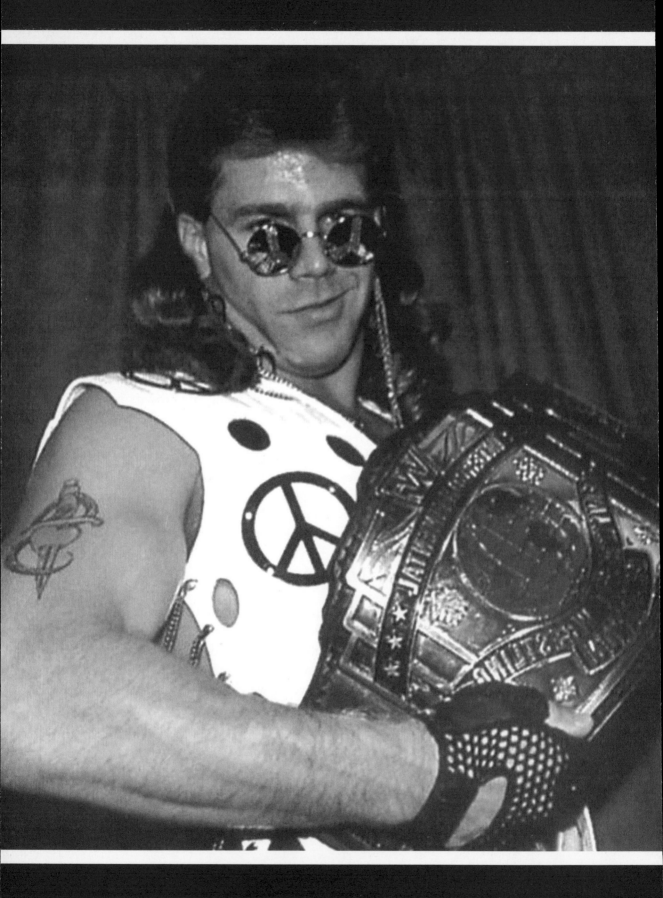

Shawn Michaels

March 25, 1995

He is probably the most controversial world champion of modern times, and Michael Hickenbottom's refusal to do jobs is legendary, yet his work rate is in a class that few will ever be able to touch. Working his way up from the Texas territory, he first gained notice as the partner of Marty Jannetty in the Midnight Rockers, later called the Rockers when they joined the WWF. Possibly still best known for the first ladder match with Razor Ramon, he irregularly left the ring to let his injuries heal, and, against many medical experts' wishes, still remains a major wrestling figure. This interview was done in person at the Boston Garden during the Wrestlemania 11 junket. He spoke of being trained by Jose Lothario, his dreams of success in the future, and of his father's disapproval of his career choice.

Shawn, let's shoot back to your earliest thoughts, maybe when you were a kid watching pro wrestling, what you were thinking of? About trying to get into it?

Well, I remember, it was the first time, I was about 12 years old, I got to stay up late for the first time and at the time I was in San Antonio, Texas, and it was Southwest Championship Wrestling, which was promoted by Joe Blanchard. I saw it for the first time and it blew me away. I was taken right there. From that day, I knew that all I ever wanted to be was a wrestler, and that's when I started watching wrestling on cable and started getting the World Wrestling Federation on WOR-TV. And throughout the years I can remember saying to myself that was where I wanted to go. At the time it was the World Wide Wrestling Federation and it turned into the World Wrestling Federation, and all my friends, everyone I knew, kept telling me that it just wasn't going to happen. Nobody didn't believe that I didn't have the talent or I was a good athlete, but they just figured that I had to know somebody or do something. You know, it was just one of those things that was a dream and was always going to be that way. And I just couldn't get it out of my mind. You know, I was pretty much raised to be a football player.

Football player?

Yes, I was an outside linebacker and you know, as you can tell, I don't have a problem bragging. But I was a pretty talented football player. The problem was I just couldn't get wrestling out of my mind. And it came to my senior year and everyone asked, "What are you going to do? Are you going to go to college, are you going to pursue football at college?"

This was at Texas?

At Randolph High School in San Antonio. And I just told my dad that I wanted to be a professional wrestler. My dad did a lot of golfing and knew a friend of a friend of a friend, you know how golf stuff works. And he said, "Maybe I can get you to meet with the promoter of Texas All-Star Wrestling." It had changed names at the time and over the years. So I said OK and we went. I was 17 years old when I graduated and I went and talked with the guy. He said that you had to be 19 to be a wrestler and "Your dad wants you to go to college. Go to college for four years and then come back." I thought, "Well, OK." So I went to a semester at Southwest State Texas University . . .

One semester?

One semester and I just never went to class. And I couldn't do anything but think about wrestling. I practiced and worked and couldn't get it out of my mind. Finally, after that semester of scoring a 1.4, I went back to my dad and told him that I didn't want to waste any more of his money. I had one birthday since, I was 18. I went back and told the promoter I can't, I don't want to waste my father's money and I have this obsession that I have with professional wrestling. So, he hooked me up with a man named Jose Lothario, who was a huge star in Texas and Florida. Not many people in the East know who he is.

We've read about him.

He was really good. He was one of the greatest Mexican wrestlers that ever wrestled. And he trained me. And then, it was just a matter of waiting for my 19th birthday.

You couldn't lie about that?

No, well, I mean that's not something that I did . . . . You know, it's not something I do today, and it's not something I did then. And I wanted to follow all the rules and you know, being the son of a Colonel in the Air Force, that's what you do. . . . After my 18th birthday, Jose got me booked in a place called Mid-South Championship Wrestling, which was promoted by Bill Watts at the time. And I broke in there.

Who was your first fight?

My first match was against Art Crews. A guy named Art Crews. Yeah, you know, where is he now?

Did you win?

No, I lost my first match. Then the next night I went to a 15-minute draw, and the next night I won. And after the first one, everyone commented that I was a natural. I remember people saying, "Kid, you're going to make a million dollars in this business." And they were right. . . . Thank goodness. But I mean, 10 years later, I'm looking at my first main event at Wrestlemania. My first World Wrestling Federation Championship match. And, win, lose or draw, it's a dream that's come true, and I'm probably the happiest guy on earth. It's been a long, hard road. It hasn't been easy, it hasn't always been fun. But, it's fun now and all the hardships, all the hard times, all the starving, all the bad people I've had to deal with, good people, medium people, you name it. You know I've seen them all. But, I wouldn't trade the life that I have now with the life that I've led for anything in the world because it's been quite an adventure.

Was there a big break at one point?

I would say there's been a couple. The first one I think would be when I went to the AWA. And I tagged with a guy named Marty Jannetty. Marty and I, to this day, I believe he and I were just about, well I believe that we'll go down as one of the best tag teams in the history of wrestling because we were innovators. We started something in tag team wrestling, you know as far as action, excitement, you know, flash that wasn't really around in wrestling. I was around 20 and he was about 24 or 25 and we were two guys doing something we loved, running around and chasing girls. You name it and we were doing it. And that was our first time to have big exposure to the wrestling world, through ESPN, and that's why I would characterize that as my biggest break. Then we got a tryout with the World Wrestling Federation and progressed here. I'd say my second biggest break that some may disagree with but was a decision that I made on my own, was splitting with Marty Jannetty. You know, it didn't make me the most popular guy, but boy it's been lucrative to say the least. It also was a time that I was a very young man and he helped me a lot, we were good friends. But the dream that I had in my mind was to be a single, successful wrestler on my own. Stand on my own two feet. And to make Shawn Michaels a household name. It wasn't something that was really negotiable with Marty, it was something that I had to do on my own. And again, like I said, it wasn't popular with everybody but I think it was the right move. I think there are a lot of people who will agree that, whether they like me or dislike me, since that time I've become one of the top stars in this sport. And, you know at 29, I think it's just the beginning.

You know, almost a year ago to the day was the ladder match.

Yes.

That had to be another great milestone.

It definitely was. It was a match that was set up, but it wasn't hyped and I don't think a lot of people expected it to be what it was.

You're absolutely right.

Thank you. And I knew in my heart that it was going to be a match that stole the show. That it was going to be the match that everyone remembered. But I think the WWF and the bosses thought — it hadn't been done regularly and it was sort of a risk. It was the WWF taking a chance and one of those things that you threw in the air, and see if it works, and it worked. It was probably the best thing that has happened to me. It was a losing effort, I didn't walk out with the Intercontinental Championship, but it's a match that'll go down in history in the minds of wrestling fans. And for me, that's important. Again, Shawn Michaels is a cocky, arrogant guy on TV, but the fans of the World Wrestling Federation know exciting them is what I do. It's what I try to do and what I live for. I love to hear them scream, I love to hear them yell. And that's why I say at Wrestlemania 11, it's going to be oh, after all the Hollywood stars, after everything's done, just like last year, I'm going to make sure the fans of the World Wrestling Federation and everyone that tunes in, the one thing that they're going to take from Wrestlemania 11 is the performance of Shawn Michaels. Whether it be a win, lose, or draw situation, I'm going to give them a show. I'm going to risk life and limb because that's what I do. I love this sport, I love what I do, it's like an addiction. It's an addiction hearing the people yell and scream and if I gotta risk life and limb to do it, then I'm going to do it. It's what I enjoy and that's where I get my gratification from.

You're doing a great job, and you'll probably be wearing the belt soon.

I hope you're right. One thing I am is the designated pain-in-the-butt of the WWF. If it doesn't happen at Wrestlemania, you can bet that I'll be causing some trouble to get my chance.

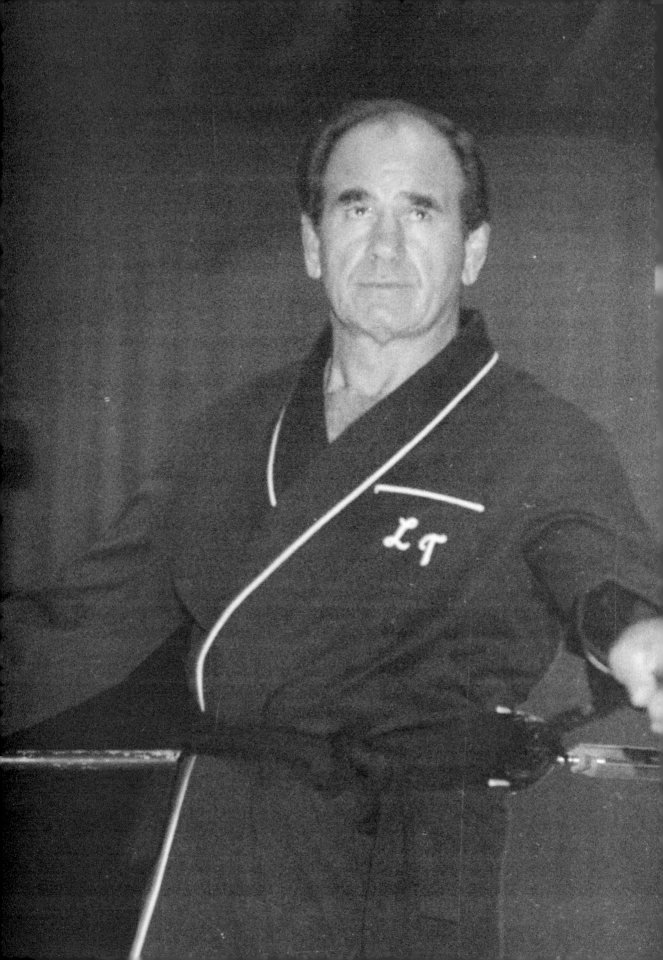

Lou Thesz
May 6, 1995

One of the best and most fascinating interview guests on the show, Thesz provided a remarkable retrospective on wrestling from the 1930s, through his first retirement in the 1950s and right up to the late 1980s, when he made a series of special in-ring appearances. An old school scientific wrestler himself, he was candid about the business, even while making it quite clear just how hard one had to work to be successful in it, and seemed as happy to talk about promoters as about his wives. Thesz never wrestled in the WWF, but he held belts in the NWA, AWA, WWA, and MWA, and worked all over the world as a wrestler, and eventually fought in a number of boxer-wrestler matches. Known as Mr. Catch-as-catch-can, this was the first of three appearances on the show.

We have with us today Mr. Lou Thesz, originally from Missouri, talking to us today from his home in Virginia. Thanks for coming on, sir, it's an honor to have you on today. You are the epitome of what pro wrestling is.

Well, I've been around a long time, maybe that's it.

What are you involved with, in wrestling, these days?

I'm working with a group in Japan — I spend about one week of my month over there — UFW International. We're not only advertising, but producing martial arts wrestling. We get some of the Olympic winners from Russia, the United States, wherever, and we teach them martial arts. Because in amateur wrestling, bone breaking or punishing holds are not permitted. Nevertheless, we teach them — not to make a big point of this thing — we teach them how to hurt people, because pin falls do not count — one must concede or one can't continue.

How does that differ from the early days when you were learning the game?

Not a great deal. A little bit before my time, about 700 B.C., they had a thing called pancratium. My coach, George Tragos — he was coaching Missouri U at the time and I was living in St. Louis, where I was reared — he took an interest in me. We went to various schools and wrestled the heavyweights, to check us out and see what we could do. But he was a wonderful coach, and after I became a pro wrestler, I met the real greats, like Ed "Strangler" Lewis and Ray Steele and Ad Santel — you know, the real goodies. They were knowledgeable, very generous, magnanimous people that would share their wares with you, and the experiences they had. You could not pay these people to do that. They just wanted to perpetuate wrestling. And that's what we did. I enjoyed all of it, and I'm just sorry I can't do it again.

Lou, in 1937, you were 21 years old, and you defeated Everett Marshall in a great match for the National Wrestling Association title.

That was an association composed of athletic commissioners that were chosen by the governors of each state. They had a lot of teeth, a lot of power, and they illustrated it several times. But that was a really good organization that had a lot of credibility, and it was the real thing. When I won the title, it was, in all aspects, the undisputed title of the world. That's where all the biggies came — from Europe, from all over the world, to wrestle here because they could make a little money. I learned martial arts wrestling in the gym with Tragos. He was not only a coach, but a carnival and circus performer. They would take on all comers, and they were not there to lose money. So they always had to have one good wrestler and one good boxer. He had to be a knockout artist, and the wrestler had to be what we call a hooker — someone that knew how to hurt someone. If they couldn't beat the fella by just wrestling and rolling around with him, why they would just hurt him and that was the end of the match. I was schooled in that at a very early age. I've seen a lot of people get crippled in the ring, who could never wrestle again, but that was part of it. With the development of wrestling in the United States, it got to be a show business thing. And like Hulk Hogan himself said, his matches were pre-arranged. With martial arts wrestling, they don't even have a look-in. There's not a window to see through. Because they've got to be able to compete, or else they cannot operate. They either know martial arts wrestling and can wrestle and compete, or they're out of the ballgame.

In your early days of wrestling, how long was it before you actually took your first belt?

December 29, 1937. I was wrestling four years before that.

Did your life change when you won the first belt?

Not a great deal. I was working out with the big boys then — Ray Steele and Strangler Lewis in St. Louis, and when I was on the west coast, with Ad Santel. I had some wonderful coaching. It was not a difficult transition for me, because that's what I was doing to begin with.

You've mentioned Strangler Lewis a few times. Was he your mentor?

Mentor, coach, and probably the greatest wrestler we've produced in this country. No, not probably. I *know* he was.

In the history books, he's been described as more of a defensive wrestler.

Absolutely.

But we don't see much of that now. Only the name of Royce Gracie comes to mind.

Oh he's pretty dull. It seems the Gracies' bloom will be off the bush pretty soon. There isn't really enough action there. But the man that Gracie wrestled recently — Dan Severn — he's very knowledgeable. He's freestyle, Greco and sambo. I worked with him in Japan a little bit, and taught him a couple of the hooks. Dan would be a world-beater if he just had the get-up-and-go to hurt people. He's too kind — a nice guy, a really wonderful person. But he's just a little reluctant to cripple anyone. And when you're dealing with people like Gracie, that's what you've got to do.

But would that work in American pro wrestling?

Why not?

Well, do fans really want to see people get hurt?

Well, in Tokyo, we had 47,000 people in a ballpark, with the same format. And that was without TV, only newspapers and magazines. But the people knew it was a contest, and that's why they were there.

Has anyone over the years intentionally tried to hurt you in a shoot match?

Of course. In a shoot match, you always have that risk. If you don't hurt him, he's gonna hurt you.

And you've taken some pretty bad bumps?

Oh, sure. I've had 200 broken bones, if you'll believe that. But they heal. And they heal a lot easier than tendons do. I've had separations and tendon damage.

Have you actually counted your injuries?

No, I never did. You know, if you get into competition and wrestle 6,000 times, it's difficult to remember where and when you really got hurt. It seems in wrestling if you get hurt one time, it comes in cycles of three. You hurt something then something else and something else. But you don't remember pain anyway. I've fractured the left patella — the kneecap — and the clavicles both times, the rotator cuff, a lot of problems. Cartilage separations in the chest, the sternum, and the side ribs. I had five broken ribs at one time. But those were all competition matches, and that's the way it was. You stop and heal up, and if you're crazy enough to do it, you go back again.

Could you talk about some of the other names from the past, such as Tony Stecher, Pinky George, and Ray Steele?

I worked out with Ray Steele constantly. We played handball together. We were a team. When I was 17 years of age I worked out with Tony Stecher in Minneapolis. Pinky George was a very good promoter. He was also a featherweight fighter. I lived in Des Moines, serving my apprenticeship at that time, and I would drive for him at night when he got sleepy. We had a great relationship, and we kept that up. He was a wonderful little guy. He died at about 93.

Is it true that George Tragos was a former Olympic champion?

Well, he was a three-time Olympian, twice for Greece and once for the United States. I don't know exactly what the track record is. He was a middleweight.

Have you worked any boxer-wrestler matches?

Yes I did. I had a contest with Jersey Joe Walcott in Memphis, Tennessee. David Broom was a sports editor down there. He came to the dressing room one night and asked if I'd ever be interested in a mixed match, and I said sure. I had seen Ray Steele go against King Levinsky in St. Louis, and Ray beat him in 32 seconds.

How long did it take you to win?

Fourth round. I got a little smart-alecky. I didn't think he could hurt me, because he caught me in a couple of combinations and really didn't shake me up. So I thought, well, he can't do it anyway. But that was stupid, because he could. And then he caught me flat-footed and rocked me. I went to one knee and he came in to upper-cut me, and I had just enough left to hook his ankle and throw my shoulder into his knee and take him down.

Who would generally win, the boxer or the wrestler?

Oh, the wrestler would win. If the wrestler has any kind of an idea and knows what he's doing, there's no way he could lose the match. If you're really sharp, you can go across the ring on your hands and knees faster than the guy could run, and you could take him down. I did that with Walcott. I faked him out a couple times, but once I stood him on the mat, I just climbed his frame, and of course that was the end of it.

You mentioned a few years ago that some of your favorite current wrestlers were Rick Steiner and Mike Rotunda. How does the scene look today?

We have some good wrestlers around. Gary Albright, a former amateur out of Nebraska, is the best Greco-Roman wrestler we have in this country today. I think the new talent is wonderful. I'm trying to look for some of it. I may make a trip to Europe this fall, because we're running out of talent. There are some good wrestlers over there.

What about over here?

I talked to a boy the other day. I was in Asheville, North Carolina, for a golf tournament, and I met Nikita Koloff. A very good athlete. He hasn't wrestled in the last year or so. But I talked with him and he's gonna start training again. I'd like to take him over there because he's very capable and has a lot of ability, and I want to get him a shot at it.

Did you pass through Boston often in your career?

I remember being in Boston, to fight Primo Carnera, the former boxing champion. Well, talking about wrestling competition — and please don't think this is a boastful move I'm making here — but I taught him a little bit about what really happens in contest wrestling. That was the Cardinal Cushing show for flood relief in Italy. Jack Dempsey was referee and we had Jack Sharkey there and Ed "Strangler" Lewis, and we had a wonderful time. Carnera was a big, strong guy, a circus performer before he fought. But of course strength isn't that important. You can take a turtle or a big bull and put him on his back, and he's helpless. And that's what I did with him. I dropped him on his head and knocked him out. A Greco-Roman backdrop. He weighed about 275. But even 375 wouldn't have been a problem because when you make that move, it's how you do it. You can lift 400 pounds pretty easily as you can 200.

What was your standard weight?

About 220. You've got the super-heavyweights — the 300 pounders. But I discovered that the middle-size heavyweights have better reflex than the real big guys. You have enough weight and power there. And if you've got real good speed, well, the reflex is the whole thing. The one that gets there first wins the race.

But aren't there exceptions to that rule? What do you think of Vader?

I see what he does, but I see some things that he leaves wide open inadvertently. Because he powers out of things. But when you lock a guy up properly, he's not gonna power out of anything — there's no power.

You were never really known as a gimmick wrestler. You were a standard, mainstream wrestling opponent. But what happened when someone like George Wagner came along? Did he take any of the fire away from you?

Not at all. I respected him because he was a wrestler. A lot of people didn't know that. But he was a darn good junior heavyweight wrestler. And he came up with the gimmick of Gorgeous George. He had a great mentality for wrestling and how to make money. I wrestled him a couple of times, and we had sellouts. He was just a junior heavyweight, but he had a lot of courage. One time I wrestled him in Chicago at Wrigley Field, and he had a crazy thing where he'd do a running jump and mount you from the back and take you over in a forward roll. But he didn't get the forward roll. I just kept him going out of the ring, his head hit the typewriters and he came up and he had a face full of blood. But he had the guts to get back in and try to finish the match.

So what do you think of Lord Lansdowne?

I think he was the originator. Man, you've done your history. I think George copied many of his things from Lord Lansdowne. And had a lot more success. But I think Lansdowne broke the ice for that sort of mentality, and George took it and ran with it and did very well with it.

Let's talk about your book on pro wrestling. It's in its second printing in Japan. Will it ever comes out in the States?

I talked to the CEO there, and he's going to explore the Japanese bookstores here and see if he can bring it over and sell it here.

What's the book about?

It's about wrestling. It's written by Koji Miyamoto, who is my business manager. I've known him since he was 17 years of age, which makes that about a 20-year relationship. Wonderful guy.

There's supposedly something in the book about you and Bruno Sammartino.

Well, I wrestled him only one time. That was in Toronto, and I beat him there. Of course, he didn't publicize that because they didn't want it to come out in the New York papers. They were still using him as the champion. But there was no count out, I just pinned him. And that was the end of that. Bruno is a wonderful guy, very strong, and a great weight lifter, but not really a sophisticated wrestler. He was a so-so worker. But I'm not talking about the working or the business matches. I'm talking about contests. If you get two names like Sammartino and myself, that should be a contest. The people are buying a ticket. Give 'em what they're paying for.

Any comments on Ric Flair, who just "retired" again?

Oh, I don't know how many times Ric's gonna retire. He started as a wrestler in Minneapolis, and had very, very good coaching up there. But since then, why, he went to work for various groups — wcw, whatever. He's a great athlete and I think he's a great guy, we had a good relationship and everything. But again, like Gorgeous George, he's a moneymaker.

Didn't you once accuse him of doing too many repetitive moves?

That's right. When it gets repetitious it's like a broken record. Who on earth is gonna see the same movie 10 times? I can't handle it. I see the movie once, I'm finished with it.

What caused your retirement in the late '50s?

Oh, I get negative at times. If I don't get what I think is a square shake from some of the promoters. In the NWA I didn't think they were booking me right, because they were running me in a lot of tank towns where there was no money, and I was embarrassed to be there and they had bad rings, and you get no sleep and no money. It got to be a situation where you just have a belly full.

So after 20 years it was enough?

Well, I knocked off for a couple years and I was swimming and sailing and skin diving and having a ball. I was working harder than I was at wrestling. Money wasn't a problem then. I had a real good apartment house and some land. I never played the stock market, but I made some money in the real estate business.

So a few years go by, you go to Japan and win a month-long tournament, and come back and you're bigger than ever. Why did you get back into it?

Ego. Itchy feet. You know, you get to the point where you say, "What am I doing? I devoted my entire life to this thing, and now I'm sitting on my duff and doing nothing." And I was much happier working than I was loafing.

After the Japan tournament, you came back to the United States and took the belt from Buddy Rogers in 1963. Were you treated any differently by the people in the business at that point?

Yes. We had a meeting of the minds because I was participating in my booking. In the beginning I was not, because the NWA champion was booked by the president, Sam Muchnick, who did a great job most of the time — but not all of the time, not enough to suit me. They moved their pencil about a half-inch, and you go out 5,000 miles, and I didn't like that part of the situation. After I was participating in the booking, I liked it a lot better.

At that time, were you looked at as the elder statesman of wrestling?

Oh yeah, even then. But that translated into a lot of respect. When you drop names like Ed Lewis, Ray Steele, Ad Santel — those are the inside people in wrestling that everybody knows. They could cut the mustard. They were the people that knew what they were doing out there. They could cripple you or whatever. Once you were associated with those people, then you get that kind of respect. Of course sometimes when you go to foreign countries, you get tried out a lot. They'd try their wings with you and see what they could do. But that's OK.

Let's bring up a couple of names from the past — Dick Hutton and Jack Brisco.

Both of them are great wrestlers out of Oklahoma. Both are unbelievable guys.

They say Jack Brisco was destined for greatness but he didn't have charisma.

Oh, I don't know. I don't agree with that. They said the same thing about Hutton, but it isn't true. A lot of people think if people don't bounce off the ropes and do a lot of choreographed tumbling, they're not colorful. But let's say if you were to do a critique on a great painting, even if you're not well versed in art, you could look at something and say it's good. You don't know why it is, but it is. And it's the same in wrestling, when they see a match with some really great moves, if they see some things that are surprising, maybe a little bulb will go on over their head, and say, maybe this is OK.

What's your opinion of Pat O'Connor?

He was a very good wrestler.

He had a match with Dick Hutton once.

Dick was the best heavyweight mat wrestler I've ever seen. He would float like a middleweight on the mat. We wrestled some contests in Texas. We liked each other, but we were watching each other like a hawk. He did a thing called the dipsy-do switch right in mid-air. He would switch from one side then switch to the other. I told him one time, you did it once, but you'll never do it again. And about five years later he caught me in it again.

Your impressions on Bronko Nagurski in the '30s . . .

Great athlete, mediocre wrestler. He was not a wrestling student. He once hit me with a tackle and knocked me over the top rope in Houston, Texas. It was nine feet to the concrete floor, I hit it with my left knee and the kneecap was fractured. So I was out for a year. It didn't cost me much — just a couple hundred thousand.

How about Jim Londos?

Great wrestler. Just not big enough for Ed Lewis. He was supposed to be a St. Louis hometown boy, but everybody knew he was from Greece. He was a good wrestler, not as good as he thought he was, but a very good wrestler.

Walter Kowalski.

Very good man. And a great competitor. He had a lot of courage. Gene Kiniski was the same sort of guy — a big roughneck. Pretty much the same style. He'd run over you like a tractor if you didn't watch him.

Didn't Gene Kiniski take your last title?

Yes, he did. But I have a lot of respect for him. He doesn't mind facing the barrier. Gene would look you right in the eye and say let's go.

Where do you see the future of the American wrestling business a few years down the line?

Well, you said the right word — business. You talk about all these sports we have, anytime you sell a ticket it's business, it's not a sport. Nevertheless, I think it can get only so bad, then it's gotta get better. That's what's gonna happen. Right now, people are very interested in the Ultimate Fight down in Tulsa, and other matches like Combat Wrestling. It's actually martial arts wrestling. It seems to be generating a lot of interest, and that's what I'm working with in Japan, and I'll continue to do it. This show business thing, this choreographed tumbling they're doing, is not gonna last. Because people know it's not a contest. And rather than having 10- and 12-year-olds for an audience, maybe we'll get some adults back that wear black ties.

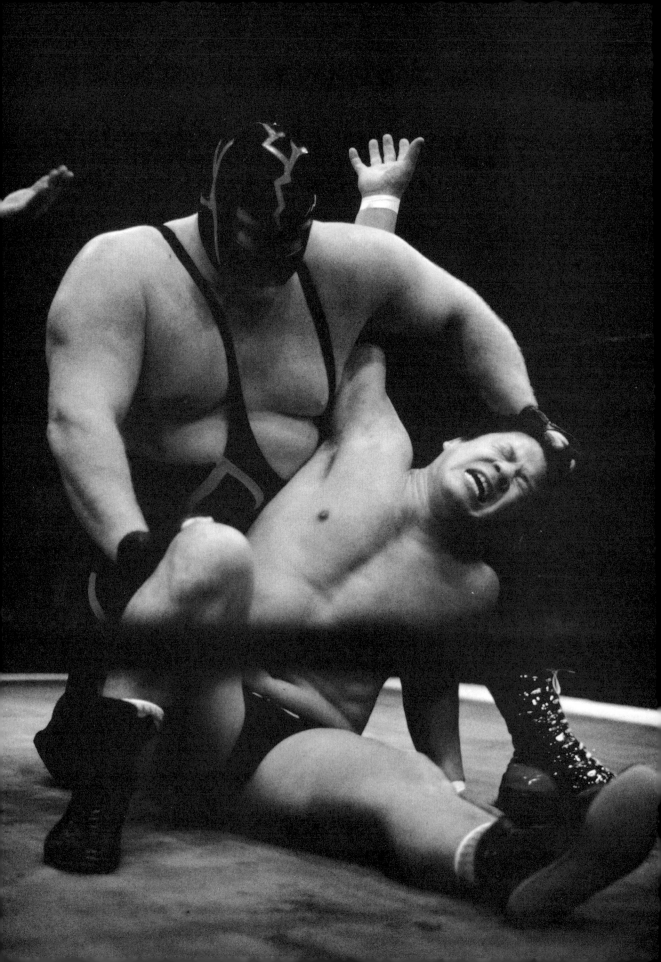

Vader

July 13, 1995

Leon White will go down as one of the most prolific world champions of all time. He's been world champ on three different continents and has probably wrestled for more promotions worldwide than anyone else in the past 20 years. In this relaxed interview, he talked about his early days in the AWA and his training with Brad Rheingans, and revealed some information about his former football days, about a totally different career that he was even then involved with, and told a terrific story of where the name Vader came from.

Vader, welcome. How are you?

I'm feeling fine. You just introduced an 11-time world champion on three different continents. In 1990, I simultaneously held three different world titles on three continents. That's a feat that no man has done. Now I know that Ric Flair's been 11-time or 12-time world champ, but he hasn't done it on three continents at the same time.

You were CWA world champion. You might have been New Japan and WCW.

And UWFI and UWA in Mexico.

Let's go back to your earliest days in wrestling. You were working for Verne Gagne and your first ring name was Baby Bull.

Ancient history. . . . That's right.

Then "Bull Power" Leon White. What led up to that? You played football at the University of Colorado, but how on earth did you get into this game?

Well, since you mentioned football, yes, I live today in Boulder, Colorado. I was recruited out of inner-city Los Angeles. A highly sought-after recruit. I got recruited from over 100 schools: Nebraska, UCLA, Notre Dame, FC, Washington, Washington State, and the list goes on and on. And I fell in love with the Rocky Mountains and the blue sky and no traffic, or none as compared with inner-city Los Angeles. And I came out here to Colorado and was a two-time All-American at the University of Colorado. Graduated as the captain of the team. Went on to the Los Angeles Rams in the first round. I was the 17th pick in the first round. My rookie season, we went to the Super Bowl and played Pittsburgh, at the ripe old age of 21. So yeah, it was a lot of fun and brings back some good ol' memories.

You lasted about four years with the Rams? Is that right?

Actually, I was only active three years and then I ruptured a patella tendon. But I had a five-year contract and I hung around for five and they paid me for five and it was a guaranteed, no-cut, no-trade contract coming out.

Nice deal.

Yeah, but [the accident] was against the Dallas Cowboys; it was on a sweep and I ruptured the patella tendon. Although the knee has come back and is strong as it's ever been, my ability to run a 4.8 second 40 yards at 325 pounds was gone.

Still, you had the ability to get into a different sport. Did you have any wrestling background at college?

Actually, somewhat. I wrestled in high school. I was in what we called the Watts Invitational, which was basically all of Los Angeles County, which encompasses about 600 high schools. People probably remember that [Watts] from the riots. I lived through that but my memory is not so good. But anyway, junior and senior year I won that. Although my background is not in amateur wrestling, it's more street fighting and, of course football.

When you were a kid did you watch wrestling?

To be honest, I never was a great wrestling fan. I watched football and some wrestling. I grew up on the Los Angeles Rams, they were my heroes and then becoming one later in life was a great thrill.

So cross us over here on how you became a pro wrestler.

Well, I finished my contract with the Rams and at this time I had a healthy knee and came back to Boulder. I had a degree in Business from the University of Colorado and I went out and obtained a real estate license. I'm a licensed broker in the state of Colorado. I built some town homes and homes and a car wash, and a few other things that I owned and operated, and to be very honest with you, I got bored stiff. I was gaining a lot of weight and becoming way out of shape and becoming a real businessman. But I decided to sell everything. The home, the car wash, condominiums, everything. I went off to Brad Rheingans' wrestling school in Minnesota.

Who did you train with besides Brad?

Brad was the coach and there were a few others who aren't in the business now, so aren't worth me mentioning.

But you got most of your training from Brad?

Initial training, yes sir.

And then it was off to the AWA?

Yep, the old AWA when they still meant something and still drew a crowd and were a good organization to work for.

Can you tell us about your first match?

I think it was so horrible that I've tuned it out.

Do you know who it was?

Don't know who it was or where it was.

When did you know that you were going to make it in this business?

I think when I was working for the AWA and got an offer to go to Europe. I was over there for two years.

Was this for Otto Wanz?

Yeah, for Otto Wanz, and I became CWA champion four times and we — me and my wife — had a lot of fun in Europe and drank a lot of beer and I wrestled a lot of big, tough men, and I learned how to wrestle.

So you got a lot of learning in Europe?

Yeah, we wrestled seven days a week for two years straight.

Was it a completely different style than the States?

Yeah, it's somewhat different, but wrestling is wrestling. I don't care where.

Then you met a guy named Inoki. There are some differences in New Japan. How did you get involved with him?

I got recruited, like in college, by Mr. and Mrs. Inoki. Masa Hatori came over and bought my contract from Otto Wanz, which is kind of unheard of today in wrestling. I got a nice contract and a bonus for leaving and it was like a trade in football.

Where did the name Vader come from?

Believe it or not, back in the 14th century, Japanese villages used to send their #1 warrior from each village separately, and whoever came back won the dispute. As the legend goes, Vader fought someone from another village for 72 hours straight on an island that they swam out to, and they died at each other's feet. Vader was an Emperor's warrior, he got that title. When Inoki saw me fight, he gave me the name and it stuck. So it has some meaning in Japan rather than the *Star Wars* thing.

At one point, Mr. Perfect was supposedly trying to bring you and Scorpio into the WWF. Do you think you could work the style of the WWF?

I think I'm one of the best athletes in the business today. Certainly one of the strongest. Bam Bam Bigelow is probably the only other big man who can compare with me. I've proven it everywhere. I've held five championships in Japan and I don't know another American who has done that except for Stan Hansen, and he was with Baba. I've shown my diversification with all the groups and know so many styles, so yes I can fit in anywhere.

Are you still with the UWFI?

Yes I am. They pay me to fight and I'll go.

Where did you learn to do the moonsault?

To be honest, it was the first time I did it in a match. It was the first time for someone over 400 pounds.

You did some damage to your wrists, though. How are they?

I broke my wrists, but they're 100%.

How's Harley Race feeling?

He ran into a wall, but is feeling better. . . .

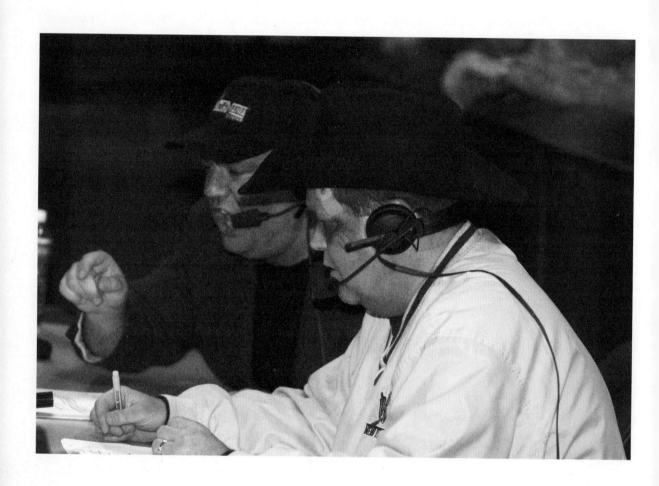

The Announcers

Long gone are the days when the excitable, but not very well informed, Dennis James would announce radio broadcasts of wrestling matches from New York, supposedly breaking carrots into the microphone from time to time, pretending it was the sound of someone's bones snapping. He certainly added some character, but things jumped to another level when Vince McMahon Jr. started announcing from ringside for his father's WWWF. Vince added both color and knowledge to the strange profession of calling the action and providing commentary to a sport that wasn't actually real.

In later years, Gorilla Monsoon retired from the ring but took up a seat at the mike, driving fans crazy by mispronouncing words and repeatedly accusing villains of not knowing the difference between a wristlock and a wristwatch. But there have also been the outspoken Jesse Ventura, the hilarious Bobby Heenan, and the infectious Joey Styles calling the shots or doing the color.

When interviewing announcers, it became clear that they were champing at the bit to tell the truth — to explain what went on behind the scenes and, to some extent, how challenging their job was. They provided some of our best interviews and most revealing moments.

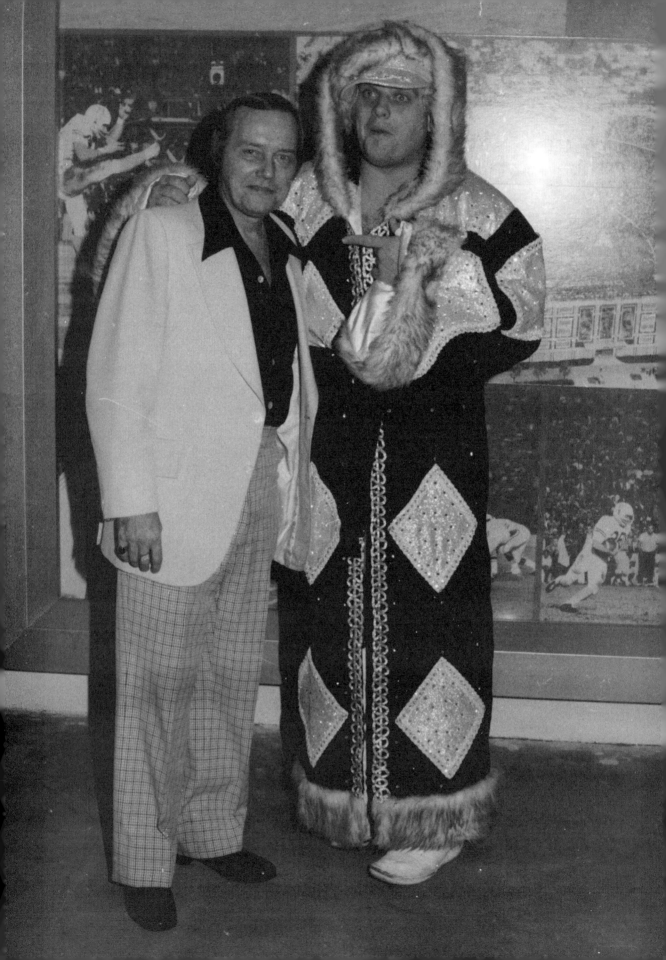

Gordon Solie
November 6, 1993

Solie will forever be remembered as the "Dean of Wrestling," the announcer who knew the name of pretty much every move ever put on a wrestler, even though he insisted on putting a French spin on the pronunciation of the word "suplex." He came on the show right at the end of his tenure with WCW, which was a time when he wasn't exactly thrilled with how the business was headed. But during his peak, he was one of the best. Anyone wanting to learn how to make an "OK" match sound great should pick up the Ultimate Ric Flair DVD Collection and listen to his call of the Flair vs. Race match from Starrcade. In this interview, he talked about his early days in the business and his respect for Lou Thesz, among others. He went into stories about his favorite wrestlers and matches, as well as his love for race cars and dogs. Of course, he also revealed some of his favorite trademark clichés.

Gordon, the earliest reference to your announcing career we could find was in Tampa in 1950. Are we on the ball?

Yeah, well I began ring announcing in 1950, some 43 years ago. Good lord that's a long time.

How did you get into such a strange profession? What was the beginning of it?

Well, I was a radio broadcaster and I used to have a 15-minute sports show. I would tell Cowboy Lutrell, who was a promoter in Tampa, that I'd be glad to have a wrestler or two on the show every week. So, lo and behold he called me one day and said his ring announcer quit and asked if I was interested. I said, "Yeah, what does it pay?" and he said, "$5 a night." And I was making 50 bucks a week, so that was a 10 percent increase, so I grabbed it.

And how long was it before you got into basically what you're doing now?

Well, of course television didn't really exist in Florida at that time. I began my television career in 1960. And that too was a long time ago, come to think of it.

So you started in Florida, but have also gone national. Has it been a bit difficult traveling all of this time?

Well, it's interesting. I have done a lot of traveling. Of course, then in 1969 or 1970, I started doing wrestling in Atlanta. Then of course, Turner put the station on the satellite in '72. So I was the first to go nationally and internationally, as a matter of fact.

Internationally. How far has your voice been heard?

All around the world.

Before we get more into wrestling, what is your connection with auto racing?

Oh, well, I've owned a couple of speedways, with partners of course. I also used to announce automobile daredevil shows and automobile racing. So, wrestling and racing kind of go together as far as I'm concerned.

Have you ever been behind the wheel?

Oh yeah. Not as a professional, however, purely as an amateur.

How about in the ring? Have you ever gotten in the ring with anyone?

Yes. I used to work out quite regularly with the late Eddie Graham and Coach John Heath. I felt to intelligently try to describe wrestling action, I ought to know or at least have a sample of what it feels like.

How does it feel?

I got hurt every time. Heath broke my nose one day. But I felt that it was well worthwhile because if I say, "That's putting a lot of pain on the deltoids," I'll know what that pain is and I felt that was very important.

Who were your favorite announcers to work with?

Buddy Colt was always a lot of fun to work with. The fellow that I work with now as a co-host, Larry Zbyszko, I enjoy. We do the syndicated wcw Pro for Turner Broadcasting. I used to enjoy working with a young lady named Barbara, that does our Spanish language shows. Roddy Piper was another one that I enjoyed working with.

There was that Don Muraco—Roddy Piper angle where Piper came to your aid from a Muraco attack during the glory days of Mid-Atlantic Wrestling.

Yeah, well it was Georgia Championship Wrestling. That was on Channel 17 and I think we were already on the satellite because shortly after, *Entertainment Tonight* came down to interview me about what was going on.

Who made the call to acknowledge that other leagues existed on the Wrestling News Network segment of the Power Hour during 1989?

Well, it wasn't necessarily my call. It was my suggestion and at that time, Joe Pedicino was producing the segment and Jim Herd was the Vice President of wrestling. We discussed it one day and said that Ford admits that General Motors exists, so why shouldn't we if we're going to have a news segment.

If we could go back and describe wrestlers from the golden years versus today, what's the difference?

Probably one of the classic living examples of superior catch-as-catch-can wrestling would be Lou Thesz. There was a difference in the way the sport was approached then than there is now. It's not wrestling's fault, necessarily, it's a social change as well. For example, when Lou Thesz would come to town he would be immaculately dressed in a business suit. I can remember calling Pete Norton, who was the Sports Editor for the *Tampa Tribune*, and say that Lou is coming into town next week and he'll be here for a week. That's what Lou would do — visit different territories to spend a week meeting the best challengers that were there. And Pete would say, "OK. Tell Lou to call me as soon as he gets in and I'll set-up a golf game at Polasea Golf & Country Club," which was the best club in town. On today's market, you don't see too many wrestlers with the exception of Lord Steven Regal, who are so immaculately dressed, if you will. But I think that's also part of our social structure. I can remember getting on an airplane and everyone was perfectly dressed. Now they get on with cut-offs and tank tops, you know.

You're still dressed well on television, aren't you? You're one of the best-dressed announcers around.

Well, my wife dresses me every morning.

There are a lot of problems facing the world of wrestling, and obviously we keep hearing rumors of this federal investigation of Vince McMahon and his company. How out-of-control is drug and steroid abuse, as far as you know, in the wrestling world today?

Well, obviously there has been some and I'm sure there is still some. I would not care to comment on the situation with Mr. McMahon. I don't feel that it would be fair of me to make any statement judgmentally at all. Obviously, some people became involved with steroids several years ago, but we must bear in mind that at that time it wasn't illegal. Consequently, a lot of young stars that I knew were taking steroids but nobody thought anything about it. It was a perfectly natural thing to bulk up. But then it became illegal and scientifically we began to discover the side effects of taking them, and frankly, unless they can eliminate the deadly side effects, I feel they should remain illegal.

Is there any way to keep them out of the business?

It's up to the individual. If a person is bent upon driving down the highway at 100 miles per hour and risking an accident, it's hard to control the individual.

What about re-educating the audience about going with smaller individuals rather than larger ones.

Well, the trend has been set with larger wrestlers, but who knows since wrestling is cyclical. There are some outstanding wrestlers currently in Mexico that are doing well. So you never know.

What promotion has been the most fun to broadcast for?

Well, Florida Championship Wrestling was a lot of fun. I always had a good time with Continental. Of course, Georgia Championship Wrestling. And I'll exclude wcw as I'm thoroughly enjoying myself right now.

Who has been the greatest wrestler you've ever seen and the greatest champ you've ever seen?

Eddie Graham was probably one of the greatest wrestlers that I've seen. As far as champions go, Lou Thesz and Dory Funk Jr. and Jack Brisco. And I wouldn't like to go into today's champs.

We won't talk about the Flairs?

Oh, Ric's great. He's a great athlete and has broken all records.

So why do you call it a "supley" and not a suplex?

Because that's how it originated in France, as "supley."

OK, we should listen to the Dean. Where, by the way, did you get that nickname?

I think it came out of a newspaper article where they likened me to Walter Cronkite. So, I called the paper and said that I was extremely flattered but I'm not sure how Walter would take it.

You never heard from Walter?

No, he never called me.

Are you a contemporary of Dennis James?

Dennis was ahead of me.

He was before you?

Yes, and I always thought that he was exactly what a wrestling commentator shouldn't be.

Should not be?

Right.

What were the basic differences between you two?

Oh, he'd take celery sticks and carrots and that kind of stuff and he'd put sound effects in. He didn't treat the sport with any kind of reverence whatsoever. I always thought Jack Brickhouse was the greatest wrestling announcer going.

He worked out of Chicago?

Yes.

Did you ever work together?

Yes. Jack was down a few years ago for wcw and we were doing segments for Chicago, and it was a real pleasure to sit down with the gentleman because he's outstanding in all ways. He's just an upstanding fellow all the way.

As far as today's announcers, what are your thoughts on Lance Russell?

He's great. We did the 900-line together in wcw and worked in Memphis back years ago.

There are so many parallels between the two of you that it's uncanny. What about Joe Pedicino?

Joe is an extremely likable guy. I thoroughly enjoyed working with him on the program *Pro Wrestling This Week* until we agreed to disagree, because he got to the point where he thought that he was bigger than the show, which wasn't the case. Physically he was pretty big, but. . . . I liked Joe, but professionally we drifted in separate directions and I might say, without any degree of satisfaction but as a degree of fact, that it wasn't too long after I left the show that it folded.

What about Jim Ross?

Oh, Jim's a great guy. I'm delighted for his new opportunity.

Do you still speak with him?

Well, not really. I don't feel that it's necessarily a good thing to speak to a rival, simply because, well you may slip and say something that you don't mean to say or what have you. So, no, we don't communicate at all.

How about Jesse Ventura?

Well, Jesse is just a dynamic personality. Mayor of Brooklyn Park, Minnesota.

Is he likable behind the scenes, though?

Oh, yeah, this is a very, very intelligent guy. I thoroughly enjoy discussing things with him because he is interested in so many things and he's done so many things.

And your newest cohort, "Mean" Gene Okerlund.

Gene, of course, I've known for 25 years. I frankly have to feel that Gene is probably one of the greatest commercial announcers that I've ever heard. He has a style and a delivery and a voice that really is superior.

What are your thoughts on Tony Schiavone?

Tony is a fine young guy, and one of the hardest working I've seen. He's excitable and carries that excitement over the airwaves as well.

What are your thoughts on Ted Turner?

A visionary. When I first went on the air at Channel 17 before the satellite I saw him more regularly. Ted is an extremely loyal person and wrestling has always done well for him and I have to admire him. He was years ahead of the networks with putting the channel on a satellite, CNN News, 24-hour news station. He's a trendsetter and I really admire him.

Will we ever see the return of 2-out-of-3 fall matches?

I sure hope so. I think championship matches should be 2-out-of-3 falls for one hour.

Why aren't they around anymore?

Well, we became an instant gratification country in the '80s and I think that's what it was. People may not have had the patience to watch the 2-out-of-3 falls.

Well hopefully they'll return. Some personal questions. We've heard that you're an animal lover. How many pets do you have?

When I lived on the lake at Lake Keystone, we always had six or seven or eight dogs and a cat, and of course at one time I had a black woolly monkey that used to put on a show for the people on the lake. Every Sunday I'd look out and there'd be about seven or eight boats just sitting offshore watching Monty as he performed, and he used to put on some great performances. He'd swing from tree to tree and all that kind of stuff. But since we moved over here — my wife became ill several years ago, so consequently we sold our place on the lake and moved into a small townhouse. Because of restrictions here, I gave my macaw to my son.

That was Quick-Draw Macaw?

Right. Then we have one dog left. She's 17 years old.

What other sports have you announced for?

I've done boxing. I've done baseball. I've never done basketball. I've never done hockey. And of course, I've done auto racing all my life. I thoroughly enjoy that. My prime has always been wrestling, though.

What are your favorite clichés?

"He's so quick, he's sudden!" "No question about it." "Now his face is a crimson mask."

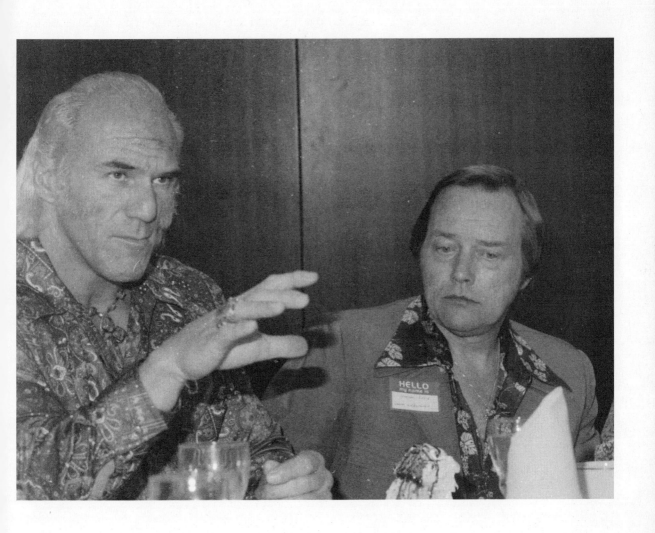

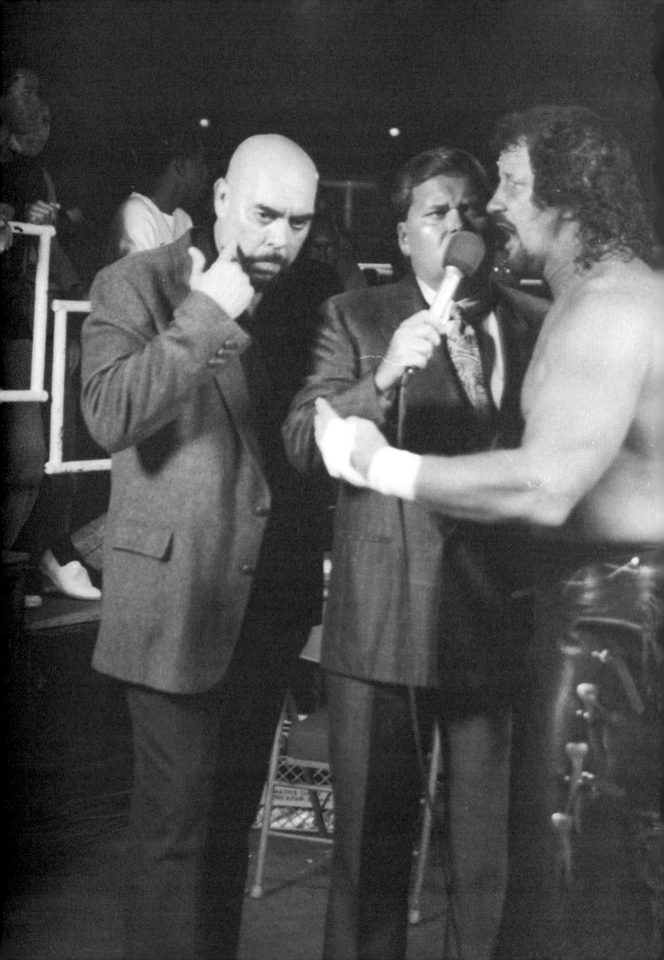

Jim Ross
June 11, 1994

Without question, Jim Ross is the greatest wrestling announcer of all time, with an incredible knowledge of performers' histories and an insightful understanding of the sport. In this interview, conducted shortly after he left the WWF due to differences with management, Ross spoke about Mid-South Wrestling, how he broke in and his relationship with Bill Watts, and the possibility of his becoming a football announcer if there were no wrestling offers. He also discussed being fired by Vince McMahon in the early 1990s and the details of that conversation. Ross let out some deeply personal information about his battle with Bell's palsy and his attempts to overcome the disease. Open to talk about anything, he was forthright about other announcers, his favorite performers, and some great stuff about working with Jesse Ventura.

Jim Ross, thanks so much for joining us. We've only had a few announcers on this show. We usually have the wrestlers themselves but the announcers definitely offer a different perspective. We all know who you are, but could you give us a very brief history of your broadcasting career?

Sure. I got started out in Oklahoma, working for Mid-South wrestling, which became the UWF. I actually got into wrestling in 1971 right out of college, working for Leroy McGuirk. He was the promoter there in Tulsa. I think I was probably a gopher for my first job. Mr. McGuirk was, unfortunately, blind, so I did a lot of driving for him. I also worked in PR and things of that nature. Then there was a guy doing interviews in Shreveport who called in sick and I stood in for him. Bill Watts was the boss and liked my potential and that's where my broadcasting started. But before I got into wrestling, I was at the college radio station working my way through school, doing basketball, football, and baseball games. I've done other things since wrestling, but wrestling is my first love and since that time in the early '70s, I've done wrestling to some degree until this past January. That's when I came down with Bell's palsy, which affects the facial nerves. I had paralysis on the left side of my face, I had terribly slurred speech.

That's not good for a broadcaster.

I couldn't sleep. I had to tape my eyes shut so they wouldn't blink. It was just a real bad situation, but I'm getting over it and I think by the 1st of July I should be as good as new.

Gordon Lightfoot had Bell's palsy a few years ago.

Oh, really?

Yeah, he had to stop performing for a while. So you're pretty much on the road to recovery?

Yeah, I hope to be fully recovered in 30 days. I've had it since January.

What offices are you looking at for broadcasting?

Well, the wrestling scene is pretty cut and dry. You either work for WWF, WCW, or regionals. I've had conversations with just about everyone, but quite frankly I'm looking at other options. I've had meetings with the Atlanta Falcons — in 1992 I broadcast one of their games and I did the Peach Bowl that year as well. So I may do some more football this year. I've talked to a couple of radio stations about doing some talk radio. I did a radio show on a big 50,000-watt station, WSB, for quite some time here in Atlanta. As a matter of fact I'm meeting with those folks next week. So I'm looking at other options outside of wrestling. I'd like to get back in wrestling. I'm trying to explore the whole gambit of things to create as many opportunities as possible, once I'm well enough to get back to work.

What's the difference for you in announcing for football and wrestling?

Well, as far as I'm concerned, the way I prepare, absolutely none. I prepare just as diligently for a wrestling match as far as looking at backgrounds and trying to trace the history of guys and find fun facts and background information as I did with football. When I was broadcasting football, my primary role was to host a 2 1/2 hour pre-game show on the Falcon radio network and to anchor the half time.

Two-and-a-half hour pre-game?

Yeah, and we did it live from the stadium that we were playing in. So during the week, I'd go to practice and interview the players and have taped interviews and I'd have a lot of live interviews. We'd have Paul Tagliabue and Hank Stram and Kenny Stabler and people of that nature. I really didn't prepare any differently. I tried to read about as much as I could about the game that I was going to broadcast or the matches that I was going to do. I tried to come up with info that would be interesting for the fans and I kind of role-played. I always considered myself a fan of wrestling. And I love the business. And football's the same thing. That was a passionate thing that I was interested in as well. So, heck, I didn't prepare any differently. It was a matter of doing a lot of research and coming to the broadcast ready to do a good job.

Were you as much as an excitable boy doing football as you are doing wrestling?

Absolutely. Absolutely.

How serious have talks gone with World Championship Wrestling and Eric Bischoff as far as returning to that organization?

We've had some very pleasant conversations. Eric and I had about three conversations regarding my situation and the fact that there might be an opportunity somewhere down the road to come back to WCW. I think I would term the talks as "positive" and "cordial." Nothing is etched in stone and there has been no job offer. There has been some good dialogue and I think the door might be open therefore somewhere down the line. I think the thing is, I'm not trying to get the cart before the horse as they say. I need to get well. Once the paralysis is completely gone, then I'm going to get very aggressive and find something in wrestling or broadcasting in general. The talks have been very pleasant. We've got a lot in common. We worked together there when I was in wcw. I understand some of the problems there and the challenges he's faced with as the executive producer. So, we've had some good conversations that I'd term "positive" and "congenial." They've not offered me a job but they're nice enough to talk with me about the possibility.

There apparently seems to be an on-air problem between you and Jesse Ventura. Where does this whole thing stem from?

Well, a lot of that was blown out of proportion to a certain extent. I was in a very unique situation right as I was leaving wcw and as much as I was the V.P. of Broadcasting, and part of my area was that I was in charge of the announcing talent. Jesse had a problem, rather Bill Watts had a problem with Jesse. I don't think Jesse had a problem with Watts. But because Watts had whatever animosity toward Jesse, it was basically vented back through me. When Jesse did something that Bill didn't like, Bill would come to me and say, "Your guy's messing up" or "Your guy's this and that." And it was a darned-if-you-do, darned-if-you-don't situation. I felt like at times that Jesse didn't prepare as diligently as I thought that he should. And I may have been wrong with that analogy. He's a very busy guy, obviously with his own radio program going and he's doing movies and then mayor of Brooklyn Park, Minnesota, and all that stuff. I guess because of my workaholic nature and the fact that when I was working at wcw, I was really consumed with the business and with the product. Jesse may have had a healthier outlook on it than I did. He had a lot of diverse interests going and I didn't really have that. I had wrestling and I worked in a little football and talk radio. But basically speaking, I may have been wrong in my analogy that Jesse didn't prepare as diligently as we felt like he should. But I think probably part of the problem, and I don't want to pass the buck here, it's not like I'm wimping out, but I think that Watts created a wedge there between himself and a lot of people and if you were the conduit between Watts and that particular individual, then obviously you were going to get some of that steam on you, too.

Now if you were to go back to World Championship Wrestling today, would there be an on-air feud between you and Jesse?

Absolutely not. I know that I'm more professional than that. And I know that Jesse's more professional than that. We have some philosophical disagreements. I don't agree with his views in politics, but that doesn't mean that he's wrong. I don't agree with his philosophies on gun control or some of these types of things. We have a difference of opinion there and oftentimes when the media gets wind of two guys working together having a difference of opinion on certain issues, it makes good reading and listening. Jesse's said some things on some broadcasts in my direction that I thought didn't need to be said or were out of place. In retaliation, I said some things on Radio WWF that were childish, so looking back on the whole situation, it was a regrettable ordeal. But I don't think at all if the opportunity ever presented itself to go back to WCW that there'd be a problem. Our goal and our job is to go out there and broadcast to the best of our ability and convey what we are seeing and try to be as prepared and spontaneous and exciting as possible.

Looking back over your whole career, is there any one announcer who you think you really clicked with? Really felt good working with?

Well, I've been real fortunate, guys that I've had some real good partners over the years. My first job was as a play-by-play announcer. I worked with Leroy McGuirk, 'cause I mentioned that he was blind, and the guys that follow wrestling know that Leroy got blinded in the early '50s during the height of his wrestling career. So Leroy was my color analyst.

You're kidding.

No, absolutely. So in order for me to interact and interface with him, I had to be very descriptive. I had to tell a very vivid story and it was almost theater of the mind. I had to be more graphic, I had to be more descriptive, I had to be more exact in how I was calling the matches so that Leroy could get involved in the darned thing. So that was an interesting early education. I worked with a lot of guys I really liked working with. Probably my favorite partner that I've worked with over my career that I felt most comfortable with was Bobby Heenan. It's a subjective thing as far as the viewers are concerned, but I felt like from my standpoint that I was most comfortable working with him. We meshed well on a personality basis. I think he's one of the most quick-witted, one of the most naturally funny guys that I've ever been around. But oftentimes, because he is so funny and you sometimes have a smile on your face, sometimes his knowledge of the business is overlooked. He's got a great knowledge of the business because of all the years in it. He's a lot more astute than sometimes he's given credit for. I like working with Jim Cornette. I thought Jim Cornette was a very good analyst. Paul E. Dangerously was at times extremely good, especially when he stayed focused on the matches. He has a great mind — very, very intelligent.

I noticed you just said at times he was focused.

Well, I think at first you've got a young guy who hadn't done it before and you get in the heat of battle sometimes on a live show, I mean we all have the potential to digress. I've done it many, many times and I have a lot of experience. I think it's a natural thing, it's not a slam on Paul. It's just a fact that when I first started broadcasting pay-per-views and Clashes with him, he was a very young kid, in his early 20s and didn't have a wealth of experience in that particular role. But his spontaneity, his wit, his insight and intelligence certainly were very, very prevalent. Like any other young broadcaster, sometimes you have to be reined in to keep your focus on what you're seeing, to not be talking about things that you're not seeing. It's very confusing when you're talking about something entirely different than what the viewer is watching on the screen.

Have you ever, even for a moment, been at a total loss for words — either because something maybe really horrible happened or something so funny occurred that you lost control?

I never really lost control from a comical standpoint because I think in the early days when I first got started, everything was taken so seriously in the territory that I was in, out in Mid-South. It was kind of a blood and guts, in-your-face type of wrestling territory. And because of the mindset of the wrestlers at the time, where they were making money on what they drew, it was imperative for their issues to be clearly established and clearly defined and communicated to the viewers, so that would hopefully translate into ticket sales for them. I would have had a very short career if I had not taken my job very, very seriously. So, I don't think I've ever broken up. I've laughed afterwards and I wanted to laugh probably when I saw some things, but I really tried to bite my tongue and I didn't go that far. I have been to matches where, like for example some matches with Cactus Jack where he executed some maneuvers that were completely out of the blue, completely spontaneous that quite frankly I didn't know how to call.

What was the reason for you leaving the World Wrestling Federation a couple of months ago?

Well, when I went to the WWF after having several talks with Vince McMahon, it was made clear to me that he wanted me to be just as I was. He didn't want to change me, because I wasn't going to change my persona or my character, shall we say. I was concerned about that because I felt that, after being in broadcasting all these years, that all of a sudden to be a completely different individual and the whole nine yards . . . well, I just didn't understand why that would need to be. And he agreed with me at that point in time. But somewhere during the year, around the fall of last year, the word came to me that he wanted me to become a cowboy and wear a hat on the air and the string tie and the cowboy jacket and boots and all this other stuff. I guess he thought that every Oklahoman dresses that way. And that's not true. So, I resisted that. And one thing you learn, I mean Vince is the boss. The buck stops with him. He makes the decisions. If you choose not to do what he wants you to do, then he'll make other arrangements for you. And that's his prerogative as the boss. I mean, that's anybody's prerogative. If your Program Director at your station wants to do something else, well that's what he's going to do.

Was it an amicable split though, from Vince?

For the most part, yes. I try not to live my life in such a negative vacuum, looking at the glass half-empty instead of half-full. For the most part, it was amicable. A lot of his people were very, very supportive and were very saddened to see me leave. But the way that it all came down I felt like it was dehumanizing. That was my opinion of it. Now, I was sick in bed, I was having these migraine-like headaches. Like I said, I was having to tape my eyes shut to sleep. It was embarrassing. My face was disfigured and I didn't want anything to enhance that. Maybe that's why my career may be in radio. But be that as it may, my face was disfigured and I had a lot of problems with my mouth because I was drooling and I had to carry Kleenex in my hand. It was real embarrassing and I didn't want to be seen in that mode. And I was called on February 10th to come in and continue conversations on me staying with the WWF. I had several meetings with their people about my contract being extended, so I thought it was a continuation of those talks. I'll never forget it for several reasons. There was a horrible snowstorm that day, just a terrible snowstorm. As a matter of fact, they closed down Madison Square Garden; the public transportation in Stamford was suspended because of the snow. I lived 12 miles from the wrestling office and I drove and it took me an hour to get there. And I got there and the meeting lasted between five and ten minutes. He just said that he's decided to go in a different direction with his announce team and "You're not going to be in my plans; so, consequently, I'm not going to renew your contract."

So you got a little severance pay there?

Yeah, you know, I got a couple months severance and went about my business.

Quick question before we get into real specifics. You mentioned when you were a WCW vice president you had other work to do besides announcing. What was that?

I was in charge of the production department. The production people reported to me. I was managing the hotline, plus providing talent on Saturdays on the hotline. I was writing a monthly column for the magazine. And I was doing the Clashes and pay-per-views and doing two hours of weekly television.

So you kept busy?

Yeah, I kept pretty busy. I think I earned my keep, as far as that's concerned. But I think that was part of my downfall as far as I accepted too much on my plate. There's a fine line between ambition and stupidity. I think my decisions bordered on stupidity. I should have backed away from some of the responsibility, but you know, you hate not to take responsibility when it's offered to you. You want to help the company and make it get better and, given the opportunity, I took advantage of the situation. At the time I thought it was the right thing to do. Hindsight's always 20/20 as we know, and if I had to do it all over again, I would've declined some of the responsibilities. You know I came to wcw as a play-by-play guy. As the old cliché goes, that's what brought me to the dance. And I would rather, if I had to do it all over again, I would rather be just a talent, an on-air talent, and/or a producer. Those are my first loves. The other things were assigned to me and again, I should've probably said no. I didn't. And it was a problem in that respect. I just took too much on and I didn't handle it very well. I really wish that I had rethought that whole situation and I didn't. At the time I thought that I was making the right call.

Did you learn how to say no by the time you went to the WWF or did the same thing happen there?

Well, I probably learned to say no a little bit, but it's very difficult to say no to Vince.

Well, what were your responsibilities there?

I produced and formatted Mania and All-American TV shows, I hosted Challenge, I did International Superstars on-air, I worked on the hotline, I launched Radio WWF, and I did voice-overs for Coliseum home video. I stayed busy there, too. From the time the radio show launched in August or July or whenever that was, until I got sick, I worked six days every week. The guys listening to the radio are saying, "What's the big deal? I worked that many hours and my dad's worked that many hours his whole life." So, I'm not crying on anyone's shoulder, but in broadcasting, it's very difficult to maintain quality and be able to prepare and plan with that type of schedule, with that many diverse products that you're responsible for. I was very busy there as well. It's a general consensus within the business that there's not an over-abundance of people with product knowledge that can translate that to a television product or radio product or what have you. It's not a matter of that I was so talented, it's just a matter of there's not that many talented people that had wrestling expertise combined with broadcasting background in the business right now. There's a big void there.

Jim, you mentioned Radio WWF. Can you give us some background to what happened with Randy Savage and Hulk Hogan with the words exchanged [where Savage went on a semi-shoot diatribe on Hogan about Liz, among other stuff]?

Well, the week that that occurred, I was in Las Vegas getting married. When I came back from Vegas with my new bride — we got back on Saturday, Saturday morning — the show had already been formatted for that night. Vince had decided that he wanted the show to be real "cutting edge" was his exact term. So he said that Randy was going to be my guest and he wanted Randy to be real cutting edge and all you had to was just follow him.

So it was Vince's idea?

Absolutely. It wasn't Randy Savage's idea, and it sure wasn't my idea.

So these weren't legitimate feelings from Randy Savage, but planned by Vince McMahon is what you're saying?

Well, McMahon was the catalyst who wanted to expose that part of history. But when Randy was given the opportunity to speak, it came from his gut. That's how he felt at the time. I was not in the WWF at the time when all that stuff went down. I was on the outside looking in. I read about it, I heard about it but I wasn't there to know about the whole scenario of what happened and behind-the-scenes of the personal side of the Macho Man and the Hulkster. That was something that I'd only heard from secondhand information or hearsay. But Randy spoke from the heart — he has some strong, strong feelings on the matter, but it was Vince's idea to bring it out. All of us there were looking with wide-eyed amazement as to what was going down because we knew we were into something that was going to be very controversial. . . .

And personal.

So very personal it probably didn't have a place on a public forum, quite frankly. Both guys deserved to tell the story if it was going to be told at all. It was unfortunate that Hulk did not get the chance to come back with a rebuttal, his side of the issue. It was a real uncomfortable situation. I regret being a part of it. It was not a highlight of my career in the WWF, I can tell you that.

Jim, we're fast running out of time, so here's the most important question of this interview. Are we ever going to see a Jim Ross wrestling doll?

I don't think there's any demand for a little fat Caucasian doll. I'm doing fine, I have an offer to the fans who want to write and I'm responding to their mail via audiotape. I always try to answer fan mail, and this is a form of a customized hotline where people write me and send me fifteen bucks and I'm going to respond to them honestly, openly, and give them a forum to vent their own frustrations or ask questions or whatever. That's what I'm doing here today. I'm doing lots of recordings and things are working out real well. I think good things are going to happen to us if we have the right mind-set.

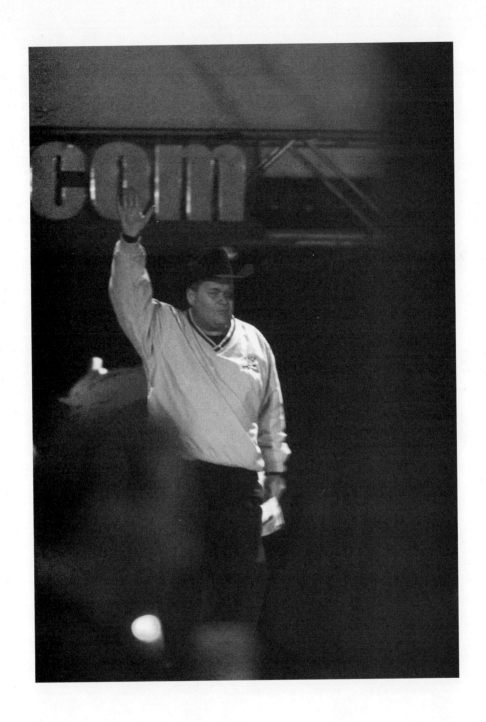

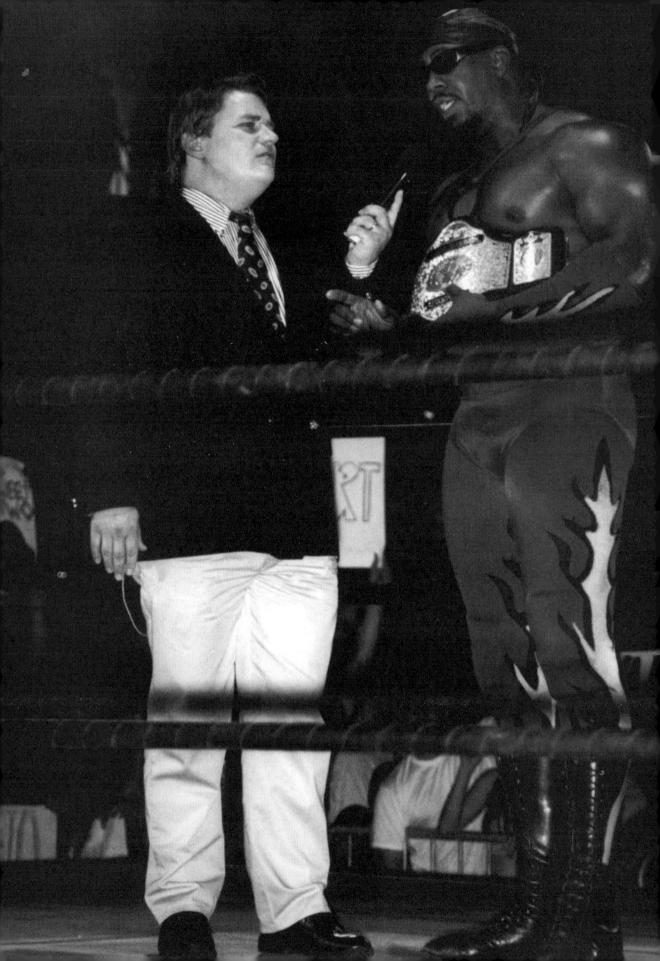

Tony Schiavone
May 24, 1995

During the 1980s, Schiavone was one of the top wrestling announcers around, and was great even when he had the tough challenge of hosting the TBS wrestling shows with David Crockett, who was arguably the worst color commentator in wrestling at the time. He went on to work for Turner at WCW until the late-1980s, when he decided after a contract dispute with boss Jim Herd that it was time to head north for the WWF. In this rare interview, he talked about how he broke into the business, the challenges and difficulties of the job, who he admired most in wrestling, why he really left WCW, why he left the WWF, and even predicted the death of Cactus Jack on a live TV broadcast due to his wild style.

Tony Schiavone, where are we talking to you from today?

Well, I'm in Sioux Park, north of Atlanta. I'm on duty as a baseball coach today. I'm on the board as well, so my whole day will be from 10 a.m.–9 p.m.

So you're a man that never rests?

Except for Saturdays from 6–8 that I broadcast wcw Saturday Night.

The number one burning question from our listeners is what does your last name mean?

Okay, that's a real last name. My family, my father's family settled — they're an Italian family and I'm a second-generation American — in Rosetta, Bangor, Pennsylvania, which is north of Allentown. The name is Shavone (rhymes with sha-phone), the proper pronunciation. My relatives call it Shavone. But my father was transferred from the Lehigh Valley area in Pennsylvania down to Virginia and for some reason, people in the south mispronounced it and called it Schiavone. And it stuck. My father is kind of a laid-back Italian anyway, and didn't want to change it. So for all I know, my father's family, and of course my children now, we're the only Schiavones in the entire United States.

Do you know what it means in Italian?

I think it means "used to be a baseball announcer, now wrestling announcer to the day he dies." I think that's the proper . . .

Let's get personal now. How old are you?

I'm 36.

And what did you want to be when you grew up?

From when I could remember, I wanted to be a baseball announcer. It started probably in the 4th grade.

And you were doing that some time ago?

Yeah, as a matter of fact, when I graduated from college in 1980, I sent my tape to many minor league teams and was hired by the Greensboro team.

By a man named Jim Crockett?

Actually, Jim Crockett came a little bit later.

Go ahead. You tell the story.

OK. Greensboro team, a guy named Tom Romanesco, who went on to work in the Padres minor league system and now he's a scout for the Mets, they hired me to do the Greensboro Hornet games in 1981 and that was a Class A Yankee farm club. A year later, I was hired by the Crockett family to do the Charlotte O's games. And I spent four years doing those games. They were Baltimore's Double-A affiliate. So I was a minor league radio announcer for five years and of course, halfway through I started doing wrestling part time and, well, here I am.

Well you ended up having one of the strangest jobs in the world. Do you agree?

Yeah, not many people do it, thank goodness. It helps the longevity of the job.

How did the switch happen?

Well, the switch happened in 1983 at the very first Starrcade. Ric Flair was going to wrestle Harley Race for the NWA world heavyweight title, and they needed someone to go to Ric Flair's home and do an interview with Ric Flair. I'd always told the Crocketts, "I can announce wrestling. Heck, anybody can."

Wrong. You're wrong.

Well, I know. That's what an announcer on the way up and wanting to do well says. You portray this confidence. So they told me to go to his house and do the interview and I was like scared to death. I never had met him before, and I knew of him. So anyway, I went to his house to do the interview and they liked it. This was at the end of 1983, and they had me do some part-time things and by '84 it was part-time wrestling, full-time baseball. And I was getting more money doing wrestling parttime than I was baseball fulltime. So I said, my family's getting larger, so I went with wrestling. I went with the money.

How big is your family?

I have five children.

Then we hope you make good money with these guys.

Yeah, it's a good living. It's a good living and it's a — I'm not going to say it's a great job; the announcing part on TV's a great job, but, you know I have to work with formatting the shows and have to live and die with the ratings, so it's a high-pressure office job during the day. So it has its wear and tear.

Before we get into that, when you were getting into it full time, were you listening to the other guys out there like Vince and like Boyd Pierce? Were there any mentors out there for you?

Yeah. I think the person that I listened to was Bob Caudle. I grew up in the Carolinas and Virginias and I knew Bob, and I remember the chance that I got to announce with Bob for the first time. It was a big moment for me.

Were you watching as a kid?

Not really as a kid. I started watching while I was in college in the late '70s. I worked part time, and on Saturdays I'd take my lunch break at my home and Mid-Atlantic Championship Wrestling would be on, so it was probably in the late '70s when I started watching and became a big fan.

There's less travel now due to more studio work. Is life generally easier in the business now?

No, it's not. I don't travel as much as I used to, but I still have office work. And I hate office work. I really do. I put a lot of time into it. I work long days.

You work as a producer?

Yeah, I work as a producer, which means I work with the production company in formatting all the shows.

Directly with Mr. Bischoff?

Yeah. Right under Mr. Bischoff.

We'll get to him in a moment. You seem, career wise, to be following Ric Flair around a little bit. NWA, WWF, WCW — back and forth, back and forth. What were the circumstances for you going to the different federations?

I'm going to be very honest with you. I was with the Crocketts and the Crocketts, so to speak, were going belly up. Vince, of course, went nationwide and everyone had problems. They [the Crocketts] were being purchased by Turner Broadcasting. That was the end of 1988. Turner Broadcasting, in the process of buying this company, hired Jim Herd to run the company. Jim Herd had a meeting with me in late 1988 and told me that I'd be making the same amount of money as Jim Ross and told me that I'd be on his television shows. Well, first of all, it didn't matter how much money I made compared to Jim Ross. But the fact was that I found out later that Ross was going to make $50,000 more than me a year. The fact that he did not tell me the truth, well, it didn't upset me. I just wondered, you know, about this guy.

This was Herd you're talking about?

This was Jim Herd. Anyway, about the same time — I wasn't under a contract — I got a call from Vince McMahon, and I went to work for him in '89. Then after a year with Vince McMahon — and let me tell you it was a great year. I know there's been a lot of bad things happening to him, but I had a tremendous year. He was good to me and good to my family. And I think a lot of him as a matter of fact.

A lot of people do.

So I got a call back from the Turner people, Jim Herd and Jim Barnett. They offered me a job, they also offered, after I would fulfill my contract, to do all they could to get me into baseball, which is what I always wanted to do. So I went back to work for him and I had some rocky years and I realized that maybe I misjudged Jim Herd. He was a pretty good guy. But I've been working here since 1990. My contract ended in 1993 and I was renewed for three more years. Nothing really came about with baseball, but that's OK.

Were there any really major differences in the working environment between Vince and Turner?

Oh, yeah. For instance, with Turner, you are a small fish in a big pond, as far as wrestling is concerned. There is not enough. I've often felt this, I've felt that sometimes it feels like we're fighting a losing battle. And that's when I'm depressed and get negative about it. Because with Vince, that's his only thing, except for the time he spent on bodybuilding. All of his efforts and time were spent on wrestling. As a matter of fact, when I gave my resignation, he told me that he'll always do better in the wrestling business than Ted Turner because wrestling "Is all I do." And he had a pretty valid point there, although we're starting to make some headway with wcw. But we had a bigger staff and more time to do editing on the shows up there. Of course I was up there at a time when he had a lot of money, and things were going well. Now things have changed. My office job was a producer of Coliseum Home Videos. And I had a secretary and an assistant! And I was a videocassette producer. Here I am a Supervising Producer and I don't have either one. You had more numbers, he had more people, it was a bigger operation and I came down here and when I came back in 1990 to be very honest, I wanted to kill myself. I thought, "Gosh, what have I done?" But it's panned out.

So how has Eric Bischoff changed the TV product in the past year?

Well, first of all, he worked out a deal with Disney. And he got us going to Disney and it's been a great relationship for us. Also he's probably allowed people within the company to make decisions on their own. That was never the case with Jim Herd. He made every final decision. With Bill Watts, he made every final decision. Therefore, it was one man. Eric has let people under him, who are in charge of different facets of the corporation, make the decisions, do things. If nothing else, he's made the working atmosphere tremendous. Eric's forte is deals. He's the one that constructed the deal with Disney. He just recently got us back on track with New Japan Pro Wrestling. He just recently went to Sweden and got a deal there. So he has been the man to do that for us. I think he's a great guy to work for, too.

We'd like you to talk about the differences and styles with your broadcast partners. Do you work bits out in advance or are they ad-libbed?

No, it's all ad-libbed. I've been very fortunate to have guys like Jesse, the funniest guy in show business, and now Bobby "The Brain" Heenan. We discuss before we go on the air what we have to promote. In other words, if Slamboree is coming up, we have to promote what is coming up for Slamboree, the matches and so forth. We never discuss what he's going to say and what I'm going to say.

You seemed pretty shocked every once in a while.

Yeah, he's great. He's absolutely great to work with.

Are they all fun? Is there anybody that you don't like working with?

No. I like working with everyone, as a matter of fact.

And you'd be a good politician, too.

Yeah.

Whose wrestling work do you really admire?

Well, I admire Flair's. I always have because he and I have been very close friends, and he's the greatest one, but to be very honest with you, the man that I admire most in this sport is Hulk Hogan. I came from the Crocketts and went to work there in 1989. And I never in my life, and never in my life since then — maybe with the exception of Starrcade last year, when Flair walked into the Charlotte Independence Arena — I've never seen a crowd reaction for anybody like Hulk Hogan. Now they can say that Hulk Hogan is, in terms of some of your fans, not the greatest worker . . .

He's not the greatest worker.

Yes he is. Because, who's been the biggest star in our sport? It's him.

You're absolutely right. Let's rephrase my question. What about in-ring ability?

OK, in-ring ability. It's Flair, it's Steamboat, and to me you can't get any better than Dustin Rhodes right now.

Yeah, boy he takes some chances.

He really is a natural. He really is.

What do you think the future is for performers like Cactus Jack? Man, he's so reckless.

Well, I've told Cactus Jack this, but I think we're going to see the death of Cactus Jack on pay-per-view. It's going to make for good TV. And I'll call it as best I can. I don't know why he does things like this.

Your thoughts on Sid Vicious?

I have nothing to say, with the exception that if I had those looks and talent, I'd still be in the business.

OK. Enough said. You mentioned that you're a close friend of Flair's. Weren't you friends with Nikita Koloff?

Yeah, Nikita and I were very good friends.

Anybody else that you're close to in the business?

Yeah, if I had to say that I had a best friend in the business, Eric Bischoff would be one, but for longevity, I'd say Arn Anderson has been my closest friend.

We wish we could see a little bit more of him.

The thing about Arn Anderson is, and you only see one side of him — the vicious, very determined athlete. But he is without a doubt the funniest man I ever met in my entire life and that includes Bobby "The Brain" Heenan. Arn Anderson could make it as a stand-up comedian. And you don't see that. He just kills us.

Alright, can you share any thoughts on today's wrestling fans? What do you see out there when you're so close to them all?

Well, I see two levels. Level number one is wrestling fans who appreciate what we do, who love the sport for what it is, who have been with it for a long time. Regardless of what you think of the sport, it's been a force in the entertainment world for years. But to be very honest with you, I have some sort of animosity toward fans who criticize the direction that we sometimes take. Let me give you an example. We were in Chicago and during some of the matches and some of the endings of some of the matches, there was a sign held up. It said, "Who booked that?" Now I'm saying that if I was just an announcer, that wouldn't bother me. But I'm in the office every day and I would give any fan this challenge: I would pay any fan whatever money they wanted to come in and sit down and try to help us book something for one week. In a week's time, they would hang themselves in the shower. There are so many variables that you wouldn't believe. This guy doesn't want to go there and this guy can't go here and this guy's contract says he needs an off day after he comes back from such and such a place. It's not as easy as people may seem to think. And now that we're with Disney, we have to satisfy that "Main Event on TV" thing, which drives me crazy. And so, all of a sudden all of your matches have already been seen on TV, what else do you have to show them? It's a very difficult business and there seems to be a lot of fans on the outside that would like to rag us and our decisions about putting this man against this man. And to be very honest with you, we spend hours and overnight sessions on doing this and we just don't throw names against the wall to see who sticks.

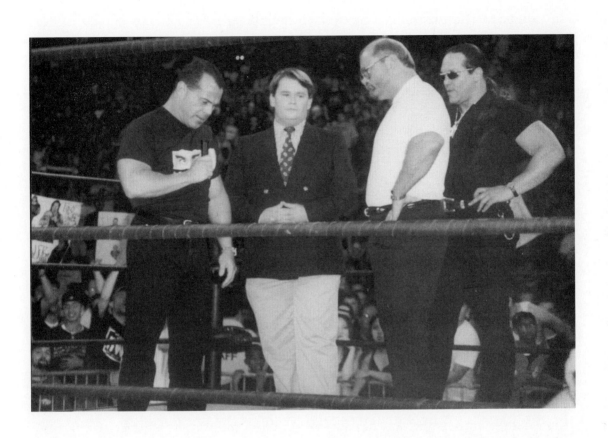

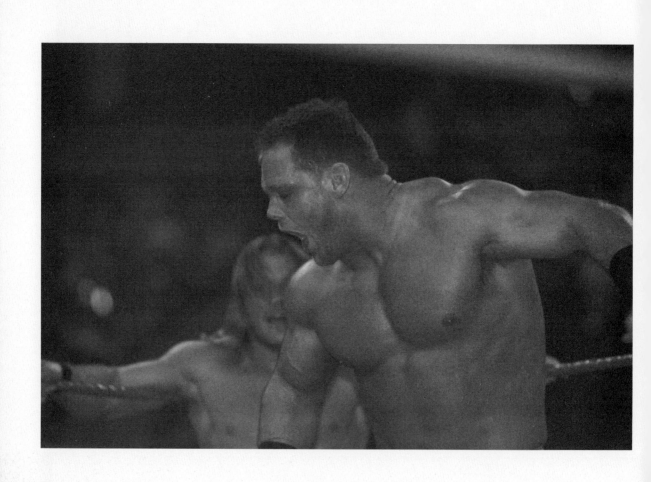

The Wrestlers Part 3:
December 1995–January 1997

The show's final year was fabulous, both in the studio, and in the world of wrestling. Remarkable strides were being made, especially late in 1996, as far as getting fans back in the arenas. Even though wcw was still outscoring the wwf in the weekly tv wars, wwf was definitely out of its doldrums. Business was looking good, and over the next couple of years, Vince McMahon would once again be leading the pack.

It was thrilling for us to find that someone as protective of the business as Bruno Sammartino had always been, turned out to be an open book once we got him on the phone. Chris Benoit was one of our toughest interviews, simply because he hadn't done many of them, but he and the other wrestlers who had been coming up through the rough-and-tumble ecw ended up being some of our most interesting guests. They all knew that they were part of a group that was making history by literally changing the scene with a different style of wrestling. Some of the best fun we had was during one of the show's last interviews, with Sandman, who we actually woke up from a deep sleep and put on the air.

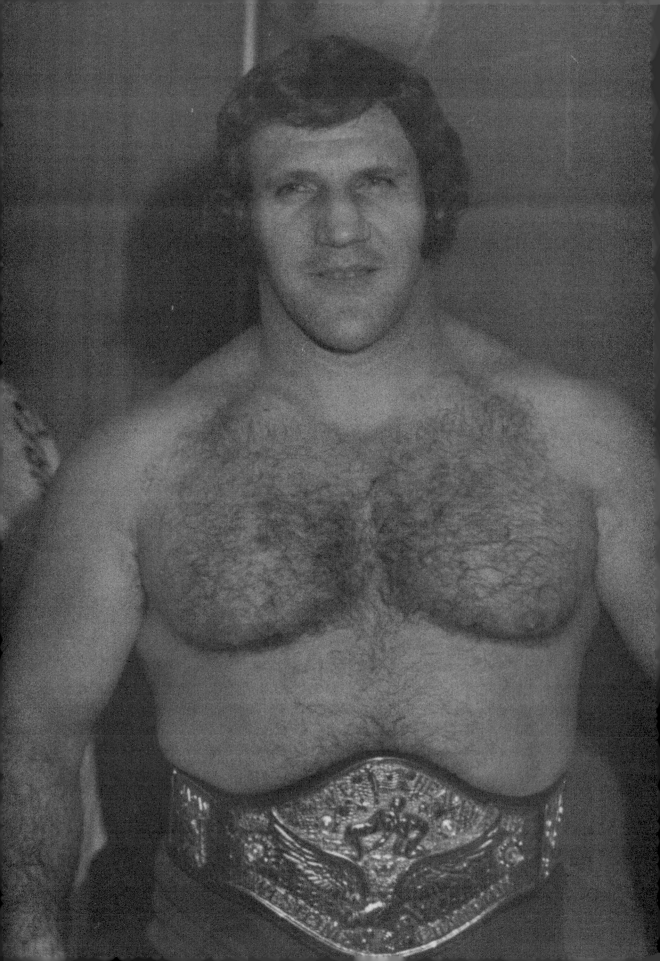

Bruno Sammartino
December 2, 1995

Bruno had already been out of the business as an active wrestler for about 14 years when he came on the show. But he was never at a loss for words as far as his opinions of the business — which at that point he didn't have a lot of respect for. From the time he first held the heavyweight belt in the WWF in 1963 (at one point in the '60s and '70s he wore it for close to an eight-year stretch) he was a well-respected champ and an idol of the blue-collar crowd. A couple of major points in his career included having his neck broken in a 1976 match with Stan Hansen, and a huge feud with his protégé, Larry Zbyszko, in 1980. Bruno was a bit skeptical about coming on the show at first — he wasn't booked through any organization; we called him at home to ask for the interview — but after a long phone chat the day before the broadcast, he decided that both we and the show were valid. He really seemed to enjoy himself on the air.

Mr. Sammartino, it's a great, great honor to have you on. Do you have any specific memories of Boston?

I really did love Boston. I had some great matches there. I don't know how many times I fought Kowalski in Boston. But each time for me it was quite a thing, because I had the utmost respect for that man. He was one of the best-conditioned wrestlers that I've ever known. This guy didn't know what getting tired meant. So it was a great challenge for me because I prided myself to be in good shape all the time. I wrestled Kowalski in Boston a number of times, and each time, for me, it was a memorable bout. I don't think I ever had what a fan might call a boring match. And in Boston the fans were absolutely fantastic. When I'd go into the ring, the ovations were great. But even afterward, after the matches, I would go to the North End — I think it was a place called Cantina Taviana — the owner came from Europe, too. He'd keep the place open and it was just great. I came to Boston once a month for many, many years. I had other great bouts there, too. I remember Tanaka, one time, and a cage match with Stan Hansen after I came back from my broken neck. I wrestled Ivan Koloff there, Prince Maivia one time. One time Monsoon and I broke the ring and they had to hold up the whole show for a couple of hours 'til they were able to repair it.

There was a George "the Animal" Steele match involving a lot of tables.

George was known for that sort of thing.

And a great fight against Don Leo Jonathan at the Boston Garden.

Yeah, that's another guy that I was quite impressed with. He was extremely agile for a guy who was 6'6", 320 pounds. He was very strong, very agile — quite an amazing guy.

Do you recall fighting at Fenway Park?

Yeah, I remember a big fight with Kowalski at Fenway.

Was working outdoors instead of in an arena a very different experience for you?

Well, I did more of that than you would think. Here in Pittsburgh, we had Forbes Field before they built the new stadium. And we used to wrestle there every summer. In New York, we did Shea Stadium a couple of times. In Montreal we used to wrestle outdoors and in Toronto and San Francisco we wrestled in the ballpark. So it wasn't such a rare thing.

What was your favorite arena or territory to wrestle in?

Well, I told you how much I loved Boston, and I mean it, but Madison Square Garden, I liked a lot. Madison Square Garden, first of all, had the name and the reputation. And to headline there, you always got a bit more notoriety as far as the papers and what have you. The place was always jam-packed and I was fortunate because the fans received me very well. So when you had 22,000 people indoors like that, and they were that vocal, it was quite an experience. I would say that was number one. And number two probably was the Boston Garden.

You once said one of your favorite fights was a good-guy-versus-good-guy against Pedro Morales. Does that still stick out in your mind?

Yeah. Promoters, for whatever reason, never wanted a match with two good guys because they would not go out there and be rough with one another. But I believed the fans would really appreciate if they put in two guys like that, and hopefully they would have a great match. So when the opportunity came with Pedro Morales, we went for one hour and 17 minutes of pure, clean, scientific wrestling. It seemed to me that the fans really loved it; we gave them nothing but action for all that time. And it was very satisfying for me because I didn't have too many opportunities to have that kind of match.

There were so many different styles, even before your time. You just mentioned a scientific match. You did scientific wrestling really well, but you could also get into the brawling aspect of it. Was there ever a point where you wanted to just do scientific?

As far as I was concerned, I didn't have the choice to do what I wanted to do. What I mean by that is that if I wrestled against Pedro Morales, of course you're gonna see a scientific match. I wrestled against Bobo Brazil — that was a scientific match. I wrestled against Argentina Rocca — that was a scientific match. I wrestled against the Mighty Zuma, from Argentina — that was a scientific match. But, when you're pitted against someone like Bulldog Brower, how are you gonna go in there and have a scientific match with him, or with George "the Animal" Steele? Kowalski used a lot of holds. He was like a machine that never stopped. But he was rough, so you have to get rough, too. So I wrestled according to my opponent. If my opponent was, say, Hans Mortier, he was rough but he liked to wrestle a lot. So we wrestled. If I wrestled somebody who was a brawler, then I was a brawler. Would I have liked some more scientific matches? The answer is yes. But as I got older, unfortunately, it seemed as though the styles had changed, and there were more brawlers than scientific wrestlers. I think I would have preferred them but I don't think I had the choices to go that route. I had to go with what was given me. Hansen was a rough-house type of guy, Bruiser Brody was rough. When you're dealing with these kinds of people, you can only have a certain type of match.

How would you compare wrestling in the United States back in the '60s and '70s with Japan and Europe?

I was in Japan last year. They bring back some of the so-called superstars of yester-year to make appearances. I've gone back I think three times in the past few years. I like what I see there because their style of wrestling is basically what it used to be here in the States in the '50s and '60s and '70s, and that's why I think wrestling has remained so popular in Japan. In fact they're very choosy now as far as who they bring from the States. Before they used to bring an awful lot of guys over. They would never have Japanese vs. Japanese. It was always foreigners, whether they came from Europe or the United States, against the Japanese. But now they're having fewer and fewer of the Americans coming over because of the style which has changed so dramatically here. And they don't want too much of that.

Didn't you work with Giant Baba back in the '60s?

I don't know how to describe the matches with Baba. I had some long ones; one time I wrestled him for over an hour. He chopped a lot but he used a lot of wrestling holds, too. Not a lot of quick stuff because he was so big and tall. But he used to put on wrestling holds a lot. I liked wrestling him.

What was the reaction to you like over there? Were you the heel?

Not really. When I went there, of course, if I wrestled Baba, the Japanese wanted to see him win the match. Yet I have to say, with good feeling, that of course they wouldn't cheer me like they cheered Baba. But they would be very polite and applaud. Of course the applause when they introduced me wouldn't be anywhere near what it was when they introduced Baba. But I was not booed when I was there. They treated me well.

What was your opinion of Rikidozan at his height? Did you see him at his peak?

Yeah, but the first time I went to Japan, I was a rookie. And he was toward the end of his career. As far as his wrestling — maybe it was because it was late in his career when I saw him — at that time he didn't show me a whole lot of wrestling maneuvers. He was using a lot of chops, and he liked to grab guys and try to throw them out of the ring, that sort of thing. But I can't judge him because I didn't see enough of him to know what he was really like.

Then how do you explain his popularity?

Well, things change as you get older. Somebody wrote about me in one of the newsletters and suggested that all I ever did was brawl, that I couldn't do anything else. This was obviously written by somebody who maybe saw me toward the end of my career with some of the people that I was wrestling at the time. I'd hate to think that anybody who saw me from the '50s, when I started, thought that's all I ever did. Of course that wouldn't be true.

A few days ago there was a question in the _Boston Globe_, asking what you were doing these days. They wrote that your middle name is Leopoldo, you were born in 1935 in Abruzzi, Italy, moved to Pittsburgh in 1951, and that you were an 80-pound teenager who began lifting weights and developed into a professional wrestler. What are your earliest memories of being interested in wrestling?

First of all, about the 80-pound stuff . . . when I was born, I was big. I weighed over 11 pounds. But the reason I was so small is that I spent 14 months during World War II, along with many people in my village, hiding in the mountains. We went through heck, and many people didn't make it. We were among the lucky ones who survived it. But that was the main reason I was small. But I always loved wrestling. I first saw it in Italy — not professional wrestling, it was Greco-Roman. And I fell in love with it immediately. So I did a little bit over there as a kid, but when we came over here, I went to language school for about six months, then I went right to high school. Unfortunately, the high school didn't have a wrestling team, and I always tried to get guys on the mat. So what happened was that one of my teachers was friends with Rex Barry, a wrestling coach at University of Pittsburgh, and he arranged for me to go and work out with his wrestlers. So when I was in high school I used to walk from my school to the Pitt Field House, which was about a half-hour walk. And that's how I got my start, working out over there. Meanwhile I watched it on TV, and was fascinated. Back in those days, there was a lot of wrestling — guys like Frankie Talaber, Ruffy Silverstein, Ed Francis, Lou Thesz, Verne Gagne. And these guys did an awful lot of wrestling. It was quite different back then. I lifted weights to gain size and strength, and then I became fascinated with that, to where I did wrestling Monday, Wednesday, and Friday, and lifted Tuesday, Thursday, and Saturday. And I started competing in weightlifting, too. I did Olympic and power lifting, and in fact I set a world record in 1959 when I did 565 on the bench.

How did you get hooked up with Capitol Wrestling?

I went to Oklahoma City, where I competed for the Northern American Weightlifting Championship. I don't know if you ever heard of Bob Prince. He used to be the voice of the Pittsburgh Pirates. He had his own television show, and he had known me from before, when we went on his show a couple of times to give a little amateur wrestling exhibition. And he invited me a couple of times to give a weightlifting exhibition. So when I won the contest in Oklahoma and he heard about it, he brought me on his show. At this time I was a big kid, I weighed about 265–270. So when I did that he asked me if I was still wrestling, if I was still going up to Pitt and working out with the wrestling team. Now while this was going on, a gentleman by the name of Rudy Miller, who represented Capitol Wrestling — that was before they became the WWWF — was in Pittsburgh for some live studio wrestling. He caught me on this television show and he started inquiring about me and I was contacted. I came down to the studio a week or two later and met him, then he asked about my wrestling background and if I was interested in a career. I told him I was and they flew me to Washington. I worked out with a few guys, and Toots Mondt and Vince McMahon Sr. and Phil Zacko came to watch me work out to see what I had. I guess they liked what they saw, and for the next few months I stayed there and trained, and that's how I started.

Did you really get worked over to see what you could do?

Well, yeah. They tried to beat the heck out of you, but I could take care of myself. I don't think anybody beat the heck out of me because I was a big kid, in good shape — I was strong, young and, you know, I'm not gonna tell you it was a breeze, but I wouldn't tell you they beat the heck out of me either.

Who was your first professional opponent?

A guy by the name of Jack Vansky.

Did you win?

Yeah.

What was the difference in the way the office was run between Vince Jr. and Vince Sr.?

In those days they had what were called territories. Vince Sr. was the promoter in the northeast. And there were others in California and other places throughout the country. They would each run their territory and then they would lend talent. For example, Sam Muchnick might call Vince McMahon Sr. and ask if he could have Bruno Sammartino on such and such a date. And Vince would cooperate, unless that day was the Boston Garden or Madison Square Garden — then he'd say, "No, but I can give him to you on this other date." And that's how I wrestled in different parts of the country. They cooperated. But I was mostly with Vince McMahon. That's what went on in those days. Jr., in my opinion, tried to become the only promoter, and he went against everybody in the other territories. And he was able to get television in those territories when he hooked up with Dick Ebersol at NBC. Then he got dates that were running against the other promoters, and in doing so, he may have succeeded in overexposing wrestling in a lot of these cities to where people started getting turned off. As a result, I think it killed wrestling all over the place. They were given too much — because whoever had the territory was still trying to run his own business and shows — and McMahon was coming in as opposition to them. And then the wrestling got more and more bizarre, with all the nonsense that goes on. I think, in general, people got turned off and as a result, one at a time all the territories went down the chute. And I don't think there's any way anybody can start something up now and make it. I don't think it can be done. As long as you have McMahon staying in the business, wrestling will remain dead.

How do you think it should work?

I think McMahon and Ted Turner should both fold up, get out of the business completely, because they're not in the wrestling business. They're in a bizarre cartoon business. I don't know what to call it. If they'd just get out of it and there was no wrestling for a couple of years, then the business could start up again, but back like it was years ago, when guys came in with their real names. Most of the people had their own names. Bruno Sammartino is my name. Dominic Denucci, Tony Parisi, Hans Mortier. You had Big Bill Miller, Don Leo Jonathan. You know what I'm saying. Now who do you have? The Million Dollar Man, the Macho Man, Diesel. You know, all these names are a joke. They've gotta get away from all the garbage, from the painted faces and all this ridiculous other nonsense, and get back into basics, get back into wrestling. I think it would take time, but I think people would come back again. People don't come out because they don't like what's out there. So quit giving them what's out there. In my day we used to pack the arenas. So that would tell you that people like that better.

Almost everyone watching these days knows that wrestling is predetermined. Do you think they have to be retrained to believe that wrestling is real for it to work again?

If I wrestled Killer Kowalski, people came out because they believed the match was going to be a match, and it was gonna be for real, and somebody was going to see who could win. They respected him as being a real tough guy. They thought I was pretty good, they thought it was gonna be a heck of a contest. Do you remember when Zbyszko crossed me and all that? People wanted to kill him. After Stan Hansen broke my neck, people wanted to kill him. If people thought that it was just a show, then the interest wouldn't be there. And that's what's happening now, nobody believes anything today.

Maybe that's why people are booing Hulk Hogan now.

He's getting booed because people finally have had it. They know the guy's not a wrestler. This guy was nothing but a steroid freak. He had a seven-minute routine out there where he'd kill the first five minutes by pointing to his ears and to the audience — begging for a reaction, I guess. Tearing his shirt, flexing, with a steroid body. And then what did he give you as far as wrestling? Did you ever see him go an hour draw with somebody the caliber of a Kowalski or a Jonathan? He would have died five times during that hour. He was a cartoon character for the kids. But then the kids grew up and went away, and people are looking at him and saying, OK, enough already. Get lost. But nobody's listening. They still use this idiot. And he's a clown, not a wrestler.

In your prime was there ever a point where you were in the ring and tempers got out of control?

Oh, that happened a lot of times. Are you kidding? Somebody would get beat up more than the other guy. It's as simple as that. I was fortunate enough that I'd come out on top. Sometimes maybe it wasn't on top, but maybe it came out pretty even with the other guys. Maybe some of the other guys thought they had the edge, but in my heart I feel that I always came out OK. But that happened a lot. No matter what anyone wants to think of it, when guys went in there, it was pretty rough. You've seen many guys and you can see on me that I have two of the worst cauliflower ears you've ever seen. I didn't get them in my amateur days. I got them in professional wrestling. And my nose has been busted 11 times. I did it all while I was wrestling. You should see how crooked my elbows are.

Give us the list of injuries.

OK, the nose has been busted 11 times, everyone's amazed at the way my ears look. My jaw was cracked, I don't know if there are any ribs I haven't broken or cracked, the fingers on my right hand have all been broken, I broke my collarbone, both of my knees have had surgery for cartilage and ligaments. And of course I had a broken neck, which was the most serious injury. I've had a fractured vertebrae in my lower back. That's the bones; if you want to talk about cuts and bruises, I've had a million of those.

Could you talk about the Stan Hansen incident? What exactly happened?

I broke the sixth and seventh cervical vertebrae. I came back to the ring six months later. I didn't plan on coming back for a long time. But here's what happened: Do you remember the match they made between Muhammad Ali and Antonio Inoki? Well, Vince McMahon got involved as far as pay-per-view in the northeast, and they had to come up with big, big bucks for those rights. But the advance on the fight was a disaster worldwide. It was one of the biggest bombs as far as promotions. And Vince called me and said, "Bruno, I've gotta get your match with Stan Hansen in Shea Stadium because this thing with Ali and Inoki is a dud, and we're gonna go under with what we had to commit to." I said how the heck am I gonna do that? Well, I had been out of the hospital maybe a week. I talked to my doctor and he told me I was out of my mind. He talked to Vince McMahon and said, "Do you understand what this guy has just gone through?" He did this on his own, and he was furious. And McMahon said to me, "Bruno, if we don't do this match, we're done. That's how serious it is." So I did come back for that match. I wrestled him at Shea Stadium. And this is fact — not bragging. The only place they did business in the northeast with the closed circuit was when they had me and Hansen, along with Ali and Inoki. But everyplace else in the country and around the world, it was a total disaster.

We've got to bring up Larry Zbyszko. The story was that you taught him everything he knew and then he turned on you. Your thoughts looking back on it today?

Well, I don't know if I taught him everything he knew. This is a kid who went to Allegheny High, considered one of the top wrestling schools in the country. He went undefeated there and then went on to college on a scholarship. He was a terrific wrestler, and I did work out with him professionally. As far as when that happened with us — and this was near the end of my career — I thought the matches, considering the time in my life, were good. Certainly the fan response was unbelievable. We drew around 45,000 people in Shea Stadium. And keep in mind, this was just a local promotion. When I wrestled him at Shea Stadium, on the same night Baltimore was playing the Yankees — they were battling for the pennant, so Yankee Stadium was almost full. And the Pittsburgh Steelers were playing the New York Giants at Giants Stadium in an exhibition game, all on a same night. So to draw 45,000 people would tell you how much interest there was in that match. In fact, everywhere we went with it, we turned people away. I thought they were pretty hard, good matches. And as far as Zbyszko, despite that time when he was very unpopular in the matches, I think he was one of the most underrated wrestlers. People now talk about this guy and that guy. But in my opinion, Larry was as good and better than most of those so-called top guys. I'm talking about people like Ric Flair and Bob Backlund.

What do you think of people like Flair and Backlund as far as wrestling performers? Do you like any of them?

Years ago I think Flair, yes. But the mistake that a lot of us make is that sometimes we don't know when it's time to get out. It's time for Flair to get out. Years ago, I wouldn't have taken anything away from Flair. He gave you a lot of action, worked hard in the ring, but I think his time has passed.

How old are you now Bruno?

I'm 60.

How did you know when it was time to get out?

When I broke my neck, I considered not coming back. But I didn't like what was going on. They kept promoting Stan Hansen, calling him "the man who broke Bruno Sammartino's neck" and "the man who retired Bruno Sammartino." I didn't like that. I didn't like to go out that way. So I came back. But when I did, I didn't have the intentions of staying there long. I just wanted to wrestle some more and then get out on my own. But they were building the Meadowlands in New Jersey, and they asked me if I would open that. They had construction problems and it took a long time to complete it. So I wrestled there on October 4, 1981. That was to be my last match. But then the Japanese found out I was retiring and they asked if I would come in for a farewell tour. So I wrestled at the Meadowlands on October 4 — I fought George Steele — then on the morning of October 5, I took a plane out of Kennedy, went to Japan and spent 10 days going to all the major cities, and that was it. I was retired, I came home, I was done. At that time I was 45 years old, but the difference between me and Flair, is that there was no doubt that I wasn't the guy

I was 15 years prior. But I was a guy who kept myself in great shape. I worked out all the time at the gym, I was not a smoker or a boozer. I never did those things, and that helps. But that's not to say that I shouldn't have gotten out a few years earlier. Maybe I should have.

Would you like to be working in wrestling in any capacity now?

The only way I would work with another organization right now is if somebody could show me they would start a new league in the way I would like to see it. Then, if they would say Bruno, we'll let you call the shots, yeah, I'd be interested. I'd like to go back and clean everybody up, have people coming in with a pair of tights, a pair of boots in the ring. I wouldn't have any paint on their faces, I would use their real names, and I'd want guys who can go out there and give people good wrestling action, not acrobatics like doing triple somersaults from the top rope. I'm talking about good wrestling action. It would take time and patience, but I think eventually people would start coming around.

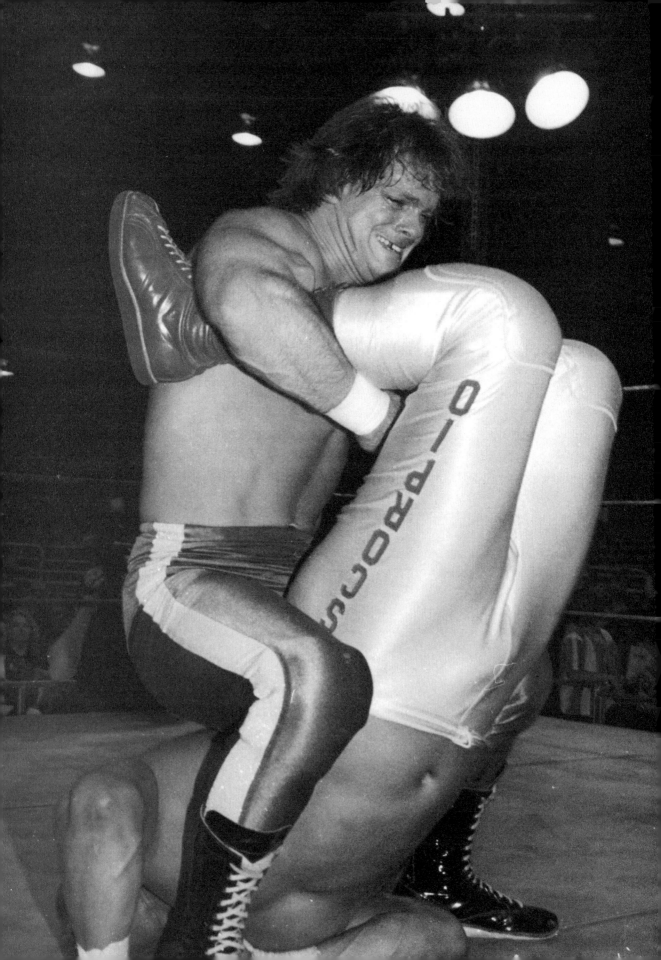

Chris Benoit
December 16, 1995

The Canadian Crippler has consistently been among the top technical wrestlers in the business since entering the scene through Stampede Wrestling in the mid-1980s under the training of Stu Hart and the Hart family. Before really catching on in the States in wcw, he was a major star in Japan under a mask as the Pegasus Kid. At the time of the interview, he had just jumped from ECW to wcw, where he became one of the Four Horsemen. He hadn't done many interviews and was regarded as quiet and very protective of the business. He at first seemed uncomfortable, but eventually opened up to discuss training and working in Japan, junior heavyweight wrestling, and the idea of educating fans to appreciate technical wrestling in the States.

What year did you actually break in to the business, Chris?

December 1985, with Stampede Wrestling.

And Owen Hart came in in 1986?

Yes, I believe so. When he broke in, I was in the New Japan Pro Wrestling dojo at the time. So I wasn't on the circuit then for Stu.

When did you know you wanted to be a professional wrestler?

Probably about 12 or 13. It was the first time I had ever been to a wrestling match, and I was really impressed by the Dynamite Kid. When I saw him I thought to myself that I'd really like to be like that.

Did you ever work with him in training?

He never ended up training me at all, but I had the pleasure of wrestling him a couple times.

Was that a big thrill for you?

Yeah, it was. It ended up being in two small spot-show towns working for Stu Hart at the time. But it didn't matter. It was just a pleasure being in the ring with him.

Did you win?

I can't remember.

Many people said Jushin Liger was too small to make it in the business. Did you ever feel you were too small?

No, I never felt that way. A lot of people sure told me that, but I never felt that way. I was always confident about myself.

You've worked with Sabu before. You're about the same size and are probably fairly equal in skill in the ring, but your styles are quite different. Was it difficult to work with him?

Not really. Sometimes when you get two wrestlers that have two totally different styles, it really makes for an interesting, competitive match.

Who are you most comfortable working with right now?

I enjoy working with everyone. I enjoy that challenge.

You fought Steven Regal recently, and that was a great match.

Yeah, I really enjoyed that.

Are you more comfortable on the mat or in the air?

Both, really. As I said, I really enjoy wrestling all different styles. I've wrestled Steve Regal a number of times in Japan, and we've twice had matches that've gone over 20 minutes. And we only used the ropes once. It was all mat work the entire match, and I really enjoyed that.

Were you called the Pegasus Kid the first time you went down to Mexico for EMLL?

Yeah, the first time.

Where did the name Pegasus Kid come from?

When I finished my year in the New Japan dojo, they sent me to Calgary for a couple years. Upon bringing me back they figured I needed some sort of identity change. I sat down with Tokyo Joe, one of the agents from New Japan Pro Wrestling that lives in Calgary, and we just kicked around some ideas and came up with that one.

And how did that name make the transition to Wild Pegasus?

I don't know.

Is there anyone in the sport that you'd like to wrestle that you haven't had a chance to yet?

Anyone that I haven't wrestled. I truly enjoy challenges and wrestling someone with a different style that I haven't done yet, and trying to have a really good match.

Have you seen Rey Mysterio Jr. yet from AAA?

Yeah, for the first time at the last J-Cup. Incredible! Truly incredible.

You won the first J-Cup two years ago. What do you think that meant in Japan, to have an outsider come in and win the first tournament? Were you cheered?

I was cheered. With the Japanese fans, there's really no good guy or bad guy. They're more interested in watching a competitive match than the persona of a wrestler. They're more interested in their technique and ring ability. They'll cheer both wrestlers. If I'm wrestling Liger and I do a good move, they'll cheer me, then two minutes later Liger'll do a good move, and they'll cheer him. They've really got a different mentality than the North American fans. They've been educated differently.

You've had a long and colorful history with Liger. You're kind of a heel here. But what is he?

I'm not sure how much the average wrestling fan would really recognize him. Surely, all the so-called hardcore fans would know him, but just when he comes out, his ring presence is so spectacular. I'd imagine he's automatically turned a good guy.

You mentioned the dojo earlier. Can you briefly give us an idea of what goes on there?

They're pretty militant, pretty strict, with their training and diet. It's totally different than any training center that you'd find here in the States. The wrestlers live there and eat there and sleep there and train there. It's really amazing to go over there and watch the way they run their camps.

When you come out you're obviously a much-improved wrestler. Are you also physically and emotionally in different shape than when you went in?

Oh yeah. It instills a lot of self-discipline in you to go through something like that. I think you come out a lot more confident about going into the ring.

What was the difference so far this time working with WCW compared to a couple years ago when you came in for a short while.

There's lots more communication now between the wrestlers and the so-called office. It's unbelievable right now. Last time there was really no communication between us. I was still going back and forth between here and Japan, and that was the big problem. Now we're keeping an open line of communication, and so far it's going really well, and I'm really happy.

How long are you under contact for?

Right now it's sort of on a trial basis. But we're getting ready to discuss more long-term plans.

How would you compare working in Stu Hart's dungeon as opposed to the dojos in Japan?

I was living, eating, and sleeping in the New Japan dojo, whereas to go into Stu Hart's dungeon, I had to make my way to Calgary, then find my own accommodation and food. I guess you can concentrate a lot more on what you're doing when you're in the Japanese-style dojo.

You've been in the business now for about 10 years. But you haven't had that much exposure in the States. Any idea why you're so much more popular in Mexico and Japan?

I guess it's just the course my career took. I was fortunate enough early on to have the opportunity to go over and train in the New Japan Pro Wrestling dojo. And from there I guess it just snowballed and I ended up having most of my career over there.

But you're here now. How did you get hooked up with Paul E. Dangerously and ECW?

I started doing some independent work in the United States for Dennis Coraluzzo. I met Paul E. once years before, and through talking to different wrestlers, ended up getting hooked up with him and Tod Gordon.

Did working with ECW help to develop a character for you?

Most definitely. Having wrestled in Japan for so many years and having spent most of my time there and in Mexico, and especially being under a mask for a while, I never had the opportunity to work on a so-called persona. So Paul E. really helped me bring that out.

Did it take you a long time to get it straight?

I didn't feel like it was so much developing the persona as it was gaining confidence in doing interviews.

Why did you leave ECW?

A better opportunity.

How did that happen?

I was approached by wcw. They started a working relationship with New Japan Pro Wrestling, and that's how we started discussing the opportunity

So now you commute from Edmonton to Atlanta?

Yeah. I go there about once a week. Hopefully, if things work out well, I'll be relocating.

What other wrestling offices would you like to work with?

I'm quite happy with my situation right now with New Japan and wcw. I hope things work out. I feel like I've got a lot of goals I've yet to accomplish, and I'd like to do that before I think about anything else.

Could you share a couple of those goals with us?

My biggest goal right now would be to really establish myself a lot more in the States.

It seems to be working, now that you're one of the Horsemen. How did that come about?

I've known Brian Pillman for quite a while, and I've been to Japan a couple times with Arn and Ric Flair. We started talking about the idea, and it grew from there.

Have you fought Flair one on one?

No, I haven't yet.

Do you plan to?

Not right now. I'm feeling comfortable being on his side.

Some people say Flair has been doing the same act for years. What are your thoughts on his contributions to wrestling?

He's a major talent. Anyone who says that about him or any other wrestler, they're really uneducated when it comes to knowing what it takes to go in the ring and actually have a match. Once you actually start doing it, you appreciate everything so much more.

Do you still get butterflies before you get into the ring?

I do. When I don't get butterflies, I kind of get afraid. Because when I do have them, that's when I have my best matches.

We've seen both Shane Douglas and Steve Austin leave WCW upset recently. They're good workers. They're great workers. Have you ever felt they might not use your talents to the extent that you would like?

I don't really think about that. Everyone has different reasons for doing different things in this business. Right now I'm happy with where I am and I'm happy with my position.

How long do you think you could stay an active wrestler?

Until I stop enjoying it. I really love what I do. I love all of it. When that goes away, I guess that would be the beginning of the end.

Are there any wrestlers currently in Japan that you think would work well in the United States?

There's a ton of wrestlers over there. But it's a totally different style. A lot of Japanese wrestlers come over here and it takes them a while to establish themselves because of that change in style and the change in what fans expect to see. Fans in the Sumo Palace in Tokyo expect a totally different match than, say, fans in the

Omni in Atlanta do. So it's just a change over, it's to get accustomed to a different style.

How important is it to have a collegiate background for pro wrestlers today?

The more experience you have, the better off you'd be. There aren't too many schools throughout the United States right now that have a sensei that is knowledgeable in all areas. There's only a handful of them, and there are so many schools around that probably shouldn't be in that business. The wrestling business is really flooded with a lot of athletes who are aspiring to make a name for themselves, but who haven't had the proper training and aren't quite ready yet.

What happens when you happen to meet some new people who don't know you and you tell them you're a professional wrestler?

I guess it's like everything else. You have some people who don't enjoy watching football, and some who don't enjoy watching hockey. You can't expect everyone to enjoy every sport.

But doesn't wrestling have a stigma? Have you had to explain what you do?

Oh yeah. Lots of times. If you meet someone on a plane, the first question they ask is whether or not it's fake. And I say no. I say it's easy to sit in your chair in front of your TV and say, "That's fake, that's easy, I can do that." But once you're in there it's a totally different ballgame.

What are your resolutions for 1996?

I'd like to establish myself a lot more in the United States and the wcw in particular.

As a Horseman?

Most definitely. We all work hand in hand.

Was there any point in time that WWF was looking at you?

Yeah, earlier this year I wrestled dark matches on three of their TV shows.

Was it interesting to you?

Yeah, for a brief time.

Why did you go with WCW instead?

I feel a loyalty toward New Japan Pro Wrestling. And obviously going to wrestle for the WWF I'd have to sever some ties. But with WCW and the working relationship they have with New Japan, and the way things are run there, I just felt more comfortable with the business decision to go to WCW.

You said something earlier about the fans in Japan being more educated as to how wrestling works. What do we have to do, what do you have to do, what do the promoters have to do, to help educate American audiences?

I wouldn't say they're more educated, but they're educated differently. Over there, they're accustomed to watching more mat work, while over here you start hearing the "boring" chants. To bring another style to the United States will be a slow and long transition.

So the change has to be within the ring, not the audience?

Yeah, I'd say so. If you look at a Japanese pro wrestling card and an American pro wrestling card, the difference is in the ring. And that's what educates the fans.

You're fighting Liger at the next Starrcade. Is he the Chris Benoit of Japan?

No, everyone's got a different style. One thing that really bothers me is when you hear someone saying, "Oh, *he's* the greatest wrestler, or no, *he's* the greatest wrestler." You can't pick the greatest wrestler because there are so many different styles. How can you compare someone in the States who's considered the greatest wrestler to someone in Mexico? They're two totally different styles. There's no greatest wrestler. It's who you personally enjoy watching the most. To pick one guy and say he's the greatest wrestler is ludicrous.

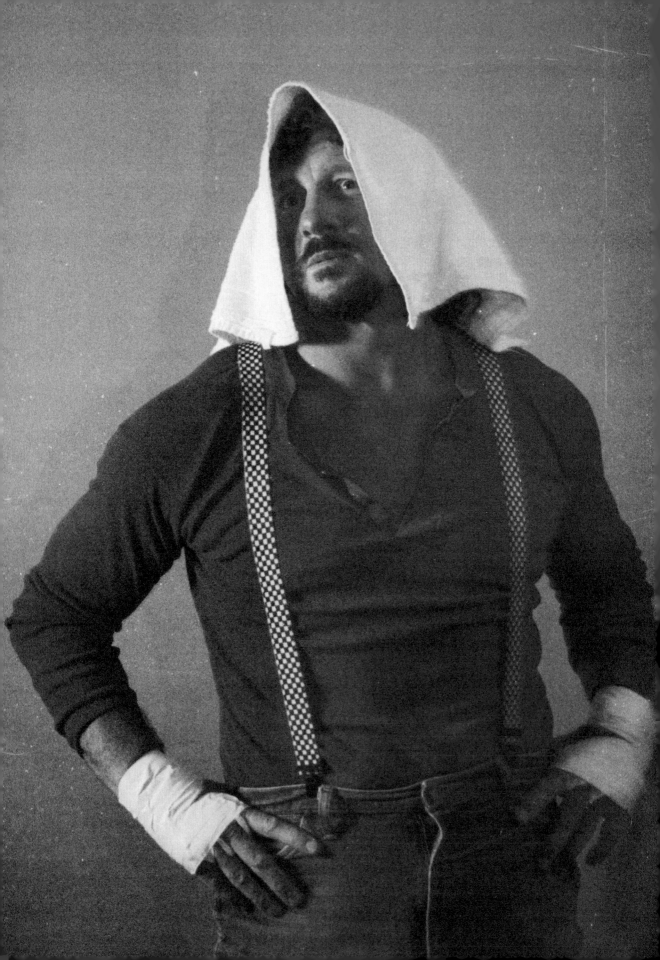

Terry Funk
January 6, 1996

It's safe to say that by the time Terry Funk came on the show, he knew a little bit about the wrestling business. He had already been a pro for 30 years, holding titles down south as far back as 1971, and grabbing a number of them in different groups over the years. He was, along with his brother, Dory Jr., a second-generation wrestler, after their father, Dory. Speaking from his home in Amarillo, Texas, Funk got a little argumentative, rather confrontational, on the subjects of hardcore wrestling and junior heavyweights. Though generally easygoing, Funk seemed to like answering the questions with questions of his own, which he then answered. At that point, he was wrestling for ECW, where his brawling style was a perfect fit. But at the age of 51, he was still saying that he had just retired . . . again. Incredibly outspoken about what's good and bad in the business, he had recently done a moonsault on TV.

Hi Terry, thanks for coming on. You're still the champ.

That was a long time ago.

You're from Amarillo, the helium gas center of the United States. So did you used to breath the helium and speak with a high, funny voice?

Well, I've done it a few times. I think probably every kid in the whole country has done that.

People remember you from so many matches. What stands out in your mind as one of the greatest matches you've had?

That's difficult, because it's always a matter of who you're wrestling. I've been able to adapt to different styles and done it throughout the years. I can claim that I've worked with some aggressive or crazy wrestlers, like Abdullah, Sheik, fellows like that. If you're talking about class wrestlers, there's Jack Brisco, probably one of the smoothest, slickest wrestlers around. He was also a wonderful technique wrestler. I also wrestled Thesz many years ago when I first started, and he was good. I can't determine or designate one match as being the most outstanding. In Japan I've wrestled everybody from Choshu to Inoki to Baba to God only knows who. It's a difficult question. There's a lot of great ones I've wrestled.

Was your first match with a guy named Sputnik Monroe?

That's absolutely true.

Could you tell us what was going through your head at your first professional match? And did you win the match?

It was a 10-minute time limit match and I didn't win it. But I lasted the 10 minutes so I considered it a successful match. It was in Amarillo, Texas, and I thought I was doing well, but evidently I wasn't because my father ran down to ringside, saw it and said, "Terry, you'd better get up off your ass and get to doing something." I leaped up and did my best, and the fans thought my father really energized me. But they didn't know that I was more afraid of him than I was of Sputnik Monroe.

Did you ever have butterflies in those days?

Absolutely. You know, I still get — not butterflies, but I have a little bit of nervousness. And I think that's good. I think if you lose that nervousness, you lose that desire to be the best.

How would you compare the promoters in Japan with the promoters here in the States?

It's basically a set deal there, but business has changed so much. I'll give you an example of what happens here. In years past, you would go into a town and do your best and hope you drew a lot of money. If the crowd was big, the wrestlers got paid a percent of the gate. That has changed through the years. All of the organizations have come along and now pay people a lot off a contract. In Japan, you also get paid by contract. You agree to the amount of money you'll be paid ahead of time. So as far as the wrestlers are concerned, the promoters are about the same all over. But the way the promoters have treated their business, the way they have protected it, the way they have loved it, is definitely different in Japan. In Japan, we're looking at a very wonderful style of sport that is thought of as athletic competition. In the States, because of wcw and wwf proclaiming themselves entertainment — and entertainment is an important thing in our profession; we have to have entertainment in all sports — but I think it's gone to the extreme due to the companies running the profession right now.

Speaking of extreme, there's Extreme Championship Wrestling, which has taken over the hardcore world. Some people say you're the godfather of hardcore wrestling. And in the storyline right now, you passed it down to Tommy Dreamer.

What do you mean I passed it down to Tommy Dreamer? Did you hear me say I passed it down? I didn't pass it down to him. I never have passed anything to anybody. That's what they want you to assume that I've done. I have a great deal of respect for Tommy Dreamer, but I haven't said that to anybody. I'm setting you straight on that.

Will wrestling become more hardcore?

That depends on what you mean by hardcore. I think that a hardcore fan is a connoisseur of wrestling. I think a hardcore fan has an intelligence of the sport. I think he knows what is good and knows what is bad at whatever style it might be. If it's the Ultimate Fighting style, he knows who's good and who's bad, because he lives, breathes, eats, and sleeps wrestling. If it's a violent style, he likes that style. Don't proclaim a hardcore fan a violent-styled fan. We get confused over what a hardcore person is. You better examine what it was when it originated, and not what you assume it is. It's not a bunch of guys just going out there and doing stupidity. And hardcore wrestlers are ones that go out there and put out 100 percent at whatever style they might be performing. It does get risky, but I'm not saying you have to be a hardcore idiot, that you have to believe in blood. In order to believe in hardcore, there doesn't have to be blood. It has to be good and it has to be 100 percent.

Do you think we'll be seeing more of the junior heavyweight type wrestlers getting a push in the bigger organizations?

Are you talking about somebody who's not on the 'roids?

No, somebody who's physically smaller, somebody around the 220-pound mark, rather than the 300-, 400-pounders.

If you look at the ratings, if you have a 300-, 400-pounder that can move like a 200-pounder, I think that's a wonderful situation, and I think you'll have the fans loving him. But if you've got a 300-, 400-pounder moving like a damn blob, it's not gonna be very interesting to anybody concerned. That might be somewhat of what's wrong — the laziness in some of our organizations. Now that's not everybody I'm talking about. There are some guys busting their butts in all organizations, and doing a great job. Unfortunately, sometimes the guys that are getting the push aren't the guys that are producing in the ring. Right now you're seeing a conversion of it because they have to bump ratings. The way you do that is by having action and the best show. They're starting to understand that they have to produce something, they've got to give those people something to make them tune in. And unfortunately, again, our total numbers have gone down. Do you know why? Because of a lack of that initiative that's out there. There has to be more competitiveness in the profession.

With the Super J-Cup in New Japan Pro Wrestling, it seems that the junior heavyweights there are drawing better than the bigger guys.

Wait a minute, the junior heavyweights are drawing money in Japan because they're having a big tournament. And they're doing big business at that tournament. So it's not a steady diet all year long. You cannot proclaim junior heavyweight wrestling the answer to what we are doing now. They are successful in Japan, and I believe they can be successful anywhere. I'm not trying to proclaim all light guys better than the heavy guys. That's B.S. Nor am I trying to go ahead and say heavyweights are better than light guys. It's just the desire to want to give the people what they deserve for paying that buck at the gate. That's what it's about. When you've got guys who are trying to protect the contracts they have, and they're satisfied with that, and there are only so many positions open, well then you get a staleness to it.

You've been in this business so long and understand how it works. There are obviously some big problems in the major organizations as far as management. If you were running a major wrestling company today, what would your first decision be?

Who am I, wcw or wwf?

You choose.

ok, if I was wcw, I'd never come up with Monday Nitro. It's absolutely absurd. It's stupidity, you're doing automatic burnout. You're destroying wrestling fans. You might think you're not, but you are. You're running people away from the televisions, you're killing your pay-per-view, and you're hurting your sport. For what reason?

Because they're trying to attack WWF.

How do you figure that is attacking them if you're doing less numbers? It doesn't make any sense.

What if you were WWF?

If I was wwf, my first decision is not to ever go and recognize wcw by putting a couple of idiots on there and calling them Hulk Hogan and Macho Man Savage. That was absurd. I thought they were above that. They've got wonderful talent and they need to rely on the good talent they have.

Do you see anyone on the horizon that they can draw on like they did with Hulk Hogan in the '80s?

What was Hulk Hogan in the '80s?

He was drawing box office numbers.

Yes he was, but how did he get there? Was it because he was Hulk Hogan? Or because he was in the right position at the right time? He was there when wrestling became mainstream, and he happened to be the one that was put into that position. You have to understand that wrestling is not only a children's product. It was, and it did big business, and it happened. But you must remember who's buying those tickets for those children. It is entertainment for all ages, not for one age or one sex. And that's what they have to look at — the entire group of fans, then they have to give them people. They have to stop all of this absurd talent naming. They have personalities, but they have to have people. They can't have just everybody having a name and a mask and a gadget. What the hell? Why was a mutant, such as Ultimate Wrestling allowed to come forward? What did they produce? They produced names, they produced guys, they produced real people. And what did they do? They more than doubled the past pay-per-view of wcw, with Hulk Hogan on it. Why? Because they gave them something the people wanted. Something that we have gotten so far away from, that we have lost.

It seems to be a hybrid of what pro wrestling was.

We can go back to that, and there's nothing wrong with it, and it's not hard to do.

Do you see more success with Ultimate Fighting?

It's going to have trouble. You'll see their pay-per-view numbers go down in the future. You have the same people becoming involved more and more. And you have to continue rotation. How many times do you want to watch Royce Gracie against Dan Severn? It's not as interesting now as it was in the past. Or even Gracie against Ken Shamrock? I don't know why the edge is off of it, but it's off. Now don't misunderstand me, they'll continue to do business, but not like it was. It hit its peak.

Terry, are you retired from the ring right now?

Well I hope so, or I wouldn't be talking like this. What the hell, I'd have people trying to hit me over the head with a two-by-four in the dressing room. Well, I'm not going in the dressing room anymore. They're not gonna find me.

Did you ever completely recover from the accident with Lanny Poffo?

Well, I can look down at my pec, and I know it. I can look at them both and one's not as big as the other. And whenever I get into the heavy weights, my tricep on the right side doesn't work as well as my left one. It's very good, but it's not the same as it used to be. But it's not a holdback at all. I've had severe injuries. The broken sacrum in wcw was a bad one. I've had problems with my vertebras and with my back. I hope the heck I'm not sounding like Ty Cobb, but I've produced for the doggone people whenever I was in the ring, and you very seldom saw a three-and-a-half-star match.

Why did you do a moonsault at the age of 51?

I did it because I loved it, and I want to be something special. I love the business with all of my heart, I love the boys in it, and I love what I did. When I'm talking I'm trying to answer you as honestly as I possibly can. And believe me, I love the people around it, I love the fans, I love everything about the business. It's something very special to me, and it's been special to my family.

Is there any more future in your movie career?

There should be, I'm supposed to do one with Bruce Willis. Let's hope it works out.

We're big fans of *Road House*.

They've played the doggone thing enough, haven't they? I got residuals off of it, but they're down to about three bucks now. Of course, I only made about 10 when they started.

Is it true that Sylvester Stallone got you started in the movie business?

Yeah, he did. That was a long time ago. I think we made *Paradise Alley* in 1978, and then I thought people would start coming around, that I'd just sit out there and I'd be a star. But I sat out there and sat out there and sat out there, and finally I came back home to Texas.

It seems like you fought them all in the wresting business. Is there anyone you missed that you would've liked to have been in the ring with?

I'd like to wrestle Dan Severn sometime, just so I can say I wrestled him. I've got a great deal of admiration and respect for the man.

Did you ever fight Vader?

No, I never did. I was in Europe with him for a while. I respect him, too. He's got a great ability. I respect anybody who has gone out there and busted their tails and made it and proved themselves a success and never gave up their identity as an individual. Right now I admire Cactus Jack.

You guys are almost spitting images of each other.

Well, not really. There's major differences but a lot of things that are alike, too.

When we think of you as a brawler back in the '80s, there are more similarities with Bruiser Brody, but in the '90s, you're almost side by side with Cactus Jack.

Brody was a good man, another man that I admired a great deal. I wish he was around. Unfortunately, he's not; unfortunately a lot of my friends aren't around anymore. . . . They're kind of disappearing.

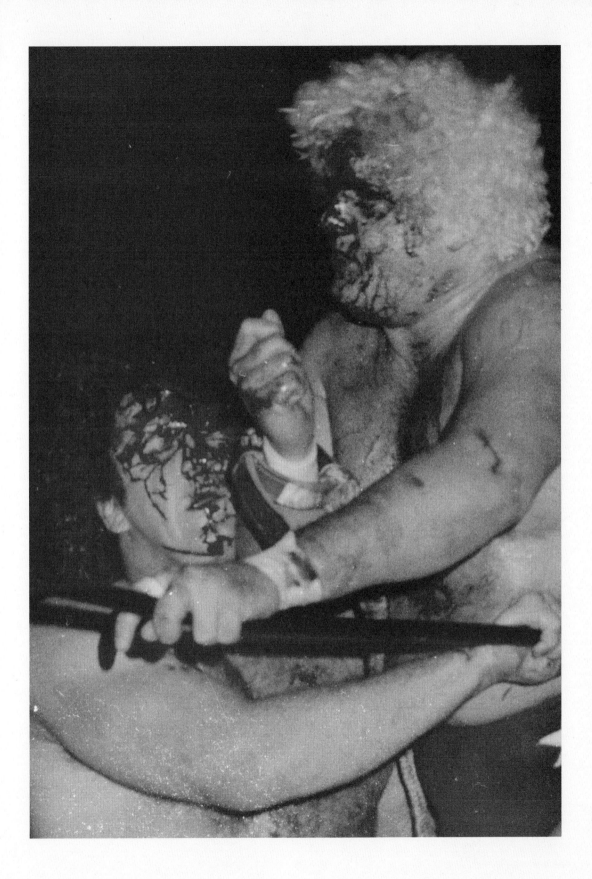

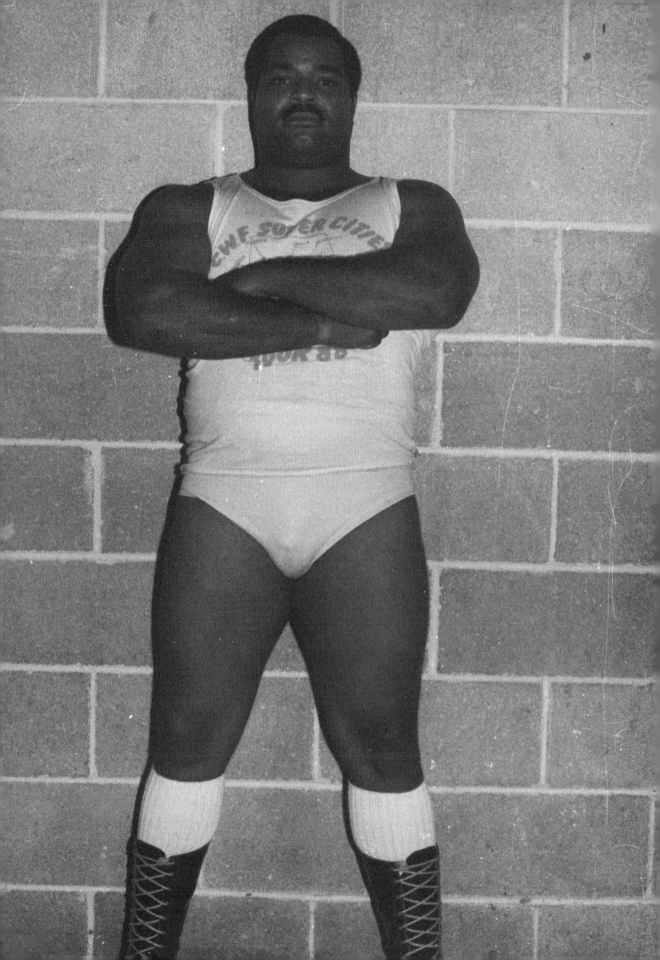

Pez Whatley
February 24, 1996

Pistol Pez wore a variety of tag team belts early on in his career, and held the NWA Southern Title in Florida a few times. But he was mostly a mid-card wrestler, gaining a little more notoriety when he took on the name of Shaska during his wcw tenure. There were a number of scheduling conflicts before he was finally able to appear on the show. But he was well worth the wait, as the long-time journeyman reminisced about his collegiate sports career, breaking in to the Tennessee territory, working for the Crocketts, racism in wrestling and thoughts on life in general.

We have with us Mr. Pistol Pez Whatley. Hello, where are you today?

I'm in Atlanta, Georgia.

Hometown?

My hometown is Chattanooga, Tennessee. But I've been down here the last three or four years.

You've been wrestling for about 20 years. Where were you before Crockett?

I've been blessed to work all over the world. Before Crockett, I worked in the Louisiana territory, up in Ohio, Florida, Canada, and got to go to Germany, Hong Kong, and Japan several times. So I got a good opportunity to swing around the world a little bit.

Pez, how did you get into the business in the first place?

Well, as you know I was a two-sport athlete in college back in the early '70s, probably before Bo Jackson had made that popular. I was wrestling and playing football at the University of Tennessee and one of my wrestling teammates, George Weingeroff, had a father named Saul Weingeroff. He happened to meet us when we were on the team and asked if we'd like to try wrestling professionally. I never thought of doing it beforehand, but it seemed interesting. We had finished our collegiate career at the time and decided to give it a shot. I played collegiate football and gave it my full shot and then tried wrestling and never stopped.

Who trained you?

When I started off, I was in Tennessee, which was Nick Gulas' territory. It was the Nashville, Birmingham, and Memphis area. I got trained by the regulars there, Karl and Kurt Von Brauner, Pepe Lopez, who got tragically killed in a car wreck, the Bass Brothers, and then The Sheik and Bobo Brazil came in and helped out, too.

So it sounds like a variety of different styles that people were training you with.

I was trying to get a hold of all the greats, and if I was going to make my mark that I would need those people and others that came in and out.

Who did you face in your first professional match?

My first match was in a Battle Royal, in Louisville, Kentucky.

Did you win?

I won my first professional Battle Royal because nobody paid attention to me. It was my very first professional match. I'll never forget it, in Louisville, Kentucky at St. Bonaventure College.

So your greatest fame came with Jim Crockett Promotions through the access of cable, on TBS. Who brought you into the NWA at that time?

Well, at that time I was in Florida working for Eddie Graham. Dusty had come to Crockett and called several times and said, "Pistol, you know I want you. You know I want you bad, but we have to work some things out." I was fortunate at the time that a few places were interested in me. But Dusty worked it out and called me and I went on up to North Carolina. But before then, I worked for Georgia Championship Wrestling when Ole [Anderson] was in charge. Ole came to Tennessee and recruited me from the Tennessee ranks because Nick Gulas and his people were trading off talent. They traded me to Georgia and they liked that I had an amateur background.

You were a face at all times until the mid-'80s, when you turned on Jimmy Valiant. Were you a heel when you first broke in?

Well, believe it or not, before that happened, Randy Savage and I and Ron Bass and Bill Ash, we all were in the same area with Nick Gulas. They were all trying to show me the traits of being a heel, so I had a small taste for it then, before going to Crockett. I had about six months as a heel, which was a short stint, before going to Crockett.

That was the territory where Randy Savage met Miss Elizabeth.

Yes. I was there when he met Miss Elizabeth. Randy and I were compadres, we worked out together all the time — our ultimate dream was to be very big in professional wrestling.

We've heard stories of territory wars from that era. We heard reports that there was a legitimate gunfight between Randy Savage and Bill Dundee over the Tennessee and Kentucky territories and stuff like that.

Well, there were some tense times and confrontations during those times as both promotions were doing particularly well and both were aggressive. It did cause tension between the two promotions and us. You know, I was with Bob Roop and Bob Orton Jr. and they were class guys who could hold their own in wrestling, so we all liked to play hard and we trained hard.

Can you verify, was a gun ever really drawn between wrestlers?

No, there wasn't a gun. What had happened was Bill went to the back of his car to get what we thought was the possibility of a gun, and Angelo Poffo hustled us out of the area because he didn't want gunplay. So, although there were people that said that a gun was revealed, there wasn't any, thanks to Angelo Poffo getting us out of there.

Have you been in real fights out of the ring?

Yes.

Were you OK?

Well, being in NCAA tournaments helped tremendously — as we know, a wrestler is better than a brawler. All he's got to do is swing his arms and you'll say "thank you" because he's giving you his body and you can take him down. Same thing with martial artists, too.

Thank you for that tip. When you went up to the NWA, did Dusty recognize how well you were getting over?

We talked about it a great deal. He was really good about that. I had been trained by a lot of qualified guys and he knew that.

When you were approached to turn on Valiant, did you agree that it was time for a persona change?

Well, I learned one thing from another professional wrestler by the name of Ronnie Garvin. One day, he said to me, "Pez, in order to make it as a wrestler and do it as a career, you've got to go both ways."

I guess that's what Pat Patterson tells people, too.

Seriously, though, if you don't experience both, you haven't done it completely. So, when I was approached with it, I was extremely excited. The territory was on fire, New York was on fire, and Verne was doing well. The business itself was very vibrant. All the boys were making money.

Was it fun?

I didn't know how it'd turn out, but it was great for me.

Did your reputation get hurt by the fans?

The black people didn't want to see it happen, they liked me the way I was. That was discouraging because I remember one time meeting fans I didn't know I had, and they told me they were very disappointed in me. But there were so many people who told me they enjoyed the entertainment that I brought to the arenas. You get mixed responses, but in the end it played out OK.

People didn't perceive this as a racial turn by the wrestling company, did they?

I'm sure some people thought that, as I was considered a very good role model at the time. When this happened, it was not accepted real well and I had preachers and churches call, and they did not like it.

What did you say to them?

I said, "Where were you when I wasn't that way? I certainly wanted to hear from you beforehand, because I didn't know you were out there." I didn't know how well I was doing as a babyface because I didn't hear from them. And when I turned, they were disappointed. You don't know until something happens to you, then you get the reaction. When Magnum got hurt, he had no idea how many people loved him until after it happened. I was shocked by the fans' response.

Soon after, the top hat came in and then you were known as Shaska Whatley?

Yes, it worked out well. I looked up the word. Shaka was actually the word that we were looking at, but that lady singer was using it, so I liked Shaska. It gave me a little bit of a difference to make me unique.

Is Pez your real name?

It's actually Pezavan. It's a French name that my father got and I don't know exactly where, but he really liked it and gave it to me.

So you became Shaska Whatley and then joined Tiger Conway Jr. as the Jive Tones in the UWF. Did you get over as well in the UWF as you did in the NWA?

Well, I thought it was good up until a few major things happened in Jim Crockett Promotions. One was the Rock 'n' Roll Express leaving, as we were heading their way. When that happened, we were about a week from feuding, but they were gone and there was a huge void.

Were the paychecks as good as in your days in the NWA?

Well, yeah, they still were, under Jim Crockett. We were looking for another great run and felt we were about to start to gel. It takes time for two individuals to mesh together. It takes time with the fluidity of putting matches together. We were wrestling at Hofstra University, in Long Island. We had a match and knew when it was over — the fans of New York are knowledgeable and they'll let you know if you're not doing well — and we felt we accomplished a major milestone when the match was over, for some reason. Well, later that evening we were at the hotel and got mobbed as well as the bigger wrestling stars. Then we knew we were doing our job and it was coming together.

In Continental, you did an angle with your son that aired on cable [FNN]. How did it come about?

Well, we were looking for a couple of components to set the territory on fire. My son was an avid fan and followed me around and the wrestlers knew it. So Eddie [Gilbert] and Paul [E. Dangerously] conceived a way to get it going. He was the defender of his father.

It came off great on TV. Did Paul give a lot of input in there?

At the time, Paul was still young, but he was very inquisitive and hung out with Eddie all the time.

There really haven't been a lot of black performers pushed in wrestling in the '80s and '90s. Why?

Well, we all live in America and there is still racism. Regardless of what business you're in. It's the same in Hollywood. I think we're afraid to sit down and communicate. I always thought it would be a much bigger angle for racial harmony than racial heat.

I'm kind of surprised that Vince or Watts never came up with a KKK-type gimmick for cheap heat.

I don't think the TV stations would go for it. They have to be particular about things like that. If you run a major business, taste and class is something you need to deal with when dealing with the public.

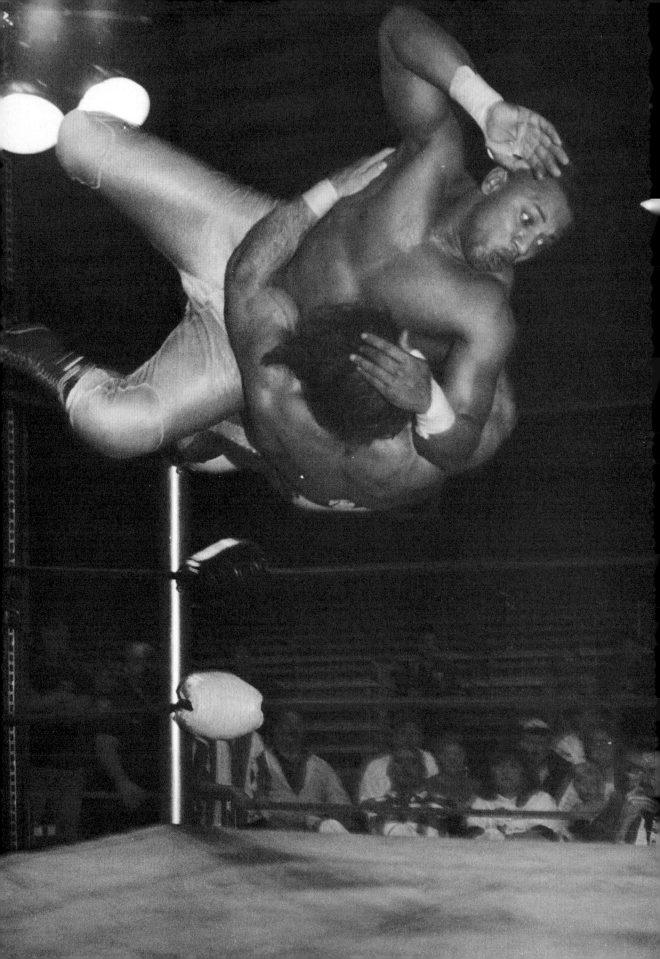

2-Cold Scorpio
May 1, 1996

Before Charles Scaggs became widely known as 2-Cold Scorpio, one of the better and most charismatic high fliers in the business, he worked his way through Rocky Mountain Wrestling, then went off to Mexico and Japan, where his style eventually developed. By the time he came to wcw in the early '90s, he was adept at both singles and tag team matches. He shared the tag title with Marcus Bagwell there, and later held the ecw tag belts with Sandman. At the time of the interview, he was still with ecw, and while he was quite happy there, he was hoping to get a shot with the wwf. Just before coming on the air, we played a tape of Bagwell making some nasty comments about him. Scorpio had no problem standing up for himself. He also had some interesting stories about personal problems with Ric Flair.

Scorpio, thanks for coming on with us. That tape was from a while ago. Is that the first time you heard Bagwell's comments?

Yeah. The conversation was never about Marcus getting fired, it was about him having heat with the other wrestlers, and I was trying to tell him. And this whole thing about doing singles, that's bullshit.

Scorpio, we have to tell you that this is a family show and need for you to clean it up a bit.

Sorry to the families out there, but I'm heated up. Marcus is saying one thing and to a certain degree, he's right. We had some words in Germany and got that straight.

Do you guys still talk?

No, we don't. I've talked to his brother once or twice and that's about it.

You're now in ECW. Is Sabu someone you like working with more than anyone?

I like working with Sabu, just like Chris Benoit. It takes a certain person to bring the best out of you. I've said before, Sabu is like The Sheik with wings. He's out there to get a good crowd response and that means sometimes taking high risks.

Have you talked with the Big Two companies recently?

Vince is just coming off that indictment and is willing to give everybody two or three chances, but doesn't want to give me that first shot.

Why is that?

I've got a problem with the WWF right now, and I don't know. They're in the business to make money and want a character to make money. I think I'm in that category right now.

But what's the problem?

Vince is the type of guy that says I've got to go home and sleep on it to think up a character before I can come in.

Is WCW's door still open?

I don't know, but I need guaranteed money wherever I go. As I told Paul E., if they come with a contract, then I'd go back. It's a good-ol'-boy system and you have to play the game.

Can a guy make a living in ECW today?

Yes, but it's up to the bookers and promoters. Paul E. doesn't really realize how much of a threat he is to the other companies. Shane Douglas and I were talking and realized that if we can eliminate some swearing, we can get some more exposure.

Juice [blood] was eliminated in ECW because of the Tommy Morrison situation, but the "Observer" said this week that the blade might come back. Any word on this?

All we heard is that in New York and Pennsylvania, there's a no-juice law. It has to be the hard way. But myself, if this is the extreme, there'll be bloodshed. As far as all through the matches, you don't need it.

It might come to commissions testing for AIDS. Boxing commissions passed a law in Pennsylvania this past week for AIDS testing. This might occur in New York.

I heard in New York, where you need an EKG, that they may do that eventually for AIDS as well, before they can wrestle, through the athletic commission.

How many shows a week do you do?

About two to three, with my 9–5 job four days a week.

Why did you get fired from WCW? Did Bischoff catch you smoking marijuana?

From what I hear, it was a setup from the get-go. Ric Flair supposedly set me up, that's what the rumor mill is. I really don't know what the lowdown is. All I know is that I got back from St. Martin and I was the only one who had to take a test, out of Ric Flair, The Nasty Boys, Arn Anderson, and everyone else that was over in St. Martin. I told everybody, what I do in my leisure time is hey, if I like to do a couple of bum butts, can't tell no lie. When I go to work and do my 9–5 and it's time to fly, I fly straight.

You seriously think Flair might have set you up legitimately?

Yeah, in all honesty, I really do believe that because I was the type of guy getting a push without them pushing me. You know, I was getting over legitimately with the people because I was doing something new.

Was this when Flair took over the booking committee?

Exactly. That was right before he got in there and then a week later, he was in the booker's spot. I really don't even know that. It could have been about how Ric Flair's old lady liked how I looked in my G-string in St. Martin.

Sounds kind of personal. Sorry to hear that. Do you want to go back to New Japan?

I'll be going back to Japan next month. I don't want to say which group as I don't want to jinx myself.

Is it Michinoku Pro?

No, but I'd like to work with the Great Sasuke. I had a match with him and Eddie Guerrero vs. me and El Samurai from years ago. He's awesome. He floats in the air and my mouth just drops.

What about Liger?

He's heavy.

What are you at?

240.

What's your schedule like?

I like to wake up at 6 and send my kids off to school at 6:45. Jump on the power ride, have a protein drink and something to eat and then it's my 9–5.

When we talked a few years ago you said that when you go to Japan, they give you a banana for breakfast.

Right, if you didn't get up and have a hard-boiled egg for breakfast, you'd have to fend for yourself. I was usually too sore for an early breakfast, so I would have a protein drink and have a banana and then get out to the ring.

Could you return to the training regimen over there?

I could do some of it. Possibly 300–400 squats, but not 500–1000 squats. Only about 150 push-ups versus 200–400.

Who do you want to work with that you haven't yet?

I've always wanted to work with Shawn Michaels. He's a hell of a talent and I respect the kid. I've always wanted to work with Bret Hart. Curt Hennig as well.

What about Owen Hart?

I've worked with Owen Hart. And he does nothing for me.

Different chemistry?

I went to Japan and he was a great high flyer, he was one of the high flyers over there. When I started high flying and I saw some high flying . . . some people shouldn't call themselves high flyers.

Does Paul fly you in every week from Atlanta?

Yes he does. I leave on Friday morning and come back Sunday. There's only a few that fly in.

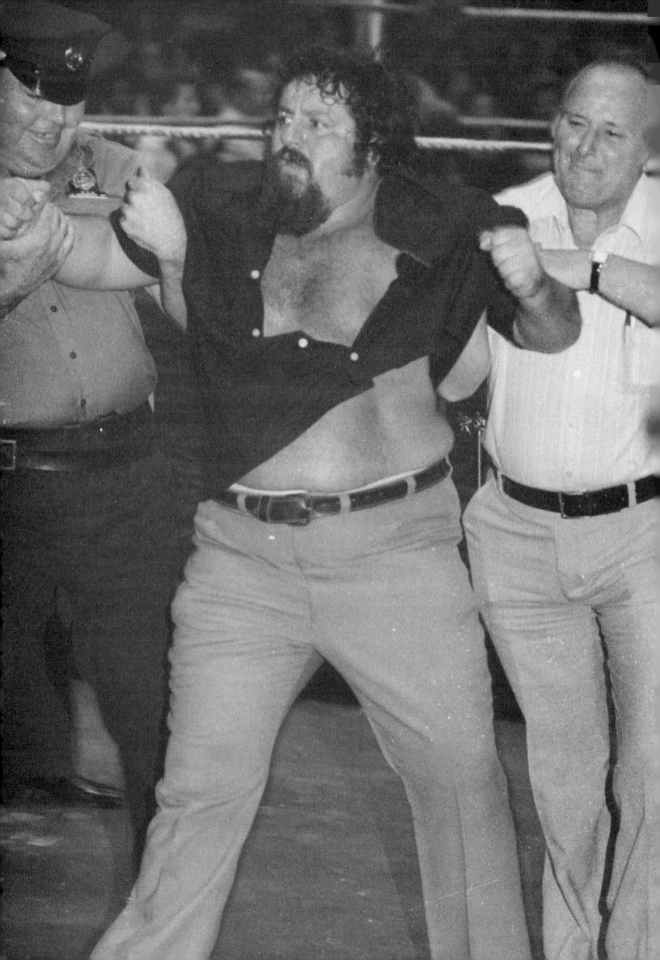

Lou Albano
June 1, 1996

Lou Albano was one of the most colorful managers in the game, using his ability to let words loudly tumble out of his mouth while turning a special shade of purple. And he wasn't one to use his looks for effect. He was more than a bit overweight, let his hair grow much too long, and in the latter parts of his career, took to wearing strategically placed rubber bands — on his scraggly beard — to make his appearance even stranger. Although he was a wrestler early on — teaming with Tony Altimore to form the Sicilians — his claim to fame was as a manager of tag teams, including the Valiant Brothers, the Blackjacks, the Moondogs, the Samoans, and Mr. Fuji and Professor Toru Tanaka. At the time of the interview, he had given up working in wrestling to try his hand at acting. Speaking from the home of one of his children, things turned slightly bittersweet, as he kept bringing up his age. His grandchildren could be heard playing in the background. He sometimes couldn't help himself from telling bad jokes.

Mr. Albano, how are you today?

Very good, thank you. You hear those children in the background? They're my grandchildren.

We didn't know you were a grandfather.

A grandfather — 11 times.

Eleven times? That's almost as many tag team champions as you had.

Just about. I had about 19 or 20 of them.

Where are you today?

I'm in upstate New York, a town called Carmel. My daughter lives here and I'm visiting. It's a pleasure to be talking with you. You've got a prestigious show; I've heard a lot about it and I'm glad to be on.

Lou, how did you break into the world of pro wrestling.

I was in service during the Korean War. Luckily I did no fighting. But they put a benefit on for the soldiers, and there was a fellow named Lenny Montana, who played Luca Brasi in "The Godfather," wrestling Arnold Skaaland. And some of the old timers were there, like Gorgeous George and so forth. I saw them, and asked them how they got into the business. I told them I realized there was a lot of theatrics involved, and that you had to learn how to fall and be a good athlete. I came out, went to the gym learned how to take my falls, and got into it. That was around 1952.

At first you were a tag team partner with Tony Altimore. How did the Sicilians form? How did you meet him? What happened?

When we got together we were the bad guys, the villains. Later we became what we call the babyfaces, the good guys. In the late 1950s we were watching "The Untouchables," Elliott Ness. We went into Chicago and we thought the Sicilians would be a good concept. We were bad guys anyway, we had tuxedo jackets on with white hats. The only mistake we made was we went in there and we were coming out with black gloves on — which is not a good thing. It signifies something bad and we were told politely to take the gloves off — which we did.

Did the Sicilians hold any belts?

Yeah, we had the Midwestern tag team belts, but never a world championship belt.

Did you run the whole circuit around the country as partners?

Oh yeah, we went all around the country and then I came back. In 1969, Bruno Sammartino suggested that I become a manager. This was in Capitol Wrestling. That's my granddaughter you hear howling in the background. Today's a very busy day. One guy's cutting grass in the back. Another is cutting a neighbor's.

Did Bruno bring you into the sport?

No, he didn't bring me in, but he asked me if I wanted to become a manager. He said I was a pretty good BS'er, pretty good talker. He said, "You never shut up, so why don't you become a manager?" So I started with Crusher Verdu, and from him I went on to be with the Valiant Brothers, Tarzan Tyler, the British Bulldogs, Andre the Giant, the Lumberjacks, the Blackjacks, I had 'em all.

In the days of Crusher Verdu, you were managing him against Bruno, right?

Yes I did. That was probably in the early '70s.

How is the business run differently now in the World Wrestling Federation as far as between the times of Vince Sr. and Vince Jr.?

I believe then there was more wrestling and wrestling ability. These guys are great, great athletes, but I think there's more theatrics involved today. I enjoyed it more years ago, maybe because I'm not doing that much anymore with the business. But I consider professional wrestlers the world's greatest athletes, to be able to take the falls the way they do, with the theatrics involved.

Did you have a lot of injuries over the years?

Oh, I broke my collarbone twice, my back twice, my hip and this and that. You can get hurt.

What is your role right now?

Once in a while I make appearances for independents. I asked for a premature release from the WWF. I didn't want to be with them anymore, and the only thing they wanted me to sign was that I wouldn't go down to Turner and the WCW, which I had no intention of doing. I'm doing some movies, and that keeps me going. I'm doing a movie called *Big Time* with Frank Gorshin and Burt Young. It's going to be a mobster comedy like in *Wise Guys* where I played the Fixer.

Didn't you make a film in Rhode Island a couple of years ago?

Yeah, that was *Complex World*, which has done well in video. It was a low budget film, kind of violent, but it was OK. I also did *Body Slam* with Roddy Piper, Tanya Roberts, and Dirk Benedict. And I did *Stay Tuned* with John Ritter and Pam Dawber. And I did the kids show, the *Super Mario* cartoon.

You're a busy man. What do you do in your spare time?

Once you hit the mid-60s, you know, it's all downhill. And I'm 64 years old.

Is there any personality out there in the wrestling business today that you wish you had under your wing in the '80s?

I've gotta say that Bret Hart, in the Hart Foundation, is an excellent wrestler, an excellent strategist in the ring. I'd have to lean towards a person like Bret Hart. Also the Steiner Brothers. They're great amateur wrestlers and know what wrestling's all about. People like that, I would've been glad to say I'll be your manager. But you know, as I said, I'm getting a little older and these guys are young fellas, and I'm sure they don't want to hang around with an old man.

You still have it, you still have the presence. When you came back with the Headshrinkers, you could still see it. You lost a lot of weight, but you were still Captain Lou Albano.

Well, I can still get out and talk and do my thing and all. But if you get into it, and get involved full time, it's a matter of getting on the road again, back and forth, and to me, it's not worth it. Occasionally I get a call from the WWF or an independent organization. Afa the Wild Samoan runs shows over in Pennsylvania. I come in and sign autographs and get a payday and walk to the ring and walk back. So it's enough to keep busy and I can do anything I want.

Where did you get the nickname of Captain?

I was captain of a Catholic high school football team called Archbishop Stepinac. I was a guard. When I came out I had a scholarship to University of Tennessee. But we might as well be honest, being the brilliant student that I was — this was in 1950, before I went in service — Jack Stroud was our captain, and we were the number one team in the nation. Today, freshmen play varsity ball, but that was the first year that freshmen could play varsity. Johnny Michaels, the All-American, pulled the cartilage in his knee, and I started five varsity games. Now, spring training is when you make the team for the following year. Well, when spring training came in, we were getting ready to go in for our finals. Needless to say, we had the finals mimeographed, and 17 of us got caught, and politely asked to retire.

It's hard to believe you would cheat.

In those days we didn't call it cheating, we called it trying to survive.

OK, it's hard to believe you got caught.

Well, it was wrong. For any kids out there listening, it's wrong to do. You might as well study and do your homework right. Especially with these computers today. If you're not knowledgeable, you can't make a living. I tried to tape something on the VCR and I gave up. That shows how stupid I am.

But you are a good role model.

I do care about the kids, I do some charity work. We raised $36 million for Multiple Sclerosis. They have a concept called the ugly bartender contest. It was "Don't be ugly like Captain Lou Albano. Let's knock out this disease." We would go around to different taverns and sign autographs and take pictures. And over a five or six year period we raised $36 million.

You sound like you're a busy guy.

Yeah, they keep me busy.

About a decade ago, on the old show *Tuesday Night Titans*, the marriage of Paul Vachon was one of the funniest bits ever done.

Right, right, a midget running around and I whacked him with a cane.

And one other time you were sitting at the desk with Vince, and he challenged you to play piano. And you walked over and played a beautiful version of "La Vie en Rose."

Well, I was lucky there. I only know one or two songs. But when you talk about midgets, there was this gal whose boyfriend kept coming home and finding her with different men. And he said, "You've gotta cut down; this has gotta stop." She said, "OK, I promise you I'll cut down." He comes home the next night, she's in bed with someone else, but she says, "I will cut down." He comes home the following night and he says, "You're in bed with somebody else." And she says, "Yeah, but it's a midget. I told you I was cutting down." And just last week, I went to the psychiatrist and said, "Doctor, can you help me? I feel like people keep avoiding me." He said, "Next." I said, "Doctor, what's wrong with me?" He said, "You're crazy." I said, "I want a second opinion." He said, "You're fat and ugly."

Lou, we're here to talk about wrestling! So you only know a couple songs on piano?

Yeah, I'm not a real pianist. I can play a couple of tunes. My mother was a concert pianist and my dad was a physician in New York. My mom was very talented, and I watched her here and there, and picked up a few numbers, but nothing where I could make a living out of it.

Over the years when you've met new people and told them you're a wrestler, what kind of reactions have you gotten?

The way I explain it is that wrestlers are the world's greatest athletes, with showmanship. I say these are great guys, big men — in my day we weren't as big as the guys today. They're in great shape. They have to perform night after night without getting killed. Occasionally they do get hurt. And I tell people it's like going to a circus. If you go to a circus, you get up, you watch the guy on the trapeze, and you say, "Whoa, he's talented. Look what he can do." You've gotta take it lightly, you've gotta go there and have fun. You've got the good guys and the bad guys. Usually the good guys win. Occasionally they trick you and the bad guy will win. But even McMahon has called it sports entertainment. And it is entertainment. But you have to realize that they're great athletes.

How did you start doing movies?

Now the reason that I got into the movies is funny. Around the early '80s, this little fella used to show up at the matches at Newark Armory. And he would say,

"Captain Lou, can you get me in?" And I would say, "Sure, grab my bag and make believe you're with me." I'd sneak him in, and later on we'd go across to the pub and have a couple beers, and we got to be friendly. And every two weeks we'd meet at the Newark Armory. He told me he was trying to be an actor but no one would use him. He said he was also a handyman and a hairdresser. And I said, "How does someone as short as you cut hair?" Well, the guy went wild. He said, "You big, fat so and so" — I weighed 300 pounds at the time — "don't ever call me short. I'm very touchy about my height. When I was a kid, I got treated like a dwarf. I hate to be called short." He turned out to be Danny DeVito. Before he was going to do *Wise Guys*, he called me up and said, "Captain Lou, you big fat so and so, come in and read for a part." I told him, "I'm not an actor, I'm a wrestler." He said, "All wrestlers are all phony actors." I went in and got the part. And Danny also got me the Super Mario cartoon. Danny owns Jersey Films, and he's become a legend.

Just like you.

Well, I don't put myself in that class. Putting me in that class is like feeding strawberries to pigs. I walked into Pepino's Restaurant near where we live a couple weeks ago, and there's Richard Gere. "Captain Lou," he said, "You're hot. I see you all over the place" — I do local commercials for a car dealership and a baseball card store and restaurants. So I said, "Yeah, I'm hot. There's only one difference between us. You do a movie and you get $15 million. I do a movie and I have to give them $200." I realize that I'm not a Laurence Olivier, and you know your place and you do your thing. I get parts to play. Someone wanted me to do some nude scenes, and I said I don't want to scare people. But I'll tell you, when I had the belly and I was 300 pounds, I did go to a doctor, and he told me to strip down, take my clothes off, which I did. He looked me up and down and told me I'd better diet. And I said, "Why, what color is it now?"

Tell us about the start of Vince Jr. doing the Rock and Wrestling Connection.

I think his father had a better concept. His father had a better territory — he never went past the Virginia border, and he went up just to Maine. Jack Louis ran it up in Maine, and then in Chicago you had Fred Koehler. In California you had Roy Shires, with Pat Patterson. In Florida you had Cowboy Ruttle. They were the promoters. There were territories. You wrestled in one area, you left and went to another area. When you talk about money, my first year in wrestling, I made like $3,000. That was in 1952. Then we went up and made 20 or 25 grand. Well, that, in the '60s, was like $90 or $100,000 today. So you were making a nice living, and guys like Sammartino, who was the champion, probably made around 200 grand a year. That was equivalent to a million today. I'm sure today with the merchandising, guys like Hogan are making millions and millions.

Did you enjoy doing the Cyndi Lauper and David Wolfe angle?

I did. That happened because I was coming back from Puerto Rico on a plane, and Cyndi came up to me and said she was a fan. She asked if I'd do her video, "Girls Want to Have Fun," and I did it and saw her at the Garden. I was the villain then, before Wrestlemania I. I looked at her and winked and said, "Cyndi, you're a nice little broad." She said, "I'm a what?" I said, "You're like other women. You're a broad. Good for having babies and cleaning house." She said, "You big, fat thing, don't you EVER say that to me." And then it was I had picked a girl wrestler — Moolah — who's like my age, 126 — to fight against Wendy Richter, who was 22 years old. And if her girl beat my girl, I had to apologize to women. Well, her girl beat my girl and I had to go on the air and say that women are at LEAST as good as men, if not, in most cases, better. When I went on Letterman's show, the women's lib picketed me, and were going "Boo, boo." And I said, "They're not yelling boo, they're yelling Lou." But later, I decided that getting out of the business would be easier, because even though it's a show, there are people that take this seriously. I thought it would be much easier for me to make a living and get around without being the villain. I started doing Multiple Sclerosis and managing the British Bulldogs and Andre the Giant. And in the latter part of my career I was handling all the good guys. For me, it's been a great experience. I've got four grown children. My oldest guy's 43, and a real estate insurance man. He's got four children. I have a daughter who's an R.N. and has four children. My son just opened a big, beautiful beauty parlor here with my daughter. He's got a little baby, and my daughter's got two.

But no second-generation wrestlers.

No, my son was an amateur wrestler, but he decided to be in the real estate business. They all do much better than I do. At least this way if I need anything I can run to them.

Lou, let's run by some names. Give us your opinion on Jim Cornette.

A very talented speaker. I've met him a few times, but don't know him real well. He does a good job talking. He's right out there and he projects.

How about Bobby Heenan?

He's excellent. I do know him very well. He made a heck of a deal down with Turner. He's one of a kind. They call him the Weasel and all that, but he's a very talented manager and commentator, just like Gene Okerlund.

How about Paul E. Dangerously?

Paul E. was my fan club president for years. He came in and started with this ECW. The only objection I can say is that it's a little too violent for kids. It's not a circus anymore. Now you're talking about hardcore, blood and glass on the floor. Nothing against Paul E. — he's a nice fellow. But it's not the kind of thing I appreciate. I like it when it's competitive, it's more or less a little amateur wrestling. You've gotta have the Cyndi Lauper deals and the guys with the blond hair, and me with a rubber band in my beard. That's fine, but not when it's overly done. I don't go for all that blood and other stuff.

Do you think he'll have success on a national basis?

I don't think they'll be real big. Because the Ultimate Fighting is having trouble in some states — it's too violent. Look at all the violence going on. You know, there is a call for good films. Look at the big films of last year and you see things like "The Lion King" doing very well. I looked at "Pulp Fiction" and "Natural Born Killers," and those just weren't entertainment.

What do you think of the Monday night wars between WCW and WWF? Do you see this as something positive for the future of wrestling?

Well, if I were McMahon, I wouldn't be running those skits saying how Ted Turner's an old man and Hulk Hogan's a has-been. All you're doing is inciting a riot. McMahon's got an old man walking to the ring saying, "Hi, I'm Ted Turner. Hulk Hogan's a has-been, and I think I'll look for another has-been." Well, let me tell you something. First of all, Hulk Hogan's not that old. He's lost a lot of his hair, his name is Terry Bollea, he was a bass guitar player, we helped bring him in. But he's still a name. It's like bringing Muhammad Ali in — the poor guy can hardly walk now. When you're talking about a Hulk Hogan, he's a name, and he's drawn money. And then you can talk about Macho Man. The guy's got a Slim Jim deal. Turner's paying decent bucks. Diesel's running down there and they've got Razor Ramon. If I were McMahon, I would avoid that. What I would've said is when Hogan's contract was through and he ran down, I would've said, "Hulk Hogan drew a lot of money for me. He's a very talented individual. I hope he can do the same for Ted Turner. There's room for everybody." And let it go. I wouldn't go against a guy that could buy and sell me tomorrow. Because I believe that McMahon has money, but I don't believe he's in the category of Ted Turner. You're treading thin water. You're looking for trouble.

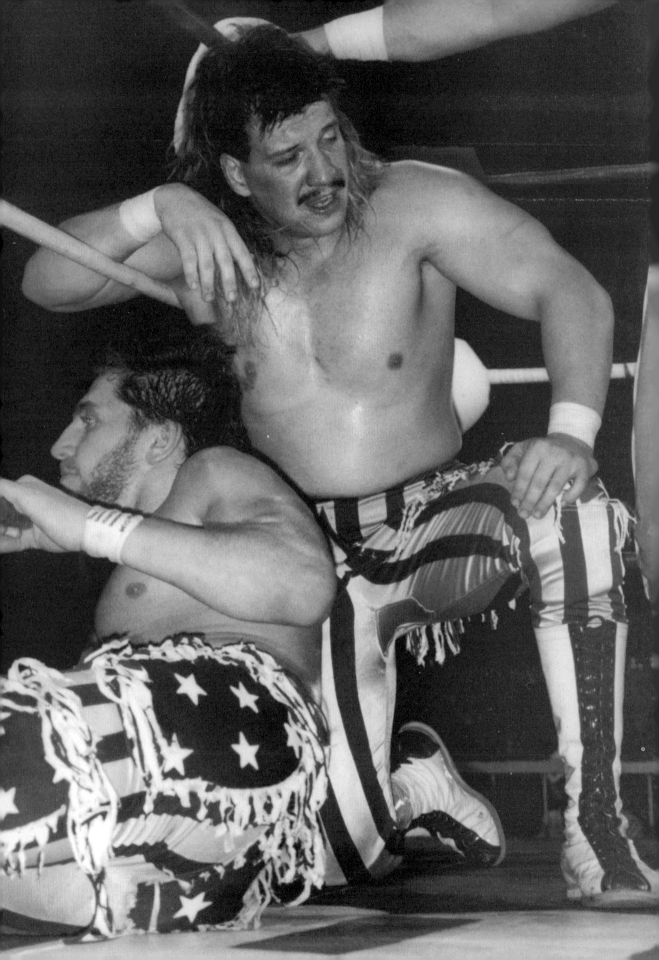

Eddie Guerrero
July 6, 1996

Second-generation wrestler Eddie Guerrero — son of Gory — is one of the most underrated performers of all time. While he'll probably always be famous for his nickname "Latino Heat," it's his versatility with many different wrestling styles that has earned him so much respect among die-hard fans, starting in Mexico, and building up a name in Japan before moving to ECW and then WCW. This interview was done in person at a WCW event in Connecticut. He was calm, pleasant, and semi-open about the business, talking about Japan, politics in Mexico and why he respects Shawn Michaels, among other subjects.

Eddie, about three years ago you were one of the most hated heels in the AAA promotion [in Mexico]. Now, it seems that you're one of the more "over" fan favorites. How has the transition been?

Oh, I'm just very thankful to God for everything that I have. I'm just glad that people like my style.

What is the difference between Lucha Libre, Japanese style, and American style of wrestling?

You've got your differences but it's basically the same. Wrestling is wrestling. You still wrestle, no matter what. It's just a little bit different style. You know, Mexico is more aerial. Japan you've got more aggressiveness and a little bit quicker style. Here in the States it's a little bit more methodical. But the thing going now in the States is that there's a revolution that's going on. You're seeing a lot of change in the style here. And I think that's the reason you've got people like Dean Malenko, Rey Mysterio Jr., Chris Benoit that people are starting to appreciate. Their type of style that they have brought in and, you know, it's a little bit different and it's giving people a little bit more action I guess.

What seems to be the problem with the commissions in Mexico? We sometimes hear reports where, for example Konnan will promote a show that's similar to the ECW-style and it'll get a little bit out of control. How strict is the commission in Mexico?

I haven't been there in over a year. But they've always been like that. I mean anything in Mexico is very strict and unfortunately their politics has a lot of strength in anything — in any kind of business. And unfortunately, sometimes it's corrupt and sometimes it's not. But a lot of times, that's what you've got to deal with. You've got to deal with a corrupt organization so you can have all of the legal stuff ready to go but they'll still want to throw something at you, which is why you'll still have problems.

What are your thoughts on the Great Sasuke in Japan?

Well, I think he's a great flier. I just finished wrestling him in Japan and he's incredible, you know. You've got your incredible fliers like Rey Mysterio Jr. and a lot of others. I don't think that I'm a great flier, I just think that I've got a little bit of everything.

They say that you're the next Ricky Steamboat.

I don't think so. I don't know. I'm just very thankful to God that I got an opportunity here and the people have received me in a positive way.

Would you say that you've taken the repertoire of Chavo, Mando, and Hector and combined them for yourself?

No, I think that everyone has their own style. I think Chavo has his own style. I think Mando has his own style. I think Hector has his own style. It's different styles at different times in the business. I don't think anyone is better than anyone else. I just think that we're all good in our own way. I mean, I still have a lot to learn. I'm still kind of a rookie here in the States if you think about it, 'cause I just started. Now you've got my nephew coming, Chavo's son, his name is Chavito. He's got a lot of talent, he just needs to get some experience under his belt. But, you know it's like what one wrestler said. "Watch out for those Guerreros. They're small, but there's a lot of them."

At one point in 1993, you and the late Art Barr were over tremendously as heels in Mexico. How is it psychologically for you, knowing that you could go out there and draw the kind of heat that you did?

Oh, I thrive on it. I loved it. It was a big change for me being a heel. And, you know, I always wanted to do it because my dad was one of the biggest heels. He was the legend over there. He was probably one of the biggest heels to ever come out of Mexico. And for me to kind of follow in his footsteps as far as being a heel over there was exciting. It was a different time in my career and I think that it did me good.

Your thoughts on the other promotion here in the United States [WWF at the time]. Shawn Michaels is the champ. Would you love to wrestle him?

He's incredible. He's fantastic. He's a phenomenal athlete and I have nothing but the utmost respect for him. You know, this is wrestling and one of these days our paths may cross and they may never even come a hundred yards from him. But if I ever get to meet him it'd be a pleasure and an honor, because he is a tremendous athlete.

New Japan Pro Wrestling is something that you've been with for a long time. Any chance of going to All-Japan Pro Wrestling?

As far as right now, no. They've been great to me. I wouldn't dream of it, unless things change. Never say never, right? But they've been like a family and have taken care of me. wcw has taken care of me, too. They're great and I love it here. For right now, I see myself here.

You've been in those Super-Junior Tournaments in Japan. Is there anybody that you've seen tapes of that made you say, "Damn, I wish I had wrestled him?"

Oh, I always wanted to wrestle Chris Benoit. Now we're against each other every night. You see talents and want to test your skills, you naturally want to lock horns with him.

What are your thoughts on Juventud Guerrera? They say he's as tremendous as Rey Mysterio Jr.

Well, you know, Juventud I think got a lot of Art's and my style from AAA and I'm glad he did. He's a good talent and I've wrestled with him and against him. He's a good kid and I wish nothing but the best.

How about Perro Aguayo Jr.? Will he go far in this business?

To be honest with you, I've never seen him wrestle. You know, if he has half the heart that his dad has, he'll be there.

In five years from now, where do you want to be? Do you want to be IWGP Junior Heavyweight champion? Do you want to be perceived as a heavyweight?

Well, a lot of people make a big thing about it. You've got your lighter weights and your heavyweights. This is wrestling. That's the great thing about wrestling. You can have a great match with a big man versus a little man. As far as seeing myself five years from now, I just want people to say that I'm a good wrestler that they enjoy seeing me out there working here. There's championships out there for me to win and if I'm fortunate enough to win one then I'm very thankful to the Lord for that.

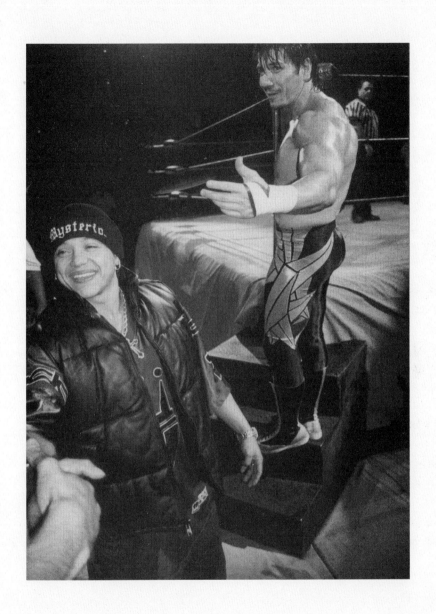

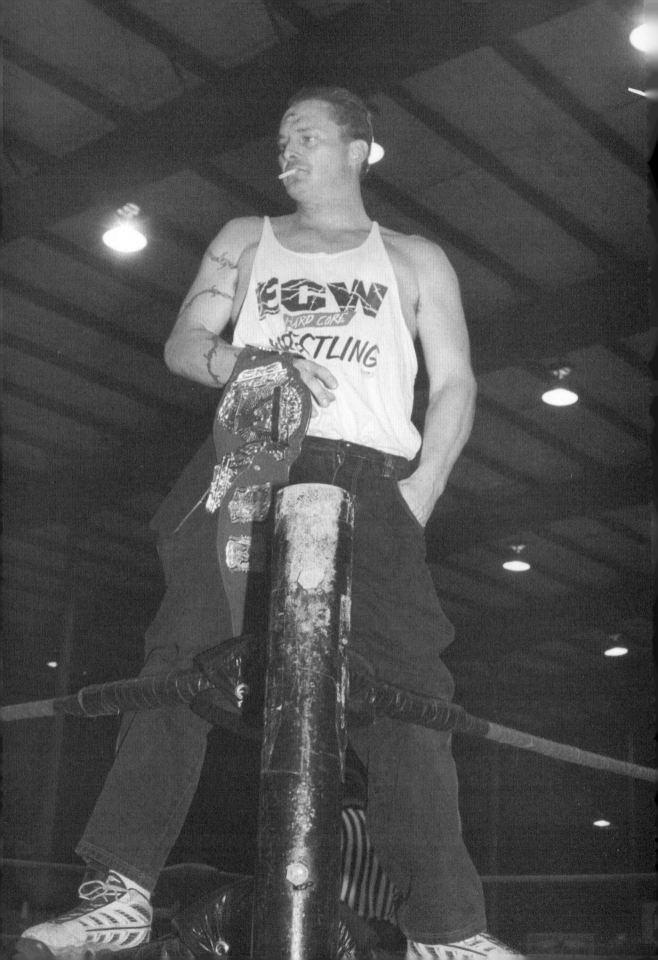

Sandman
January 4, 1997

Jim Fullington started his career on the independent circuit in the late '80s and early '90s in the Philadelphia area. He hit it big with ECW around 1992, first taking the belt from Don Muraco, then wearing it two more times over the next few years, before eventually migrating to WCW. His shtick was playing a beer-drinking, cigarette-smoking tough guy. But that all might have been pretty close to the real Fullington. For this interview, done while still with ECW, he was awakened at his hotel from a deep sleep, coughing and clearing his throat a lot, slightly disoriented. He was in town to do a show the same evening in Revere. This was shortly after Eric Kulas, a 17-year-old fan, was invited to be part of a match at the same arena, and was bloodied up and hospitalized.

Sandman, you're on the air on Wrestle Radio.

Oh, that's great. You woke me up right over the air?

We called a couple of hours ago. We thought you were awake.

Well, you woke me up then, too. What's up, guys? Who am I wrestling tonight?

It's you and D-Von [Dudley] against [Chris] Candido and Mikey Whipwreck. Who did you wrestle last night?

Raven, and it wasn't even really a match. We just kind of brawled through the building and stuff like that. It wasn't really a set up match.

Would you mind answering a question about the business now that you're wide-awake?

Yeah, now that I'm wide-awake.

Was it a big loss for you guys when Nancy Sullivan left? Was she adding much to the promotion?

None whatsoever. She's a manager, not a wrestler. You talk losses, you talk about losing one of your top guys. You're not talking about losing a lady manager. Come on!

But she is quite a looker.

Yeah. And she's getting on in years, too.

How's everything going in the organization?

The organization's going great.

We keep hearing about hassles with whether or not there will be a pay-per-view. What do you think?

I have no idea. I don't deal with that stuff. If there's a pay-per-view, tell me where, and I'll be there to wrestle. That's all.

But doesn't that mean an extra payday for you.

No, the pay's always the same.

Any aspirations to go to WCW or WWF?

I've already been offered by wwf and wcw. What the hell do I want to go up there for? They're signing people for $80–$90,000 right now. I make that in ecw and I wrestle twice a week and sleep in my own bed every night.

Were you living in Utah at one point?

Yeah, Salt Lake City. But I'm back on the east coast now. I started a construction company out there with the godfather of my son. The company's doing great, and I'm still doing some business out there. But I need to wrestle right now. That's where my heart is.

How did you break into this business?

I wanted to be a wrestler since I was about 4 years old. All my other little friends wanted to be cops, firemen and stuff like that. I wanted to be a wrestler. I was always watching wwf — George "the Animal" Steel, Tony Garea, Chief Jay Strongbow. I grew up with all of those guys.

Where did you grow up?

Right outside of Philadelphia.

How did you break in?

I went to a wrestling school. There was a wrestling school in Philadelphia. It was for the Tri-State Wrestling Alliance.

Who were you trained by?

A bunch of guys, but nobody that anybody would know. I pretty much trained myself. I just watched tapes, learned what to do, hit somebody over the head with something. It ain't rocket science in ecw.

Did Paul Heyman give you your first break?

Heck no, it was Joel Goodheart. I'm pretty much the sole survivor left from the Tri-State Wrestling Alliance. That started in Philly, then it was NWA Eastern Championship Wrestling.

Who was your first professional match against?

J.T. Smith.

What happened?

I kicked his ass.

Didn't he leave the promotion?

Yes. It was wife problems. He moved out of Virginia, it was a hassle for him driving up here. His wife's a pain in the ass, but he is a great guy.

Were you guys sad to see Scorpio leave?

I was. Scorpio's a very good friend of mine. But we all knew it was coming. You've got to understand. To me and to a lot of guys in the business, Scorpio's one of the top five wrestlers on this planet. So sooner or later, somebody else was gonna pick him up.

Will that continue to happen in ECW? Will you guys get so good that others will keep making offers to you?

A lot of guys have been offered already, but you've gotta understand that they're not offering million dollar contracts anymore. That unbelievable money isn't there right now. So pretty much the guys that are here are the guys that are gonna be staying. Frankly, everybody here has already been offered something by somebody else.

So you're wrestling only two nights a week right now?

Yeah, Friday and Saturday. It's a wonderful thing. I make a hundred grand a year and I wrestle two nights a week.

So what do you do in your downtime? What does Sandman do for a hobby?

I lay on my couch, watch television, and drink beer. My weekend starts on Monday and lasts till Friday. My workweek is Friday and Saturday night.

Are you in pretty good shape as far as injuries?

Hey, I can hardly get out of this bed to go to the bathroom, my body's killing me so bad.

What kinds of injuries have you had?

Elbows, shoulder, I blew my knee out, my back. Everybody's got a bad back in this business. Everybody's got nagging injuries. But if you want to feed your family, you get in that ring every night.

Do you think you'll be OK as an old man?

No, I'll be in a wheelchair by that time.

Have you worked against Terry Funk?

I've worked with him as a tag team partner, but not against him, though I'd love to.

It could be arranged, he won't be retiring.

Yeah, he's retired. He's retired 19 or 20 times now, every other day he's retiring. And the next thing you know they're billing "One more chance for the Funker." It's unbelievable, that guy's got more lives than Felix the Cat.

Is the crowd in Boston much different from the home crowd in Philadelphia?

Yeah, a little bit. You've gotta understand, our crowd at the ECW Arena [in Philadelphia] is totally different from any other breed of animal, than any other wrestling crowd on the planet. So you can't really judge another crowd by the ECW Arena crowd. The ECW Arena crowd is unbelievable. I love working in front of them. But Boston is pretty much the same as the rest of our crowds go.

The fans have to always be ready to get out of the way.

Absolutely, because you have to understand that sometime during the night, no matter where you are in the building, you've got a front row seat.

You sound like you're having a good time in this business.

Oh, I love this business. I'm living my life's dream.

You guys had some problems the last time you were in Revere, when a kid got in the ring, and there was a big controversy.

What was the problem there?

Someone didn't show up and some kid got in the ring as a tag team partner for somebody in a Gangstas match, and blood flew everywhere, and the guy had to go to the hospital.

But blood flies everywhere every damn night in ECW. So what's the problem?

Well, the kid was only 17.

I don't care how old the kid was. If you bleed, you bleed. I don't care if you're 2 years old or 92. You get hit, you bleed.

But should the kid have been in the ring?

He was clueless.

Do you ever get loopy and drink malt liquor instead of beer?

No, I don't like malt liquor. I like a bunch of different beers.

Is there such thing as a good local Philadelphia beer?

Not that I know of. Well, Rolling Rock is close to Philadelphia. That's a decent beer.

What's up with you and your wife, Lori? Are you marred, divorced, or what?

Technically I'm still married, but we've been separated. Our separation's been in front of the camera for nine months by now. But we've really been separated for a couple years.

How does your son like being in the business?

He loves it. You have to understand that my son is 7 years old, and for his first five years he watched his dad on TV every week.

Did you have any reservations about him getting into the act?

None whatsoever. I wish when I was 5 years old I was in the ring.

How old were you when you did first get in a professional ring?

27.

That's a little late, isn't it?

Yeah, are you kidding me? I've only been in the business for about six years.

Any upcoming tours in Japan with the IWA?

Yeah, I've got something goin'. I'm looking for like a 20-week tour over there, but I'm not sure exactly when it'll start. But Japan sucks. The country sucks. They hate us. We hate them. We can't speak the language. Might as well be on a different planet. They do pay good, though.

Do you actually sit and watch the other wrestling groups?

I watch anything and everything that I can.

What do you like out there?

I like certain different guys, but it's pretty much watching them do what we did a couple months ago. All they're doing is copying everything we do.

Is there anybody you'd like to get into the ring with in other organizations?

No, I don't care who the hell I get in the ring with.

Could you compete in UFC?

Hell, no.

Are you a fan of Roddy Piper?

Are you kidding me? Piper is the greatest. Piper, Curt Hennig, Flair — they're some of my all-time favorites.

Sandman, thanks a lot for coming on today.

Call me back in a couple hours. Wake me up when I've gotta go to the show.